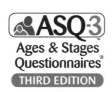

ASQ·3
Ages & Stages
Questionnaires®
THIRD EDITION

ASQ·3
User's Guide

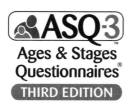

ASQ-3
User's Guide

by

Jane Squires, Ph.D.
Elizabeth Twombly, M.S.
Diane Bricker, Ph.D.
Early Intervention Program
Center on Human Development
University of Oregon, Eugene

and

LaWanda Potter, M.S.
EC CARES
Lane County, Oregon

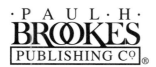

Baltimore • London • Sydney

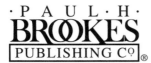

Paul H. Brookes Publishing Co.
Post Office Box 10624
Baltimore, Maryland 21285-0624
www.brookespublishing.com

Visit www.agesandstages.com to learn more about the complete ASQ system.

Typeset by Integrated Publishing Solutions, Grand Rapids, Michigan.
Manufactured in the United States of America by
Sheridan Books, Inc., Chelsea, Michigan.

Library of Congress Cataloging-in-Publication Data
ASQ-3 user's guide / by Jane Squires ... [et al.].
    p.   cm.
    For use with: Jane Squires. Ages & stages questionnaires. 3rd ed. Baltimore, Md. : Paul H. Brookes, 2009.
    Includes bibliographical references and index.
    ISBN-13: 978-1-59857-004-5
    ISBN-10: 1-59857-004-8
    1. Child development—Testing. 2. Infants—Development—Testing. 3. Child development deviations—Diagnosis. I. Squires, Jane. II. Title: Ages & stages questionnaires user's guide. III. Title: Ages and stages questionnaires user's guide.
    RJ51.D48B75 2009 Suppl.
    618.92'0075—dc22   2009004926

British Library Cataloguing in Publication data are available from the British Library.

2019   2018   2017   2016   2015   2014   2013   2012
10   9   8   7   6

Contents

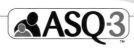

Appendixes

List of Tables and Figures

ASQ-3

APPENDIX C

About the Authors

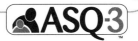

The ASQ system, including the *Ages & Stages Questionnaires®, Third Edition* (ASQ-3) (English and Spanish); *ASQ-3™ User's Guide,* the *Ages & Stages Questionnaires®: Social-Emotional* (ASQ:SE) (English and Spanish); and *The ASQ:SE User's Guide,* were developed by the following authors:

Jane Squires, Ph.D., Professor and Director, Center on Human Development/University Center for Excellence in Developmental Disabilities and the Early Intervention Program, University of Oregon, Eugene

Dr. Squires is a professor of special education, focusing on the field of early intervention/early childhood special education. She has directed several research studies on the *Ages & Stages Questionnaires®* and *Ages & Stages Questionnaires®: Social-Emotional* and has also directed national outreach training activities related to developmental screening and the involvement of parents in the monitoring of their child's development. She has investigated early identification of social-emotional disabilities in preschool children and a linked systems approach to improving social-emotional competence in young children. In addition, Dr. Squires directs master's and doctoral level personnel preparation program and teaches graduate classes on early intervention/special education.

Diane Bricker, Ph.D., Professor Emerita and Former Director, Early Intervention Program, Center on Human Development, University of Oregon, Eugene

Dr. Bricker served as the director of the Early Intervention Program at the Center on Human Development, University of Oregon, from 1978 to 2004. She was a professor of special education, focusing on the fields of early intervention and communication. Dr. Bricker has been a primary author of the *Ages & Stages Questionnaires®* and directed research activities on the ASQ system starting in 1980. She has published extensively on assessment/evaluation and personnel preparation in early intervention.

Elizabeth Twombly, M.S., Senior Research Assistant, Early Intervention Program, Center on Human Development, University of Oregon, Eugene

Ms. Twombly is a senior research assistant at the Early Intervention Program, Center on Human Development, University of Oregon. For the past 20 years, she has been involved in ongoing research studies on the *Ages & Stages Questionnaires®* (ASQ) (including the renorming for the third edition of the ASQ) and the *Ages & Stages Questionnaires®: Social-Emotional* (ASQ:SE). Ms. Twombly has provided training and technical assistance nationally, and in other countries, on the use of ASQ and ASQ:SE in social service, educational, health, and medical settings. Her areas of interest and research include the involvement of parents in early childhood and early intervention systems, cultural considerations in assessment and intervention, infant mental health, and systems of care for substance-exposed newborns.

Robert Nickel, M.D., Professor of Pediatrics, Department of Pediatrics, and Medical Director, Child Development and Rehabilitation Center, Oregon Health & Science University, Eugene

Dr. Nickel is a professor of pediatrics in the Department of Pediatrics and at the Child Development and Rehabilitation Center (CDRC), Oregon Health & Science University, and he is the medical director of the Eugene office at CDRC. He has been instrumental in the production of materials related to developmental monitoring activities, including the Infant Motor Screen (screen test/manual and videotape) and Developmental Screening for Infants 0–3 Years of Age (manual and videotape), part of a training program for primary health care professionals. As a developmental pediatrician, he attends a number of clinics for children with special health care needs in the Portland and Eugene CDRC offices and at outreach sites.

Jantina Clifford, Ph.D., Assistant Professor, Early Intervention Program, Center on Human Development, University of Oregon, Eugene

Dr. Clifford is an assistant professor at the University of Oregon Early Intervention Program, where she teaches graduate courses in early intervention/early childhood special education. In addition to teaching at the university level, Dr. Clifford provides training internationally on the *Ages & Stages Questionnaires®* and the *Ages & Stages Questionnaires®: Social-Emotional.* Her professional interests include personnel preparation, the development and evaluation of early childhood assessment measures, and issues pertaining to the healthy development of internationally adopted children and support for their families. Prior to the pursuit of her doctoral degree, Dr. Clifford served as an early childhood educator for 8 years.

Kimberly Murphy, Education Program Assistant, Early Intervention Program, Center on Human Development, University of Oregon, Eugene

Ms. Murphy has coordinated several research studies involving both the *Ages & Stages Questionnaires®* (ASQ) and the *Ages & Stages Questionnaires®: Social-Emotional.* Her recent contributions include coordination of data recruiting, collection, and analyses for the renorming study for the third edition of ASQ and serving as web content editor/coordinator of the web site designed for national ASQ data collection.

Robert Hoselton, Research Assistant, Early Intervention Program, Center on Human Development, University of Oregon, Eugene

Mr. Hoselton received a B.S. degree in computer science from the University of Oregon in 2004. He has been involved with several research studies on the *Ages & Stages Questionnaires®* (ASQ). His most important contributions include data collection and analysis for technical reports. Mr. Hoselton designed and developed a web site and online applications used for national ASQ data collection.

LaWanda Potter, M.S., Administrator and Program Manager, EC CARES, Lane County, Oregon

Ms. Potter is an administrator and program manager for EC CARES, an early intervention/ early childhood special education (EI/ECSE) program in Oregon. She received her master's degree in child development and family studies from Purdue University. Ms. Potter has been involved with several research studies on the *Ages & Stages Questionnaires®* (ASQ), including questionnaire revisions, data analysis, and documentation. She has also provided outreach training on the ASQ system across the United States. Ms. Potter is a co-developer of *The Ages & Stages Questionnaires® on a*

Home Visit DVD. She continues to provide training to child care providers and EI/ECSE personnel on implementing the ASQ in programs.

Linda Mounts, M.A., Infant Development Specialist, Regional Center of the East Bay, Oakland, California

Ms. Mounts is an infant development specialist and has worked for more than 30 years in clinical and research settings with infants and toddlers. While at the Center on Human Development at the University of Oregon, she assisted with development and research on the *Ages & Stages Questionnaires®*. Ms. Mounts is employed by the Regional Center of the East Bay in northern California, evaluating young children from birth to 3 years of age.

Jane Farrell, M.S., Early Intervention/Early Childhood Special Education Specialist, EC CARES, Lane County, Oregon

Ms. Farrell provides direct services to young children, birth to 5 years of age, who are experiencing developmental delays or disabilities. Her varied roles include home visitor, parent/toddler group teacher, early childhood special education consultant, and individualized family service program coordinator. Ms. Farrell received her master's degree from the University of Oregon Early Intervention Program in 1992. She coordinated the first *Ages & Stages Questionnaires®* (ASQ) outreach project in the country, providing training and consultation on systematic use of the ASQ in 25 states. She then took a position as an early intervention specialist in Wiesbaden, Germany, where she participated on a team that developed a full range of early intervention services for the overseas military communities, including implementation of the ASQ as a Child Find and screening system. Ms. Farrell is a coauthor of *The Ages & Stages Questionnaires® on a Home Visit* training DVD and continues to provide ASQ training throughout the United States.

ABOUT THE TRANSLATORS OF THE ASQ-3 SPANISH

Ellen McQuilkin, M.A., Professional English-to-Spanish Translator, Eugene, Oregon

Ms. McQuilkin is a native of San Diego, California, where she grew up speaking Spanish and taking frequent trips to Mexico. She later lived in central and southern Mexico with her husband, a native of Mexico D.F., and their two children. Ms. McQuilkin studied music and Spanish as an undergraduate before completing her master's degree in Spanish from the University of Oregon, where she then taught Spanish language and literature in the Romance Language Department for nearly a decade. She has worked on a variety of translation projects in social services, education, and the arts, including the English–Spanish translation of Indicadores Dinámicos del Éxito en la Lectura (IDEL), a formative assessment series of measures designed to assess early literacy skills of children learning to read in Spanish.

Pauline Mross, M.A., Professional English-to-Spanish Translator, Eugene, Oregon

Ms. Mross worked closely with Ms. McQuilkin on the translation of ASQ-3. She is the cotranslator of the English-Spanish version of IDEL and many other projects in social services, medicine, education, and the arts. She also teaches college-level Spanish language and literature.

Preface

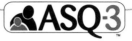

As the fields of early intervention and early childhood special education moved into the 1980s, a number of important changes were on the horizon. In particular, we, like many others, saw three significant and interrelated needs. First, there was a great need for parents and family members to become genuinely involved in the assessment, intervention, and evaluation activities surrounding their infants and young children who were at risk or had disabilities. Second, there was a clearly articulated need for tests or procedures that would monitor the development of infants who were thought to be at high risk for developing problems as a result of medical, biological, or environmental factors, or a combination of these factors. Third, there was growing pressure, spurred by diminishing resources, to find effective yet economical means to serve growing numbers of children who were at risk or had disabilities and their families. Our awareness of these problems set the stage for the development of the *Ages & Stages Questionnaires®* (ASQ; previously called the *Infant/Child Monitoring Questionnaires*).

The impetus for the development of the ASQ system came from several sources. The first source was the belief of many, if not most, scientists, practitioners, and parents that early detection of developmental problems is essential to timely and effective intervention. Second was the consistent finding that biological or medical indicators (e.g., prematurity, low birth weight, small for gestational age) are not reliable predictors of subsequent infant outcomes (Hack et al., 2005; Saigal et al., 2006). An infant who is premature and has health problems during the neonatal period will not necessarily have developmental problems at age 3 or 4 or older. Major longitudinal studies of infants considered at risk for developmental delay consistently report that socioeconomic, rather than biological, factors are the best indicators of future problems except for the very smallest of preterm babies (Brooks-Gunn et al., 1994; Hart & Risley 1995; Sameroff & MacKenzie, 2003; Werner & Smith, 1992; Werner, 2000).

A third impetus for the development of the ASQ system was the prevalent use of a multi-disciplinary team evaluation model for monitoring the development of designated populations of children. This model requires that children be brought to an evaluation center for a multi-disciplinary examination conducted by a group of highly trained professionals. Using this model, infants tend to be seen only once or at widely spaced intervals (e.g., yearly). Given the dynamic nature of development, systems that evaluate an infant at only one point in time or at extended time intervals seem likely to be ineffective in the timely identification of children who may require intervention services. Problems can arise in children at any point in their developmental trajectory, requiring that effective monitoring systems assess children at reasonable time intervals.

In addition, multidisciplinary team evaluations tend to rely primarily on professional judgment and often seek little information about the child's behavior from parents or family members. Parents were seen as the recipients of information and were expected to contribute little to the understanding of their child, except for a recitation of past health and general family experiences. In addition to infrequent evaluations and exclusion of parents' input about their child, the use of highly skilled professional teams to monitor the development of large groups of infants at risk for developmental delay is expensive. The expense is particularly troublesome given that much of the team's time is likely to be spent evaluating children whose development is progressing without problem. It has been consistently reported that approximately 30% of the infants identified with a biological or medical risk factor (e.g., prematurity) require some form of intervention (Widerstrom & Nickel, 1997). Although it seems useful to monitor the development of risk populations, it seems inappropriate to use expensive, highly skilled professionals to do so.

We believe that the development of all infants and young children should be consistently monitored; however, that elusive goal remains a challenge (Bricker, 1996; Squires & Nickel, 2003). Until the challenge is met, the development of infants and young children experiencing biological, medical, or environmental risk factors should be periodically assessed; however, the problems described above strongly suggested to us the need for change. Thus, in 1979, we began work on a monitoring system designed to circumvent, or at least attenuate, the difficulties of prediction, timeliness, accuracy, and cost. Our goal was to develop a system that was both effective and affordable. Specifically, the evaluations should occur at well-spaced intervals, the procedure should accurately identify children in need of further evaluation, the system should be easy to set up and maintain, the systematic inclusion of information from parents or caregivers should occur, and the monitoring should be economical.

These criteria set the parameters for the type of system we were interested in developing. Inspiration for the ASQ came from an article published in 1979 by Hilda Knobloch and her colleagues (Knobloch, Stevens, Malone, Ellison, & Risemburg, 1979). In this study, a 36-item questionnaire with items derived from the Revised Gesell Developmental Examination (Knobloch, Stevens, & Malone, 1980) representing the developmental period from 20 to 32 weeks was mailed to the parents of more than 526 28-week-old infants considered at high risk for developmental problems. The questionnaires were completed, returned, and scored to classify the infants as normal, abnormal, or questionable. At 40 weeks, the infants were brought to a clinic for a professional evaluation. Knobloch et al. (1979) reported that according to the professional evaluation, parents and professionals were in general agreement about the classification of the infants. The success of this study led us to reason that it might be possible to develop a dynamic monitoring system for infants and children that relied essentially on feedback from parents or primary caregivers.

By the end of 1979, a set of six questionnaires was developed to be administered to infants at 4-month intervals. The questionnaires were composed of items that asked parents or other caregivers simple questions about their infant's behavior. Once completed, the questionnaires were mailed back to a central site for scoring. It was imperative to examine the questionnaires' validity and reliability because, during the 1970s and well into the 1980s, many professionals were highly skeptical of parents' ability to accurately assess their child's development.

In 1980, we received a grant from the National Institute on Handicapped Research (now the National Institute on Disability and Rehabilitation Research [NIDRR]) in the U.S. Office of Education (now the U.S. Department of Education). The major goal of this project was to establish a monitoring system using the six parent-completed questionnaires at 4-month intervals. Infants considered to be at risk for developmental delay were evaluated from 4 to 24 months of age. Related objectives included 1) comparing the accuracy of the parental monitoring with an evaluation completed by a professional, and 2) determining whether there were factors (e.g., level of education) that predicted the type of parent who can accurately complete the questionnaires. The findings from this 3-year study were extremely encouraging. First, we found that most parents had no trouble understanding and completing the questionnaires. Second, the test–retest and interrater reliability were more than 90%. Finally, there was strong agreement between parents' classification of their infant using the questionnaires and a trained examiner's classification using the Revised Gesell Developmental Examination (Knobloch et al., 1980). Modest overreferral for further evaluation occurred, while more substantial underreferral occurred. These findings were promising enough to suggest the questionnaires should receive further study.

From 1983 to 1985, work continued on the questionnaires, largely through the monitoring of infants discharged from the neonatal intensive care unit of our regional medical facility, Sacred Heart General Hospital. It was during this time that the original six questionnaires were refined and questionnaires targeting children 30 and 36 months of age were developed. In 1985, a grant was received from NIDRR. The objectives of this 3-year project were to examine 1) agreement between parental classification and trained examiners' classification—specifically examining overidentification, underidentification, sensitivity, and specificity; 2) test–retest and interobserver reliability; and 3) cost of using the questionnaires. In general, project results supported previous findings. The agreement between parents and professionals on the classification of the infant or child was generally high, although variations occurred across intervals. Underidentification was low, while overidentification varied considerably across age intervals but was generally acceptable. Specificity was high, while sensitivity varied from low to moderate, suggesting some change in questionnaire scoring was in order. Reliability continued to be high, and the cost of using the questionnaires was found to be modest—approximately $2.50 for each questionnaire.

In 1988, we received a 2-year Social and Behavioral Sciences Research Grant from the March of Dimes Research Foundation, and in 1990, a 2-year continuation was granted. The subjects addressed by this project included 1) examining the use of the questionnaires with a group of low-income parents, and 2) assessing the effect of completing the questionnaires on parents' attitudes and knowledge of development. Results from this project suggested that low-income parents and caregivers with limited education can successfully and accurately complete the ASQ; however, the relatively small sample required caution in generalizing these findings to broad groups of parents. We did not find that completion of the questionnaires produced measurable effects on parents' attitudes or knowledge of development. Interestingly, this latter finding was in conflict with feedback we were receiving from the field. Many parents and practitioners who were using the questionnaires insisted the questionnaires assisted them in observing, understanding, and teaching their infant or young child.

Another grant to study the questionnaires was received in 1991, again from NIDRR. This project was designed to help expand questions addressed by the previous March of Dimes–supported project, specifically, 1) Can parents from extremely high-risk populations accurately complete the questionnaires? and 2) Does completion of the questionnaires affect parents' attitudes and knowledge of early development? Results from this 3-year project largely replicated and expanded our earlier findings. Parents with extremely low incomes, parents with limited educational backgrounds, teenage parents, and parents who abused substances served as subjects. These parents were able to accurately complete questionnaires on their infants and young children (Squires, Potter, Bricker, & Lamorey, 1998). Although the findings for the question on parents' attitudes and knowledge of early development were complex, in large measure we found that completion of the questionnaires did not result in significant attitude change or quantifiable enhanced knowledge of development. However, qualitative interviews reflected caregivers' enhanced knowledge of their child's current behavioral repertoire and of new games and activities to play with their child to encourage developmental skills.

After publication of the first edition of the ASQ in 1995, we began a second phase of research, writing and developing additional questions, to complete the 4 to 60 month series. In 1997–1998, the 60 month questionnaire was developed and studied. Developmental resources such as standardized and curriculum-based assessments and kindergarten curricula were used as the basis for items. After field-testing two editions of this questionnaire between 1996 and 1998, a final version of the 60 month questionnaire was completed, and concurrent validity and reliability studies were undertaken in early 1998. Work was also begun on a series of supplemental questionnaires to address missing age intervals (e.g., 10 months). These were created and field-tested to develop an ASQ system that could accommodate children of any age between 4 months and 60 months. These supplemental questionnaires—at 6, 10, 14, 18, 22, 27, 33, 42, and 54 months—were composed of empirically tested items that were taken from the ASQ questionnaires at 4, 8, 12, 16, 20, 24, 30, 36, and 48 months and filled out the series for a total of 19 questionnaires. These revisions and additions constituted the second edition of the ASQ, published in 1999.

Since publication of the second edition, wide use of the ASQ has allowed us to collect additional data, this time in community-based programs such as Head Start; Early Head Start; Healthy Start; and a wide variety of education, health, and social services agencies that screen and monitor young children for developmental problems as part of early identification systems. Specifically, Healthy Start and Parents as Teachers programs in a variety of states; public health nursing programs in New York, Washington, and southwest Minnesota; and Child Find efforts in Connecticut, Idaho, North Dakota, Florida, and Hawaii have made the ASQ an integral program component. Pediatricians, nurses, social welfare workers, and early intervention screening teams have used the ASQ as a cost-effective measure for identifying developmental delays in young children (see, e.g., Dworkin & Glascoe, 1997; Earls & Hay, 2006; Hamilton, 2006; Hix-Small, Marks, Squires, & Nickel, 2007; Magpie Trial, 2004). Many of these programs have shared data with us, which we have incorporated in our database. Gathering of data from these programs, using the Spanish translation as well as the English version, has allowed us to amass a large database across the age intervals, from a variety of families and children in diverse settings across the United States. We feel that these data on diverse children in diverse settings will improve the generalizability of our results.

To supplement this database collected, we began a web-based data collection system for the ASQ in 2004. Questionnaires from all 50 states have been completed by a variety of parents/caregivers using a research web site. To date we have more than 8,000 ASQ questionnaires completed online, to add to the 7,000 paper questionnaires collected since 2000, making our total database more than 18,000 questionnaires. Analyses of these different methods of data collection, using item response modeling, indicate few if any differences in paper versus electronic ASQ completion.

In addition to our empirical work, we have received constructive feedback on the questionnaires from parents, early intervention program personnel, and additional medical, child welfare, and early childhood practitioners. Feedback on questionnaire format and monitoring procedures from these parents and practitioners has been incorporated into the ASQ system as appropriate.

In addition, programs using the ASQ for screening and follow-up monitoring have been developed internationally; China, Southeast Asia, Australia, Africa, India, Europe, and Central and South America all have several significant projects using the ASQ with families and young children from birth through 5 years. For use in these countries, the ASQ has been translated into numerous languages, including Korean, French, Norwegian, Somali, Hmong, Vietnamese, and Chinese. We have gathered feedback from these international programs as well. We are extremely grateful for the sharing of data and experience with the ASQ from across the world, and we believe that this collaboration has enhanced the quality and utility of the ASQ.

Findings on the questionnaires have been extensively published. This list of publications is included in Appendix A of this volume. A description of data analyses and results are contained in Appendix C. As Appendix C indicates, much time and effort have been expended to examine the questionnaires. Although further work remains to be done, we believe that the current database indicates that the validity and reliability of the questionnaires for use in a variety of programs, with diverse children and families.

Based on almost 30 years of research and use, five major revisions have been made in this third edition. First, the administration age ranges specifying the age span for questionnaire administration have been widened and modified to accommodate a child of any age. In addition, the specific age range for questionnaire administration has been noted on page 1 of the questionnaire (e.g., 12 month ASQ-3, for children 11 months 0 days through 12 months 30 days) so that the age span for administration is clear to users. (It does take us a while to learn some things!)

Second, 2 and 9 month questionnaires have been added to the 19 intervals, making 21 questionnaires in the series, for children from 1 month to 66 months. While the 2 month questionnaire does not have the same empirical cutoff scores as the other intervals from the second edition of ASQ, guidance is provided about score interpretation including next recommended screening times. In addition, caregivers are given the opportunity to observe their newborn child and to practice completing the ASQ-3 early on. Thus, this edition of the ASQ includes the 19 questionnaire intervals from the second edition (i.e., 4, 6, 8, 10, 12, 14, 16, 18, 20, 22, 24, 27, 30, 33, 36, 42, 48, 54, and 60 months) as well as the 9 month questionnaire (with item content from the 10 month questionnaire) and the newly developed 2 month ASQ.

Third, revised cutoff scores have been developed for the 19 questionnaires from the previous edition, based on empirical data on more than 18,000 questionnaires completed across the preschool age span. We believe that these cutoff scores more closely reflect our U.S population of the 21st century and will assist programs in determining which children should receive a more in-depth developmental assessment for early intervention and related family support services.

Fourth, a "monitoring" zone has been delineated on the scoring summary for each age interval. This monitoring zone represents a range that is at least 1 but less than 2 standard deviations below children's mean performance in each developmental domain. This monitoring zone is meant to highlight children's developmental skills that are not below the referral cutoff score but that may need further close attention and monitoring. For example, providers may want to give caregivers an activity sheet describing fun activities that a child may do to develop certain skills, such as fine motor skills using large pencils and crayons and child-safe scissors. In addition, children whose scores are in this monitoring zone may need to be rescreened in 2–4 months to ensure that their skills remain above the referral cutoff scores.

Finally, minor changes in wording, illustration, and examples have been made to some items in this third edition. Changes recommended by users, especially related to improving clarity of items and the cultural appropriateness for diverse families have been incorporated. Additional questions have also been added to the Overall section, related to expressive language and parental concerns about behavior.

This *User's Guide* has been revised and updated throughout. Information about using the ASQ in different settings and with different completion methods has been expanded, as we have become aware of different ways the ASQ is being used across the world. Finally, a chapter containing additional family scenarios (case studies) has been added, to reflect the current diverse uses of the ASQ. We are hopeful that the expansion and revision of the ASQ system contained in this third edition will make this tool increasingly attractive and useful to programs and personnel interested in screening and tracking young children during their early years of life.

With the passage of the amendments to the Individuals with Disabilities Education Act (IDEA) in the late 1990s and later (PL 105-17, PL 108-446), and the emergence of the infant/early childhood mental health movement in the early 2000s (Knitzer, 2000), came a call for early detection of social or emotional problems in young children. In response to this urgent need, we developed the *Ages & Stages Questionnaires®: Social-Emotional*—available in both English and Spanish—and an accompanying *User's Guide*. This screening tool, meant to be used in conjunction with a general developmental tool (like the ASQ-3) that assesses cognitive, communicative, and motor development, helps identify the need for further social and emotional behavior assessment in children at eight age intervals: 6, 12, 18, 24, 30, 36, 48, and 60 months. These ASQ:SE questionnaires each address seven behavioral areas: self-regulation, compliance, communication, adaptive functioning, autonomy, affect, and interaction with people. An accompanying videotape/DVD, *ASQ:SE in Practice,* has been developed to assist with training staff to use the ASQ:SE.

We are hopeful that the increased availability of the ASQ-3 and the ASQ:SE will improve the screening and tracking efforts of programs throughout the United States and elsewhere.

Improved screening programs should result in the efficient and accurate identification of infants and young children who will benefit from further evaluation and, if needed, timely intervention.

Jane Squires, Ph.D.
Diane Bricker, Ph.D.

REFERENCES

Bricker, D. (1996). The goal: Prediction or prevention? *Journal of Early Intervention, 20*(4), 294–296.

Brooks-Gunn, J., McCarton, C., Casey, P., McCormick, M., Bauer, C., Bernbaum, J., et al. (1994). Early intervention in low-birth-weight premature infants. *Journal of American Medical Association, 272*(16), 157–162.

Dworkin, P.H., & Glascoe, F.P. (1997). Early detection of developmental delays: How do you measure up? *Contemporary Pediatrics, 14*(4), 158–168.

Earls, M. & Hay, S. (2006). Setting the stage for success: Implementation of developmental and behavioral screening and surveillance in primary care practice. The North Carolina Assuring Better Child Health and Development (ABCD) project. *Pediatrics, 118,* 183–188.

Hack, M., Taylor, H., Drotar, D., Schluchter, M., Cartar, L., Andreias, L., et al. (2005). Chronic conditions, functional limitations, and special health care needs of school-aged children born with extremely low-birth-weight in the 1990s. *Journal of American Medical Association, 294,* 318–325.

Hamilton, S. (2006). Screening for developmental delay: Reliable, easy-to-use tools. *Journal of Family Practice, 55*(5), 415–422.

Hart, B. & Risley, T. (1995). *Meaningful differences in the everyday experience of young American children.* Baltimore: Paul H. Brookes Publishing Co.

Hix-Small, H., Marks, K., Squires, J., & Nickel, R. (2007). Impact of implementing developmental screening at 12 and 24 months in a pediatric practice. *Pediatrics, 120*(2), 381–389.

Individuals with Disabilities Education Act (IDEA) Amendments of 1997, PL 105-17, 20 U.S.C. §§ 1400 *et seq.*

Knitzer, J. (2000). Early childhood mental health services: A policy and systems development perspective. In J. Shonkoff & S. Meisels (Eds.), *Handbook of early childhood intervention* (2nd ed., pp. 416–438. New York: Cambridge University Press.

Knobloch, H., Stevens, F., & Malone, A.F. (1980). *Manual of developmental diagnosis: The administration and interpretation of the Revised Gesell and Amatruda Developmental and Neurological Examination.* Houston, TX: Developmental Evaluation Materials.

Knobloch, H., Stevens, F., Malone, A.F., Ellison, P., & Risemburg, H. (1979). The validity of parental reporting of infant development. *Pediatrics, 63,* 873–878.

Magpie trial follow up study, The: Outcome after discharge from hospital for women and children recruited to a trial comparing magnesium sulphate with placebo for pre-eclampsia pregnancy. (2004). *Childbirth, 4,* 5.

Saigal, S., Stoskopf, B., Streiner, D., Boyle, M., Pinelli, J., Paneth, N., et al. (2006). Transition of extremely low-birth-weight infants from adolescence to young adulthood. *Journal of American Medical Association, 295*(6), 667–675.

Sameroff, A.J., & Mackenzie, M.J. (2003). Research strategies for capturing transactional models of development: The limits of the possible. *Development and Psychopathology, 15,* 613–640. Retrieved May 13, 2009, from http://journals.cambridge.org/action/displayAbstract?fromPage=online&aid=169351

Squires, J., & Nickel, R. (2003). Never too soon: Identification of social-emotional problems in infants and toddlers. *Contemporary Pediatrics, 20*(3), 117–125.

Squires, J., Potter, L., Bricker, D., & Lamorey, S. (1998). Parent-completed developmental questionnaires: Effectiveness with low and middle income parents. *Early Childhood Research Quarterly, 13*(2), 347–356.

Werner, E.E. (2000). Protective factors and individual resilience. In J.P. Shonkoff & S.J. Meisels (Eds.), *Handbook of early childhood intervention* (2nd ed., pp. 115–132). New York: Cambridge University Press.

Werner, E.E., & Smith, R.S. (1992). Overcoming the odds: High risk children from birth to adulthood. Ithaca, NY: Cornell University Press.

Widerstrom, A.H., & Nickel, R.E. (1997). Determinants of risk in infancy. In A.H. Widerstrom, B.A. Mowder, & S.R. Sandall, *Infant development and risk: An introduction* (2nd ed., pp. 61–87). Baltimore: Paul H. Brookes Publishing Co.

Acknowledgments

In the late 1970s, when we began to think about the need to develop a monitoring system for early detection of infants who might need intervention, we did not realize how our simple idea would persist and grow over the years. The idea—asking parents to monitor the development of their infants using easy-to-complete questionnaires—had immediate appeal to a range of parents and professionals and quickly took on a life of its own. Because of the questionnaires' instant appeal, caregivers and practitioners often saw no need to determine the questionnaires' psychometric properties and utility for a range of users. Over the years, we have been told repeatedly by an array of parents and professionals, "I know they [the questionnaires] work. Why do you need to conduct studies?" In spite of their instantaneous acceptance and strong face validity, we have felt obligated to assess the validity, reliability, and utility of the *Ages & Stages Questionnaires® (ASQ)* across a range of children and families as the ASQ has been revised over the years. We have been addressing this challenge since 1980. Although work always remains to keep the questionnaires up-to-date and relevant, we feel comfortable with the questionnaires' use in identifying with relative accuracy infants and young children who need further assessment. As with any screening tool, some under- and overidentification occurs. The dynamic nature of development and errors inherent in measurement probably make the creation of an ideal tool impossible; however, we believe the ASQ offers one of the better screening options available.

Over the 30-year span of projects associated with the ASQ system, many individuals assisted in planning and conducting data collection efforts. In particular, we would like to acknowledge Linda Mounts for her many contributions to the project; Ann Marie Jusczyk for her initial help in recruiting and testing subjects; Suzanne Lamorey, Jantina Clifford, Hyeyoung Bae, Juli Lull Pool, Ching-I Chen, and Agnes Tsai for assisting in data collection and analysis activities. In addition, we would like to thank Doris Potter for contributing her photographs to this *User's Guide*.

Thousands of infants and children and their families have completed and returned questionnaires, and many have been willing to participate in a range of testing with a variety of instruments. Without the data generated by these children and their parents, we would have been unable to examine the reliability, validity, and utility of the questionnaires.

In addition to parents and children, we have received valuable feedback about the questionnaires from professionals who are using them. In particular, we thank a variety of individuals representing nursing, early childhood, early intervention, and Head Start agencies in Hawaii, including Ginger Fink, Ruth Ota, Patsy Murakami, Roma Johnson, Gladys Wong, and Shair Neilson. For the second edition, Liz Twombly and Sue Yockelson were particularly helpful in gathering information from the field about needed revisions and additions. Jantina Clifford, Rob Hoselton, Kimberly Murphy, Paul Yovanoff, Hollie Hix-Small, and Kevin Marks contributed invaluable data collection, management, and analysis skills that made this third edition possible. Ellen McQuilkin, Paulina Mross, María Pilar Pomés Correa, Harris Huberman, Mario Peterson, and Donna Jackson-Maldonado made up the expert panel that gave feedback on the second edition Spanish translation and assisted in the development of the Spanish ASQ-3. Ellen McQuilkin and Paulina Mross also translated forms, letters, intervention activities, questionnaires, and the *Quick Start Guide.* Finally, Harald Janson, Carmen Dionne, Kay Heo, Xiaoyan Bian, Miguel Cordero, Ignacio Iriarte, and Jaime Pointe are among our many valuable international partners who have gathered data on adaptations and translations of the ASQ in international settings. They continue to devote their prodigious research skills to adaptations of the ASQ around the world.

The ASQ-3 would not exist were it not for our long-time editors and now friends at Paul H. Brookes Publishing Co. Melissa Behm, Heather Shrestha, Mika Smith, Heather Lengyel, and Paul Brookes have been at our side as we have developed the ASQ from an initial 8 paper questionnaires to an entire system containing 21 intervals, CD-ROMs, DVDs, learning activities, and electronic and web-based options. While we sometimes wince at their time lines and demands, we know that the ASQ-3 is a high-quality, multifaceted, and widely used screening system because of their expert guidance.

The success of any complex long-term project is dependent upon an array of factors, including consistent financial support, commitment from project staff, subjects' good-faith participation, ideas with merit, reasonable and practical plans of action, and luck. We have been fortunate to have had all of these.

Jane Squires, Ph.D.
Diane Bricker, Ph.D.

Photocopying Release

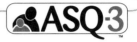

Purchasers of the *Ages & Stages Questionnaires®, Third Edition (ASQ-3™): A Parent-Completed Child Monitoring System* are granted permission to photocopy the ASQ-3 questionnaires, as well as the letter templates and forms from the *ASQ-3™ User's Guide,* solely in the course of their agency's or practice's service provision to families. Purchasers may also photocopy the supplemental materials provided with the ASQ-3 questionnaires. Photocopies may only be made from a set of original ASQ-3 questionnaires and/or an original *User's Guide.*

Each branch office or physical site that will be using the ASQ-3 system must purchase its own set of original ASQ-3 questionnaires; master forms cannot be shared among sites.

Electronic reproduction and distribution of the questionnaires, letter templates and forms, and supplemental materials is prohibited except as otherwise explicitly authorized (see Frequently Asked Questions on pp. xxii–xxiv and the End User License Agreement included with the ASQ-3 CD-ROM).

None of the ASQ-3 materials may be reproduced to generate revenue for any program or individual. Programs are prohibited from charging parents, caregivers, or other service providers who will be completing and/or scoring the questionnaires fees in excess of the exact cost to photocopy the master forms. This restriction is not meant to apply to reimbursement of usual and customary charges for developmental, behavioral, or mental health screening when performed with other evaluation and management services.

The ASQ-3 materials are meant to be used to facilitate screening and monitoring and to assist in the early identification of children who may need further assessment. The ASQ-3 materials may not be used in a way contrary to the family-oriented philosophies of the ASQ-3 developers.

Unauthorized use beyond this privilege is prosecutable under federal law. You will see the copyright protection line at the bottom of each photocopiable form.

For more information about the ASQ or to contact the Subsidiary Rights Department, go to www.agesandstages.com.

Frequently Asked Questions

ASQ·3

These are some of the frequently asked questions that users pose to Brookes Publishing. The information that follows is primarily focused on rights and permissions associated with using ASQ-3.

PHOTOCOPYING

Can the ASQ-3 questionnaires be photocopied?

Yes, the ASQ-3 questionnaires as well as the letter templates and forms in the *ASQ-3™ User's Guide* may be photocopied for use at a single physical site with all of the children served by that site at no additional charge. Purchasers may also photocopy the supplemental materials provided with the ASQ-3 questionnaires. See the Photocopying Release for certain restrictions.

NUMBER OF ASQ-3 BOXES NEEDED

My organization has many locations throughout the state. How many boxes of the ASQ-3 do I need to buy?

Each branch office or physical site that will be using the ASQ-3 system must purchase its own box of original questionnaires with accompanying CD-ROM; questionnaire boxes, CD-ROMs, and master forms cannot be shared among sites. Each physical site must also have its own copy of the *ASQ-3™ User's Guide*.

I understand that use of the ASQ-3 is site specific, but I'm not sure how a "site" is defined.

A site is a single physical location, such as an office. An organization may have various sites—for example, the downtown office, the East branch, and the North branch. The sites may be located in the same city or town, the same county, the same state, or even different states. For instance, the University of Michigan has three campuses in Michigan: Ann Arbor, Flint, and Dearborn. Each campus is a different site; the main campus in Ann Arbor cannot purchase the ASQ-3 and then share copies of it with the two branch campuses in other cities. Even on one campus, there are different sites; say, if the School of Social Work wanted to use the ASQ-3 and the School of Education also wanted to use the ASQ-3, they each, as they are separate departments located in different buildings, must purchase their own ASQ-3 box. Head Start programs are another example: Even though there are dozens of Head Start programs across the United States, and they're all part of the same organization, the main office cannot purchase one ASQ-3 box to share with all of the sites; each must own an original ASQ-3 box and *ASQ-3™ User's Guide*. Some ASQ-3 users are pediatricians with more than one office in the same town; each office must own an original ASQ-3 box and *ASQ-3™ User's Guide* rather than sharing the ASQ-3 materials between the multiple offices in the same town.

POSTING

Can I post the PDF questionnaires on the CD-ROM on my program's computer network?

The questionnaires, family information sheets, Information Summary sheets, intervention activity sheets, What Is ASQ-3™? handout, mailing sheet, Parent Conference Sheet, Child Monitoring

Sheet, and order form can be posted on your program's local area network (LAN) or intranet if *only* people in your organization at a single physical site can have access to the LAN or intranet. Employees can then print and use the questionnaires as needed from their own computers at that single physical site but can only access these items from that single physical site. Remote access from another physical site, including by virtual private network (VPN), file transfer protocol (FTP), tunneling protocols, or other means, is not permitted.

Can I post the ASQ-3 sample questionnaire from www.agesandstages.com on my web site?
No. However, Brookes Publishing encourages and permits linking from your web site to the sample questionnaire on Brookes Publishing's web site, www.agesandstages.com.

Can I post ASQ-3 questionnaires on my web site or my organization's web site?
No, posting ASQ-3 questionnaires on any web site, password protected or otherwise, is not permitted.

E-MAILING

Can I e-mail ASQ-3 questionnaires to a colleague or a family?
No, blank questionnaires may not be e-mailed to anyone for any reason. However, you may always share a *completed* questionnaire with a family in the course of your service provision to them.

Can I post online or e-mail the "What Is ASQ-3™?" document?
Yes, you may post the "What Is ASQ-3™?" document on your web site or your organization's web site. You also may e-mail "What Is ASQ-3™?" to a colleague or a family. However, when posting online or e-mailing, the document may not be altered in any way, and the copyright protection line at the bottom may not be removed or replaced.

Can I e-mail a Parent Conference Sheet or a Child Monitoring Sheet to a family?
Yes, as long as the sheet is *completed,* you may e-mail a Parent Conference Sheet or a Child Monitoring Sheet to a family in the course of your service provision to them.

Can I e-mail the letter templates and forms to a family?
Yes, after you've customized the text of the letter templates and forms from the *ASQ-3™ User's Guide* to fit your organization's and the family's needs and included the appropriate information, you may e-mail the documents to a family in the course of your service provision to them.

EXTRACTING

Can I use some of the questions from the ASQ-3 in an item that I am creating?
Brookes Publishing appreciates interest in the ASQ-3. However, you need written permission from Brookes Publishing before adapting, translating, reformatting, reprinting, or reproducing (except as covered by the ASQ-3 Photocopying Release) the questionnaires, the *User's Guide,* any related materials, or any part thereof in any way. To apply for permission, please complete a Permission Request Form online at www.brookespublishing.com.

CD-ROM

What can I do with the ASQ-3 CD-ROM?
The CD-ROM can be treated like a more durable version of the paper forms. This means you may print and photocopy the questionnaires and other materials as needed under the terms specified in the Photocopying Release and the End User License Agreement on the CD-ROM.

The questionnaires, Information Summary sheets, Child Monitoring Sheet, Parent Conference Sheet, mailing sheet, intervention activities, and supplemental materials can be posted on a local area network (LAN) or intranet. Only people in your organization at a single physical site can have access to the LAN or intranet and can only access the materials from that single physical site.

Are the questionnaires on the CD-ROM interactive?
No, the questionnaires on the CD-ROM are not fillable or interactive. The PDF files on the CD-ROM are basically a more durable version of the paper forms. You can use the CD-ROM to print the questionnaires and then photocopy them as needed.

ELECTRONIC MEDICAL RECORDS/ELECTRONIC HEALTH RECORDS

My practice/office uses an electronic medical record/electronic health record (EMR/EHR). How can I incorporate the ASQ-3 in our EMR/EHR?
Some uses of the ASQ-3 within an EMR/EHR are permitted without explicit permission from Brookes Publishing. These uses also are in compliance with the ASQ-3 Photocopying Release and the End User License Agreement for the ASQ-3 CD-ROM. Any use not described below requires permission from Brookes Publishing; to contact your sales representative or the Subsidiary Rights Department, go to www.agesandstages.com.

For instance, if your practice/office uses a paper questionnaire, asks the parent to complete it, and then enters only the child's scores into the EMR/EHR, that would not require any permission from Brookes Publishing. Or, if the practice/office's EMR/EHR has fields that identify the ASQ-3 questions by number only (*not* including the text of each question) along with spaces to indicate what the parent has marked for the answers, that would not require any permission from Brookes Publishing. Nor would the practice/office scanning into the EMR/EHR a *completed* ASQ-3 questionnaire (and/or the *completed* Information Summary sheet), as long as that completed questionnaire is not interactive and not modifiable; this is the equivalent of a practice photocopying a completed ASQ-3 questionnaire and placing it in the child's paper file or photocopying a completed ASQ-3 questionnaire to give to the parent to take home to keep for his or her records.

TRANSLATIONS

I work with a population that does not speak and/or read English. Is the ASQ-3 available in other languages?
Yes, the ASQ-3 is available in Spanish from Brookes Publishing. Other languages are in development and may be available; for the latest information, please see www.agesandstages.com.

I am conducting a research project with a population that does not speak and/or read English and I would like to use the ASQ-3. Can I get permission to translate the questionnaires myself?
Brookes Publishing is pleased to consider requests to translate some or all of the questionnaires. Please contact the Subsidiary Rights Department at www.agesandstages.com.

MORE INFORMATION

How do I get more information about ASQ-3 usage and rights and permissions?
More information is available at www.agesandstages.com. If your question is not answered by the details provided online, please e-mail your inquiry to Brookes Publishing's Subsidiary Rights Department at rights@brookespublishing.com. E-mails are answered as quickly as possible. However, due to the volume of inquiries received, please be advised that it may be approximately 4–6 weeks before you receive a response.

I

Overview of ASQ

1

Introduction to ASQ

ASQ-3

Early and accurate identification of infants and young children who have developmental delays or disorders is key to the timely delivery of early intervention services. Establishing a comprehensive, first-level screening program is the first step in obtaining needed services for infants and young children and their families. The goal of comprehensive Child Find programs is to separate accurately the few infants and young children who require more extensive assessment from the children who do not. To be useful, first-level screening programs need to assess large numbers of children and, therefore, require screening measures or procedures that are easy to administer, at a low cost, and appropriate for diverse populations.

WHAT IS ASQ-3?

The *Ages & Stages Questionnaires® (ASQ-3™): A Parent-Completed Child Monitoring System, Third Edition* (Squires & Bricker, 2009a), meets these criteria for a first-level comprehensive screening and monitoring program. The ASQ-3 screening system is composed of 21 questionnaires designed to be completed by parents or other primary caregivers at any point for a child between 1 month and 5½ years of age. (Throughout this book and in the ASQ system, the word *parents* is used to refer to individuals central to a child's life, including parents, grandparents, and other primary caregivers.) Questionnaire intervals include 2, 4, 6, 8, 9, 10, 12, 14, 16, 18, 20, 22, 24, 27, 30, 33, 36, 42, 48, 54, and 60 months of age. These questionnaires can identify accurately infants or young children who are in need of further assessment to determine whether they are eligible for early intervention or early childhood special education (EI/ECSE) services.

Each questionnaire contains 30 developmental items that are written in simple, straightforward language. The items are organized into five areas: Communication, Gross Motor, Fine Motor, Problem Solving, and Personal-Social. An Overall section addresses general parental concerns. The reading level of each questionnaire ranges from fourth to sixth grade. Illustrations are provided to assist parents in understanding the items. For the 30 developmental items on each questionnaire, parents mark *yes* to indicate that their child performs the behavior specified in the item, *sometimes* to indicate an occasional or emerging response from their child, or *not yet* to indicate that their child does not yet perform the behavior. Program personnel convert each response to a point value, total these values, and compare the total score with established screening cutoff points.

COMPONENTS OF THE ASQ SYSTEM

This section introduces the *ASQ-3 Starter Kit,* the *ASQ-3 User's Guide,* the ASQ-3 questionnaires and other key items in the ASQ system, including the *ASQ-3 Quick Start Guide* (Squires & Bricker, 2009e), training DVDs and materials, a materials kit, learning activities, the companion social-emotional screener (ASQ:SE), and the ASQ Online system.

ASQ-3 Starter Kit

Programs using ASQ-3 need this *User's Guide* as well as a box of ASQ-3 questionnaires for each site using the system. These two main components of the system are available as the *ASQ-3 Starter Kit,* which gives users the core materials necessary to start screening children using ASQ-3.

ASQ-3 User's Guide

This *User's Guide* is essential to implementing ASQ-3 effectively. It contains vital information about planning, organizing, administering, scoring, and evaluating the screening and monitoring system as well as psychometric information on ASQ-3. New to the third edition are chapters describing ASQ completion methods and settings and a chapter of case studies illustrating the ASQ in practice. In addition, the *User's Guide* contains useful appendixes designed to facilitate the screening and monitoring process. Please refer to the section at the end of this chapter called "How This Guide Is Organized" for more information about the content of each chapter and the appendixes.

ASQ-3 Questionnaires

ASQ-3 includes 21 reproducible master questionnaires and 21 reproducible, age-appropriate scoring and data summary sheets. The master set of questionnaires, available on paper and CD-ROM in the ASQ-3 box and in online completion format through ASQ Family Access, allows program personnel to select age intervals and reproduce the necessary number of copies to assess participating children. The boxed set of questionnaires also includes a brief product overview booklet and reproducible supplemental materials to support use of ASQ-3. The Child Monitoring Sheet can be used to track a child's screenings over time, and the Parent Conference Sheet is designed to organize meetings with families about screening results.

Translations

ASQ-3 questionnaires are available in English and Spanish through Brookes Publishing, and additional translations of ASQ questionnaires are completed or under development. Please visit www.agesandstages.com for current information on the availability of questionnaires in other languages. Brookes Publishing considers requests to translate questionnaires as needed for successful implementation within the community. For consideration and further information, please visit www.agesandstages.com.

ASQ-3 Quick Start Guide

The *ASQ-3 Quick Start Guide* (Squires & Bricker, 2009e) is designed for professionals on the go and is a lightweight, laminated guide to ASQ-3 administration and scoring basics. Available in English and Spanish, the *ASQ-3 Quick Start Guide* was developed to support effective implementation of ASQ-3. It provides key information for users in an easy reference format and is an inexpensive way for programs to make sure that all staff using ASQ-3 have guidance for administering and scoring even when they do not have this *User's Guide* in hand.

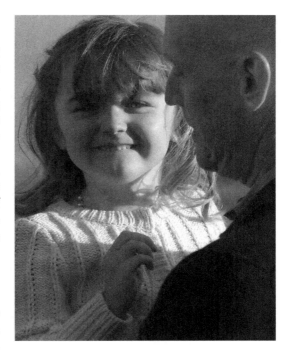

Training Materials

ASQ-3 is designed for easy use and generally requires little training, although it is important that staff be familiar with the information contained in this *User's Guide* and Chapter 6 in particular. Many programs use the available DVD training tools to introduce ASQ and show staff how to screen, score, and interpret results. Two DVDs describe procedures for using and scoring the questionnaires. *ASQ-3 Scoring & Referral* (Twombly, Squires, & Munkres, 2009) explains how questionnaires are completed and scored, highlights factors that may affect screening results, describes the referral process, and offers key ideas for building trusting relationships with families. *The Ages & Stages Questionnaires® on a Home Visit* (Farrell & Potter, 1995), which demonstrates a home visitor guiding a family through completing questionnaires for their two children, shows professionals how to successfully integrate ASQ into home visits, create opportunities for child learning, and promote positive parent–child interaction. The www.agesandstages.com web site is updated with information about additional training materials for administrators and program staff as these materials are developed.

For programs that wish to maximize their use of ASQ-3, regularly hosted seminars and customized, on-site training seminars are available through Brookes Publishing's professional development program, Brookes On Location. The seminars give an introduction to developmental screening, a detailed overview of ASQ-3, the role of parents in the ASQ-3 screening process, and specific information on how to interpret ASQ-3 scores and make referral decisions. For more information, please visit the Brookes On Location information section at http://www.agesand stages.com.

Materials Kit

Although the items needed to complete ASQ can generally be found in a family's home, some programs find it useful to gather the essential materials a family member, caregiver, or professional will use to observe a child's skills. The *ASQ-3 Materials Kit* contains the items needed to do ASQ screening at every age interval. The *ASQ-3 Materials Kit* consists of toys, books, and other items designed to encourage a child's participation and support effective, accurate administration of the questionnaires. Every item is safe, easy to clean, durable, age appropriate, gender neutral, and culturally sensitive. The kit includes a booklet on how to use the kit with the questionnaires as well as a tote bag for storage and travel.

Learning Activities

Developed to coordinate with the ASQ system, the *ASQ-3™ Learning Activities* (Twombly & Fink, 2013a; 2013b; available in English and Spanish) consist of games and ideas for interaction that address the same developmental areas as ASQ. These sets of games and interactions can be used with children who have been screened using ASQ. Each set provides parents with a short description of typical development and five to eight activities that help children progress in key developmental areas. The activities use safe, age-appropriate materials that most families have at home and encourage close parent–child interaction.

ASQ:SE

The Ages & Stages Questionnaires: Social-Emotional (ASQ:SE) takes the ASQ a step further by concentrating on the importance of considering social-emotional competence in young children. The *ASQ:SE Starter Kit* contains eight reproducible master questionnaires; eight reproducible, age-appropriate scoring/data summary sheets; a CD-ROM with printable PDF questionnaires and scoring sheets; intervention activities; and the *ASQ:SE User's Guide* (Squires, Bricker, & Twombly, 2003). A Spanish translation of the ASQ:SE questionnaires is also available from Brookes Publishing (for information on other translations of the ASQ:SE, see www.agesandstages.com). The *ASQ:SE User's Guide* describes the assessment targets; explains how to contend with the differences in time and setting, development, individual, and family/culture that may affect results; and offers strategies for using the ASQ:SE. The DVD *ASQ:SE in Practice* (Squires, Twombly, & Munkres, 2004), assists with general administration and scoring.

ASQ Online System

To help manage the ASQ screening process, online management and questionnaire completion systems are also available. Available for use with both ASQ-3 and ASQ:SE, ASQ Pro, ASQ Enterprise, and ASQ Hub form a robust online management system that supports screening administration, automated scoring, information storage, and reporting on child and program data. ASQ Pro is intended for single sites or single users, and ASQ Enterprise is intended for multisite programs. ASQ Hub is a high-level administrative account that allows state entities and other large organizations to review certain information from ASQ Pro and ASQ Enterprise accounts. Programs may purchase online management subscriptions using the keycode printed on the boxed set of paper/CD-ROM questionnaires.

ASQ Family Access is an online questionnaire completion system that enables programs to allow parents to complete questionnaires for their child online using a secure, private web site. Programs can opt for families to access the system at home or on a computer set up at a program office or clinic.

USING THE ASQ SYSTEM

The questionnaires can be used for two important purposes. First, they can be used for comprehensive, first-level screening of infants and young children. For example, parents can complete questionnaires for their child prior to a kindergarten roundup or at well-child checkups. Second, the questionnaires can be used to monitor the development of children who are at risk for developmental disabilities or delays resulting from medical factors, such as low birth weight, prematurity, seizures, or serious illness, or from environmental factors such as poverty, parents with mental impairments, history of abuse and/or neglect in the home, or teenage parents.

There is flexibility in how one uses the questionnaires. For example, questionnaires can be used at 6-month intervals, one time only (e.g., 12 months), or at a few selected intervals (e.g., 12, 24, and 33 months).

The questionnaires are designed to be completed by the child's parents in the home. Programs using ASQ Family Access can send parents a link to a secure web site to complete a questionnaire. Alternatively, paper questionnaires can be mailed to parents. Parents can try each activity with the child and observe whether he or she can perform the designated behaviors. Questionnaires are then returned by mail to a central location for scoring, brought to a primary care clinic for scoring and discussion dur-

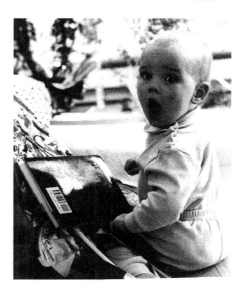

ing a well-child examination, or reported to the program electronically via the online system. Or, questionnaires can be completed during home visits with the assistance of service providers. Paper and online questionnaires can also be completed on site in waiting rooms, clinics, schools, and child care environments.

ADMINISTRATION AND SCORING

Although the questionnaires are designed to be completed by parents, ASQ-3 requires professional involvement. One or more professionals will need to establish the screening and monitoring system, develop the necessary community interfaces, train individuals who will score the questionnaires, and provide feedback to parents of children who are completing the questionnaires. Paraprofessionals can operate the system once it is established, score the questionnaires, and provide routine feedback to families of children who are not identified as requiring further assessment or monitoring. Each questionnaire can be completed by parents in 10–15 minutes, and scoring can take as little as 1 minute and no more than 5 minutes.

An ASQ-3 Information Summary sheet for each age interval is included with the ASQ-3 questionnaires. This form provides space for scoring the questionnaire as well as space to record basic information about the child and overall comments from the parents. This sheet permits professional staff to keep a 1-page summary of questionnaire results while allowing parents to keep the questionnaire for further reference about their child's developmental level.

To score a questionnaire, the parents' responses—*yes, sometimes,* and *not yet*—are converted to points—10, 5, and 0, respectively—and are totaled for each developmental area. These five area scores are then compared with empirically derived cutoff points that are shown on bar graphs on the ASQ-3 Information Summary sheet. Children whose scores fall within the white area of the bar graph are considered to be developing appropriately and should continue the screening process at regular intervals. Children whose scores fall within the light gray shaded monitoring zone ($\geq$ 1.0 and < 2.0 standard deviations below the mean) may require close attention, specialized activities, and/or repeat screening; however, scores in the monitoring zone do not indicate a need for further assessment as yet. If a child's score falls within the darkly shaded portion of the bar graph in any developmental area (e.g., Communication, Fine Motor), then further diagnostic assessment is recommended.

RESEARCH ON THE ASQ SYSTEM

Study of the ASQ began in 1980 when it was first called the Infant/Child Monitoring Questionnaires. Since 1980, a number of investigations have examined the validity, reliability, and utility of the ASQ. To examine the validity of the ASQ, children's classifications on parent-completed questionnaires were compared with their classifications on professionally administered standardized assessments, including the Revised Gesell and Amatruda Developmental and Neurological Examination (Knobloch, Stevens, & Malone, 1980), the Bayley Scales of Infant Development (Bayley, 1969, 1993), the Stanford-Binet Intelligence Scale–Fourth Edition (Thorndike, Hagen, & Sattler, 1985), the McCarthy Scales of Children's Abilities (McCarthy, 1972), and the Battelle Developmental Inventory (Newborg, Stock, Wnek, Guidubaldi, & Svinicki, 1988, 2005). For ASQ-3, overall agreement on children's classifications was 86%, with a range of 83%–88%. Sensitivity, specificity, underidentification and overidentification rates, and percent agreement values are reported in Appendix C of this book.

Studies on the reliability of the questionnaires have examined interobserver and test–retest reliability as well as internal consistency. Test–retest information was collected by asking a group of 145 parents to complete two questionnaires on their children at a 2-week interval. Classification of each child based on the parents' scoring of the two questionnaires was compared and was found to be at 92% agreement. Interobserver reliability was assessed by having a trained examiner complete a questionnaire on a child shortly after the parent had completed one. The percent agreement between ASQ classifications between parents and trainer examiners was 93% of 107 children based on the parental and trainer examiners' completion of ASQ-3. These and other reliability data are discussed in Appendix C of this book.

ADVANTAGES OF THE ASQ SYSTEM

Assessments of infants and young children's development should be done on a regular and periodic basis because of the rapid behavior changes that occur in the early years (American Academy of Pediatrics, 2001, 2006; Halfon et al., 2004; Johnson, Myers, & Council on Children with Disabilities, 2005; Nickel & Squires, 2000; Squires, Nickel, & Eisert, 1996). More cost-effective means (e.g., parent-completed tools) may be better suited for periodically monitoring early development (Chan & Taylor, 1998; Drotar, Stancin, & Dworkin, 2008; Glascoe, Foster, & Wolraich, 1997; Glascoe & Robertshaw, 2007) because professional assessments are expensive and are usually not performed at regular intervals.

The ASQ system relies on parents to observe their child and to complete simple questionnaires about their child's abilities. In addition to being cost effective, using parents to complete developmental questionnaires may enhance the accuracy of screening assessments because of the variety and array of information parents have about their children (Bodnarchuk & Eaton, 2004; Dieterich, Landry, Smith, Swank, & Hebert, 2006; Fenson et al., 2007; O'Neill, 2007). Another advantage is that using parent-completed tools such as ASQ-3 fulfills the spirit of the federal Individuals with Disabilities Education Improvement Act (IDEA) of 2004 (PL 108-446), which calls for parents to be partners in their child's assessment and intervention activities. Completing the questionnaires allows parents to gain valuable information about developmental milestones, their child's strengths, and appropriate early intervention techniques to use at home.

Flexibility is another main advantage of the ASQ system. The ASQ system can be adapted to a variety of environments, including the home, primary care clinics, child care environments, preschool programs, and teenage parenting programs. Questionnaires may be completed by parents during home visits from nurses, social workers, and paraprofessionals.

Using the master set, screening programs may choose ASQ-3 age intervals that fit their populations, program goals, and resources. For example, medical practitioners may use the 18 month ASQ interval because it corresponds to the time of well-child visits. Public health home visiting programs may choose the 4 and 8 month ASQ age intervals because they correspond to home visiting schedules. Head Start programs may use only the 48 month questionnaire, and toddler programs may choose to use the 12, 14, 16, 18, 20, 22, 24, 27, and 30 month questionnaires. The ASQ Family Access online questionnaire completion system allows parents to complete a questionnaire in their home while having results transferred to a central location to be reviewed by a nurse or office personnel and later discussed with the family during an office visit. The ASQ system is flexible and can fit the needs of diverse monitoring and screening programs. Additional advantages of the ASQ system, such as ease of questionnaire completion and questionnaire scoring, are discussed in Chapter 2 of this *User's Guide*.

HOW THIS GUIDE IS ORGANIZED

This *User's Guide* is written for professionals and paraprofessionals who plan to use the ASQ-3 system. The remaining chapters provide information on the background and use of the ASQ-3 system and step-by-step instructions for planning, using, and evaluating the screening/monitoring system. Chapter 2 focuses on the need for screening and monitoring, previous approaches to screening, problems with these approaches, and the inception and development of the ASQ system. Chapter 3 provides an overview of the ASQ system, including components and phases. Chapter 4 describes how to plan a screening/monitoring program and methods for using and scoring ASQ-3. Chapter 5 contains information on organizing and managing ASQ-3 within an agency. The essentials of using ASQ-3, administration, scoring, and follow-up, are contained in Chapter 6. Chapter 7 includes information about evaluating the system. Chapter 8 describes various completion methods for ASQ-3, and Chapter 9 discusses settings in which ASQ-3 may be used. Chapter 10 is a collection of family scenarios illustrating different settings and applications for ASQ-3.

The appendixes provide valuable supplemental information. Appendix A lists recommended readings about ASQ and developmental screening. Appendix B, a glossary, is intended as a helpful reference while both planning and implementing the monitoring program. The technical report, in Appendix C, discusses the validity and reliability research conducted on the ASQ system. Appendixes D–F contain reproducible materials useful to ASQ administration (sample letters and forms, a materials list, and parent–child intervention activities to encourage a child's development).

For up-to-date information about the ASQ family of products, please visit www.agesand stages.com. The www.agesandstages.com web site will have ASQ news and research updates, supplemental content, and basic training materials. (For answers to frequently asked questions about rights and permissions, see pp. xii–xxiv.)

2

The Need for ASQ

ASQ-3

Most people believe that the quality of life experienced during infancy and early childhood has a significant effect on subsequent development. Serious medical, biological, and environmental problems demand swift attention and remediation if maximum development is to be attained. Therefore, early identification of children whose developmental trajectory is delayed or atypical is essential in order to institute timely action to correct or attenuate problems. Early identification of children with developmental or behavior problems is predicated on the assumption that it is possible to make a distinction between children whose development is uneventful or whose problems are transitory and children who are facing serious and persistent developmental challenges. Steady progress has been made toward the timely identification of children with disabilities since the mid-1980s, and during that time, ASQ has been recognized as an integral and accurate screening and monitoring tool that has contributed to significant positive outcomes for the children whose lives it has touched.

NEED FOR SCREENING AND MONITORING

In addition to a general societal consensus that early detection of problems is a worthwhile goal, other important factors have contributed to the growing commitment by local, state, and federally funded agencies to monitor the development of designated groups of infants and young children. These factors include

- A growing population of infants at risk for developmental disabilities because of environmental conditions such as poverty, drug abuse, and neglect
- Increased emphasis on prevention of developmental disabilities and chronic illnesses
- Federal and state legal and statutory regulations addressing the need for early and effective Child Find programs

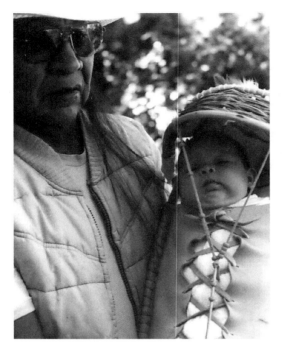

These factors have led to a growing number of federal- and state-supported programs designed to identify and track the development of infants and young children who are at risk for future problems. This growth in early identification and monitoring of risk groups has resulted in a need for reliable and cost-effective approaches for screening and monitoring programs. To be effective, tests and procedures must accurately discriminate between children who require further assessment and those who do not. To conduct comprehensive assessments of children who have no problems or children whose problems are transitory is a poor use of limited resources. To overlook children who have problems that are likely to persist or become serious is wasteful for the children, their families, and the community.

The need for effective screening and monitoring of infants and young children considered at risk for developmental disabilities and the lack of low-cost strategies was the impetus for the development of the ASQ. Other screening and monitoring procedures are reviewed to provide a context for the ASQ approach.

SCREENING AND MONITORING APPROACHES

Screening and monitoring of infants and young children have been conducted primarily by means of periodic follow up with designated groups of infants considered to be at risk for developmental disabilities. The major exception to this basic approach has been the general screening procedures conducted in the public schools with children entering kindergarten or first grade. Head Start programs have also mandated universal screening of children served in Head Start settings. Most screening programs conducted with infants have focused on populations who are at risk for developmental disabilities as a result of medical, biological, and environmental circumstances (American Academy of Pediatrics, 2006; Batshaw, Pellegrino, & Roizen, 2007; Johnson et al., 2007; Meisels & Atkins-Burnett, 2005). Screening approaches can be classified as four main types: the professionally based multidisciplinary team approach, the well-child checkup approach, the community-based evaluation "roundup" approach, and the parent monitoring approach.

Multidisciplinary Team Approach

The multidisciplinary team approach, which began in the 1970s and has been used since then, assesses designated groups of infants at risk for developmental disabilities. An example of this type of approach is screening groups of premature infants with low birth weights who meet specific criteria (e.g., Casey, Whiteside-Mansell, Barrett, Bradley, & Gargus, 2006; Shankaran et al., 2004) at designated intervals. Much of the screening conducted by multidisciplinary teams is designed to determine the frequency of problems in specific populations of infants and/or to locate predictor variables. Using this approach, infants are brought to evaluation centers at established intervals and are assessed with one or more standardized measures by highly trained professionals who usually represent a range of disciplines. Often, the children are given medical or neurological examinations as well.

Well-Child Checkup Approach

Identifying infants and young children who are at risk for developmental delays at well-child checkups in physicians' offices or in public health facilities is a second approach to screening and monitoring. Tests such as the Denver II (Frankenburg et al., 1996) and Pediatric Symptom Checklist (Jellinek, Murphy, Robinson et al., 1998) are used by professionals or paraprofessionals to assess the developmental status of the infant or young child. The tests generally used in this approach are quick to administer and can be used with young children at any age. The American Academy of Pediatrics (2006) recommended developmental surveillance at every well-child visit and use of formal, validated tools such as the ASQ at 9, 18, and 24 or 30 months of age, or whenever parent or provider concern is expressed.

Community-Based Evaluation "Roundup" Approach

A third approach is the community-based evaluation "roundup." Roundups are held so that parents can bring their infants or young children to an evaluation center for screening. Roundups can be held one to four times per year and are staffed by professionals and volunteers. Tools such as the Developmental Indicators for the Assessment of Learning–III (Mardell-Czudnowski & Goldenberg, 1998) and the Early Screening Inventory–Revised (Meisels, Marsden, Wiske, & Henderson, 1997) are generally administered by professionals; however, volunteers may assist in the assessment process. The tools used are usually easy to administer and can be used with large groups of children.

Parent Monitoring Approach

Having parents monitor their children's development is a fourth approach to screening (Bricker & Squires, 1989; Squires & Bricker, 1991; Squires, Bricker, & Potter, 1997; Squires, Nickel, & Bricker, 1990; Squires et al., 1996). An example of a parent monitoring approach is using the Denver Prescreening Developmental Questionnaire II (Frankenburg & Bresnick, 1998) in a physician's office. This tool was designed to be completed quickly by parents prior to medical or evaluation visits. Knobloch and her associates (Knobloch, Stevens, Malone, Ellison, & Risemburg, 1979) developed the Revised Parent Developmental Questionnaire for the same purpose. These measures require minimal professional input and can be used at any age. The Parents' Evaluation of Developmental Status (PEDS; Glascoe, 2005) is a third example of a parent-completed screening questionnaire. The PEDS asks parents about their general concerns in 10 developmental areas and is easily completed in pediatric and other settings. The ASQ-3 is a final example of a parent monitoring approach. Although the ASQ-3 system shares similarities with each of the tests previously discussed, it also differs in important ways that are discussed later in this chapter.

SCREENING AND MONITORING CHALLENGES

Screening and monitoring young children's development presents several challenges, which are discussed next.

Child Development

The dynamic nature of development is perhaps the first and most important challenge for the timely identification of problems in infants and young children. Development in most children proceeds at a predictable rate and in a predictable fashion. That is, most children learn to roll over before they crawl and pull to stand before they walk; however, within such developmental

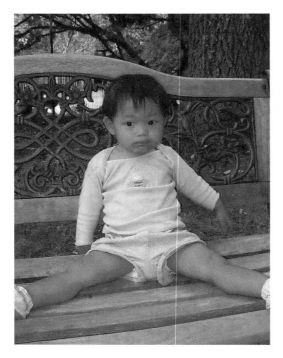

sequences, extensive variations across children can occur for a variety of reasons. Sometimes these variations do not cause concern (e.g., some children never learn to crawl but do learn to walk without problem), whereas other variations can lead to increasingly serious problems. Developmental variations do not occur at specified times. That is, children may develop difficulties at any point in time. For example, if a medical problem occurs when a child is 9 months old, then the condition may have a brief or a lasting effect on the child's subsequent development. In addition, infants raised in poverty may not show developmental delays until 2 or 3 years of age, or they may show none at all.

Because the nature of physiological or environmental conditions confronting individual children cannot be reliably predicted over time, one cannot assume that because a child's developmental trajectory is on target at 9 months, it will remain on target as the child ages. In addition, one should not assume that an infant developing poorly at 4 months will continue to develop poorly over time. The dynamic nature of development makes it prudent to screen children over time. Screening programs that assess children at only one point in time will likely overlook children whose developmental problems occur after the assessment interval. In addition, if the screening occurs initially at 4 or 5 years old, then timely identification of problems may have been delayed by, literally, years. Programs that screen children repeatedly but at infrequent intervals also run the risk of not detecting problems in children in a timely manner. Effective programs screen children at frequent intervals; however, frequent screening dictates the use of economical procedures to keep costs low.

Parent Involvement

Including parents and caregivers in assessing their children's developmental status is a second challenge for screening and monitoring programs. Screening and monitoring measures that are completed by professionals with minimal parental input do not reflect the intent of federal law or recommended practices in EI/ECSE. Beginning with the Education of the Handicapped Act Amendments of 1983 (PL 98-199), followed by the Education of the Handicapped Act Amendments of 1986 (PL 99-457), and finally with the Individuals with Disabilities Education Act (IDEA) Amendments of 1997 (PL 105-17) and IDEA 2004, federal legislation has made it increasingly clear that parents have the right and responsibility to become involved in their child's assessment, intervention, and evaluation efforts (Squires et al., 1996). Using screening systems that do not include parents in meaningful and useful ways disregards this important mandate. In addition, recommended practice dictates involving families to ensure that the rich, extensive reservoir of information that parents and other caregivers hold about the child is accessed (Sandall, Hemmeter, Smith, & McLean, 2005). Failure to gather and use parental information for determining the child's developmental status results in, at best, an incomplete assessment picture. Parents know what their children can do. An assessment that takes place outside the home in a relatively short period of time may not yield accurate results on its own because the child's full range of abilities have not been able to be assessed due to time constraints or the child being in an unfamiliar location. Including parents and their input fills in these gaps that clinical assessments might miss. Inclusion of families in child assessment activities is also a recommended practice because that involvement has the potential to assist parents in acquiring critical information concerning their child as well as to learn more appropriate developmental expectations for their child.

Cost

Cost is a third challenge for screening and monitoring approaches. Screening and monitoring large groups of children is expensive. When highly skilled professionals conduct screenings with designated target populations, the cost of frequent screening becomes prohibitive, which likely explains the reason that most of these programs screen children only once or at infrequent intervals. The cost of detecting the small number of children in need of follow-up can be very high for approaches that rely on skilled professionals. Many investigations report that less than 30% of the children in their at-risk monitoring groups required intervention services by school age, depending on the child's birth weight (Bricker, Squires, Kaminski, & Mounts, 1988; Centers for Disease Control and Prevention, 2007; Hack, Taylor, Drotar et al., 2005). For example, if a group of 100 children are screened once per year for 6 years at the moderate cost of $50 per screening, then the total cost of screening all of the children is $30,000, or $300 per child. Conversely, first-level screening approaches that employ parents to complete developmental questionnaires can significantly reduce the cost of screening and monitoring large groups of children.

THE AGES & STAGES QUESTIONNAIRES®

ASQ, initially called the Infant/Child Monitoring Questionnaires, was specifically developed to address the challenges described in the previous section. The ASQ-3 system addresses the dynamic nature of development by offering multiple assessment intervals. Inclusion of parents is ensured either by having parents actually complete the questionnaires or by having program staff assist parents in completing the questionnaires. The need for cost accountability is addressed by using parents to monitor their children's developmental progress.

The ASQ-3 system has three components: 1) questionnaires, 2) procedures for efficient and effective use of the questionnaires, and 3) support materials for use with the questionnaires. The ASQ-3 system can be implemented in four phases: 1) planning the screening/monitoring program, 2) preparing, organizing, and managing the screening system, 3) administering and scoring the questionnaires and carrying out follow-up, and 4) evaluating the screening/monitoring program. Each of these phases is discussed in detail in Section II (Chapters 4–7).

ADVANTAGES OF THE ASQ SYSTEM

Parent Involvement

Including parents and other caregivers to assess and monitor the development of their children is the primary advantage of using the ASQ system. Programs that offer screening and monitoring activities can be very diverse in terms of goals, population served, and available resources. Such diversity requires an adaptable system that involves parents. By involving parents in the reporting of their children's developmental progress, instead of solely professionals, a program has more flexibility in information gathering. The ASQ system's involvement of parents not only makes economic sense but also meets the mandates of IDEA 1990 (PL 101-476) and its amendments in 1997 and 2004, including—with the use of the ASQ:SE—the mandate for early detection of social or emotional problems in young children. Using ASQ-3 also helps educate parents about developmental milestones and their child's strengths and can introduce appropriate developmental activities to use at home.

Sound Research Base

The ASQ screening system has been tested extensively and is based on sound child development and assessment principles. Backed by 30 years of rigorous research, ASQ-3 has proved highly accurate in identifying children with developmental delays, with excellent sensitivity (.86) and specificity (.85). ASQ-3 was standardized on a large research sample of 12,695 children that mirror the United States population in geography and ethnicity and includes representation across socioeconomic groups. See "ASQ-3 Technical Report" (Appendix C) for more information about the empirical research behind ASQ-3.

Ease of Questionnaire Completion

Completing the questionnaires is relatively simple and straightforward and takes approximately 10–15 minutes. Therefore, it can be reliably accomplished by individuals with no specific training. Most motivated parents or other caregivers can complete the questionnaires without assistance, although some parents may require minimal help (e.g., interpreting some items). The questionnaires are written at a fourth- to sixth-grade reading level and contain useful illustrations when appropriate. A few parents (e.g., those with mental health problems, those who cannot read) will need substantial assistance from a professional or paraprofessional in order to complete the questionnaires. The ASQ-3 is designed to accommodate a range of strategies for completion of individual questionnaires (e.g., on paper, online, in an interview format), permitting programs and professional staff to individualize their approach to working with families.

Ease of Questionnaire Scoring

Scoring a completed ASQ-3 questionnaire is also simple and straightforward and can be accomplished by program personnel in approximately 2–3 minutes. Item scores for each developmental area are added and then compared with cutoff points provided on the Information Summary sheet of each questionnaire. For programs using the ASQ online management system, questionnaire scoring is automatic. For programs using the ASQ online questionnaire completion system and the ASQ online management system together, results are transferred electronically to the management system for scoring and professional evaluation.

Flexibility of Screening Administration

Creating a screening/monitoring system for ASQ-3 can also be adapted to meet the individual needs of communities and programs. The administration of the parent-completed questionnaires is extremely flexible. Questionnaires can be mailed to the child's home, completed online by parents at a secure web site, or completed during home visits; completed during a parent and child visit to an evaluation center, a well-child checkup, or a visit to a physician's office; or completed during a telephone interview with the parents. Some communities and programs may choose to combine strategies so that most parents receive questionnaires through the mail or online, whereas a few parents (e.g., those who cannot read) complete questionnaires through telephone interviews. Some communities may develop a system in which all physicians and medical clinics ask parents to complete questionnaires prior to their child's well-child visit.

Cost Effectiveness of ASQ-3

The ASQ-3 is a low-cost option for developmental screening and monitoring. As a one-time purchase per site, the ASQ-3 box of questionnaires does not need to be reordered. Twenty-one questionnaires, appropriate for screening children between the ages of 1 and 66 months, are included in reproducible formats on paper and CD-ROM. Using ASQ Family Access, the online questionnaire completion system, is even more cost effective because it eliminates paper and postage costs. Because the ASQ-3 is a first-level screener, results from completed questionnaires clearly indicate whether a referral is needed, eliminating time and cost associated with second-level screening.

CHALLENGES WITHIN AN ASQ SCREENING/MONITORING SYSTEM

As with all screening/monitoring systems, the ASQ-3 has some limitations and presents programs with a variety of challenges.

Organizational Requirements

Using ASQ-3 requires an organizational structure that ensures parents are receiving and returning questionnaires as directed by the program. Systems need to be in place and monitored to confirm that questionnaires are mailed or given to parents and that information is collected at the specified interval, that questionnaires are returned and appropriately scored, and that parents are given the necessary feedback. When screening large groups of children, procedures should be in place to ensure that the approach is implemented as planned. Online management systems can provide technical assistance for users and ongoing updates as appropriate to enhance implementation of the screening/monitoring system.

Need for Parent Cooperation

ASQ-3 is not appropriate for use with all families. Some parents may be unwilling to complete questionnaires or may find it too intrusive to complete the questionnaires. In addition, there are families that may experience significant chaos in their lives, rendering them unable to complete the questionnaires. Parents who have cognitive or emotional impairments may be unable to understand the use of the questionnaires. For these parents and families, alternatives are necessary.

Cultural and Language Modifications

Cultural and language modifications may need to be made with families—there is no screening tool that will work for all families, in all settings. Some items that are not compatible with the cultural norms of some families (e.g., saying "no" to children, children looking at themselves in mirrors) may need to be omitted. Language and other modifications may also be required. Although numerous ASQ translations have been undertaken (e.g., Spanish, French, Vietnamese, Chinese, Norwegian, Thai, Hmong, Somali), there will be families who speak languages and dialects for which a translation is not readily available. Experienced translators as well as community members will need to assist programs in deciding how to most effectively use the ASQ-3 with families who may present complex and challenging conditions. Chapter 10 presents case examples that illustrate how to use the ASQ-3 in a number of different family situations.

Accuracy of Screeners

Screening instruments by nature are brief and easy to administer; however, they are not always accurate. Children who need further assessment may be missed, and some children may score below the screening cutoff score who are developing typically. Ongoing periodic screening and careful evaluation of program outcomes will assist in identifying screening errors and minimizing costly professional assessments.

CONCLUSION

Involving parents or caregivers is the heart of the ASQ-3 system. The pivotal role of parents in the ASQ-3 system addresses the IDEA 2004 mandate of meaningful family inclusion. Inclusion of parents has the added feature of keeping screening costs within reason. In addition, flexibility in completing and scoring the questionnaires and implementing the ASQ-3 system provide strong reasons to consider using a parent-completed questionnaire as a first-level screening approach. The components and phases of the ASQ-3 system are described in Chapter 3.

3

The ASQ-3 System

Screening and monitoring systems should accurately discriminate between infants and children who require further assessment and those who do not. In addition, the screening and monitoring procedures should be economical because large groups of children are involved. The ASQ was developed to reliably identify children in need of further assessment and to do so at a low cost. The three components of the ASQ-3 system include the questionnaires, procedures for using and scoring the questionnaires, and support materials. The four phases of using the ASQ-3 system include planning the screening/monitoring program; preparing, organizing, and managing the screening program; administering and scoring the ASQ-3 and following up; and evaluating the screening/monitoring program.

COMPONENTS OF THE ASQ-3 SYSTEM

Questionnaires

The ASQ-3 system revolves around using and scoring its associated questionnaires. There are 21 questionnaires that are designed to be administered at 2, 4, 6, 8, 9, 10, 12, 14, 16, 18, 20, 22, 24, 27, 30, 33, 36, 42, 48, 54, and 60 months. Each questionnaire contains simple questions addressing five specific developmental areas and one Overall section that focuses on general parental concerns.

Structure

Each questionnaire consists of the following elements:

- A *family information sheet* indicates the age range intended for the questionnaire interval, asks for basic identifying information about the child and the person completing the questionnaire, and contains space for key program information. There are two sets of family information sheets. The first set is more family friendly and consists of print and PDF masters. The second set is provided as PDF masters only and are intended to facilitate accuracy of data collection.

- Each *questionnaire,* also marked with the age range for the questionnaire interval, is 4–7 pages and starts with a brief explanation and points to remember when completing the questionnaire. There are 30 questions about the child's development, written in simple, straightforward language and arranged hierarchically from easy to more difficult, and a series of 6–10 Overall questions to elicit parental concerns. The questionnaire interval is clearly marked on each page of the questionnaire.

- Each questionnaire comes with an *ASQ-3 Information Summary sheet* that is to be completed by the professional scoring the questionnaire. This page includes simple instructions as well as space for recording identifying information, item responses, and the child's scores in relation to the cutoff points.

Items

Each questionnaire contains an Overall section, which asks about general parental concerns, as well as 30 questions that are divided into the following five areas of development:

1. Communication, which addresses babbling, vocalizing, listening, and understanding
2. Gross Motor, which focuses on arm, body, and leg movements
3. Fine Motor, which pertains to hand and finger movements
4. Problem Solving, which addresses learning and playing with toys
5. Personal-Social, which focuses on solitary social play and play with toys and other children

The questionnaire items were developed by examining the content of developmentally based, norm-referenced tests and resources. Content that matched a specific test interval (e.g., 2, 4, 8, 12 months) was used as the basis for the development of specific ASQ-3 items. After the content was selected, a set of specific criteria was used to guide the writing of each questionnaire item. These criteria required that items 1) address important developmental milestones, 2) target behavior appropriate for the developmental quotient range of 75–100 for each age interval, 3) be easy for parents to observe and administer, and 4) use words that do not exceed a sixth-grade reading level. To further assist parents in using the questionnaires reliably, small illustrations are provided where possible beside the item to help convey the intent of the question. Figure 3.1 shows an item from the 16-month questionnaire. When relevant, written examples of the desired target behavior are included with the question. Throughout the questionnaire items, male and female pronouns are alternated.

6. While standing, does your child throw a ball *overhand* by raising his arm to shoulder height and throwing the ball forward? *(Dropping the ball or throwing the ball underhand should be scored as "not yet.")*

Figure 3.1.   Each ASQ-3 questionnaire features 30 simply worded questions, like the one shown here, distributed evenly across five areas of development (Communication, Gross Motor, Fine Motor, Problem Solving, and Personal-Social) and one Overall section designed to address parental concerns. Many items are accompanied by illustrations to assist parents in answering the questions about their child's behavior and development.

ASQ-3 in Spanish

The ASQ-3 questionnaires and *Quick Start Guide* are available in Spanish, and the parent letters and intervention activities (see Appendixes D and F) are also available in Spanish. The Spanish questionnaires have been field tested with Spanish-speaking parents in a variety of geographic regions of the United States (e.g., Arizona, Texas, Washington State); however, separate cutoff points have not been empirically derived. Differential item functioning analyses indicate that for the most part, English and Spanish items function similarly for young children in both languages. The ASQ-3 Spanish translation was reviewed by a panel of experts to make the translation as accurate and as widely accessible as possible for the variety of Spanish dialects spoken by families in the United States.

Other Translations

For information about additional questionnaire translations that are available for previous editions or currently under development for ASQ-3, please visit www.agesandstages.com.

ASQ:SE

The ASQ:SE is a screening tool meant to be used in conjunction with the ASQ to identify the need for further social and emotional behavior assessment in children from 3 to 66 months of age. Eight questionnaires are available, in both English and Spanish, which address seven behavioral areas: self-regulation, compliance, communication, adaptive functioning, autonomy, affect, and interaction with people. An accompanying *ASQ:SE User's Guide* (Squires et al., 2003) is also available to assist professionals in using the ASQ:SE questionnaires.

Psychometric Findings

Data pertaining to both the validity and the reliability of the ASQ have been collected on large numbers of children and families. These data are summarized next, and Appendix C contains a detailed discussion of these data.

Questionnaire Validity

The primary procedure used to examine the validity of the ASQ has been to compare children's performance on the questionnaires with their performance on standardized developmental tests. Specifically, children's classifications based on parent-completed questionnaires were compared with the classifications derived from individually administered developmental tests by trained examiners or assessment teams. In the first and second editions of the ASQ, comparisons were made using several different developmental tests, whereas for ASQ-3, comparisons were made using the first and second editions of the Battelle Developmental Inventory (Newborg et al., 1988, 2005), as well as eligibility assessments by multidisciplinary teams.

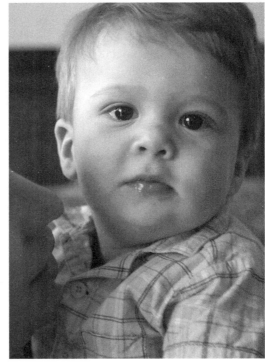

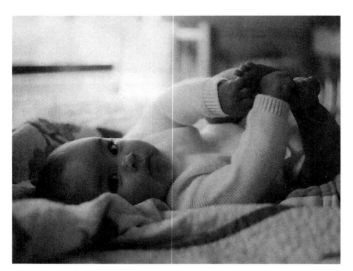

Data included in ASQ-3 have been collected since 2002. More than 18,000 ASQ-3 questionnaires have been collected on children from all 50 states and several United States territories. These questionnaires have been used to determine screening cutoff points, as well as to study validity and reliability. Combined validity findings across intervals indicate that the overall agreement across questionnaires was 86%, with a range of 73%–100%. Underidentification (i.e., children not identified as having a developmental delay by the ASQ-3 who were diagnosed as having delays on the standardized assessment) across intervals ranged from 1% to13%. Overidentification (i.e., children for whom the ASQ-3 indicated a delay who were categorized by the standardized assessment as developing typically) ranged from 6% to 13% across intervals. Sensitivity (i.e., children for whom the ASQ indicated a delay and who were categorized by the standardized assessment as having a delay) ranged from 85% to 92%, and specificity (i.e., children for whom the ASQ-3 did not indicate a delay categorized by a standardized assessment as developing typically) ranged from 78%–92%. Positive predictive value (i.e., a measure of the probability that a child with a questionnaire that indicated delay would have a poor outcome on the standardized assessment) ranged from 32%–64%. Rates of referral across the intervals ranged from 3% to 8%.

Questionnaire Reliability

Test–retest and interobserver reliability data have been collected for the ASQ-3. Test–retest reliability information was collected by asking a group of 145 parents to complete two questionnaires for their children at a 2-week interval. That is, parents were asked to complete the same interval questionnaire on their child twice within a 2-week time period. When completing the first questionnaire, the parents did not know that they would be asked to complete a second questionnaire. The percent agreement for the 145 parents was 92%. Intraclass correlations ranged from .75 to .82, indicating strong test–retest reliability across ASQ-3 developmental areas.

Interobserver reliability was assessed by having a trained examiner complete a questionnaire for a child shortly after a parent had completed a questionnaire. The parent was unaware of the comparison to be made, and the examiner had no knowledge of how the parent had responded on the questionnaire. Interobserver reliability was derived by comparing the agreement between the classifications (i.e., screened or not screened) of 107 children based on the parents' and trained examiners' completion of ASQ. The percent agreement between ASQ-3 classifications between parents and trained examiners was 93%. Intraclass correlations ranged from .43 to .69, suggesting robust agreement between parents and trained examiners.

ASQ-3 Procedures for Using and Scoring Questionnaires

A variety of options can be considered for using the ASQ-3 system. Frequently used options include mailing the questionnaires to the home, completing them on a home visit, completing them electronically, and asking parents or service providers to complete them on site at a clinic or child care center. A combination of these options also can be used (e.g., giving the questionnaires to parents during a home visit and asking them to bring the questionnaires to their next well-child visit, completing questionnaires electronically via on-site kiosk).

Several factors determine which options to use; each of these options is analyzed and outlined in detail in Chapter 5. First, resources must be considered. If personnel are available for home visits, then this may be the best option for some families, although this option will cost the program more than online questionnaire completion or mailing the questionnaires to homes and asking families to return them by mail. Second, the characteristics of the families must be considered. Some families will require help to complete the questionnaires at home (e.g., parents with mental, physical, or emotional impairments). Home visits or on-site completion may need to be considered in these cases. Third, family preference will be a factor in choosing which option to use. Some families may want to complete the questionnaires when the working spouse is available in the evenings and then return them by mail. Other families may prefer completing the questionnaires with a home visitor during the day. For some families, the options may change as life circumstances change.

Options for scoring the questionnaires are also available. The questionnaires may be scored by the program staff in their offices. Questionnaire results can then be shared with parents by telephone, by mail, or on the next home visit. The online management system scores the questionnaires and provides ASQ-3 Information Summary sheets for program staff to discuss with families. Because scoring takes only a few minutes, another option is for staff to score the questionnaires on site or during a home visit and give parents immediate feedback. Parents can then keep the completed questionnaires and program staff can keep the results recorded on the Information Summary sheets. A last option is that parents themselves can score the questionnaires using the Information Summary sheets. Again, options must be chosen based on parent preferences, family characteristics, and program resources.

ASQ-3 Information Summary Sheet

Each questionnaire is accompanied by an ASQ-3 Information Summary sheet, which has the following two purposes: 1) to assist with scoring and follow-up and 2) to provide a summary of the child's performance on the questionnaire. The ASQ-3 Information Summary sheet can be kept by program staff as a record of the child's performance on individual questionnaires so that the questionnaires themselves can be returned to parents or service providers for future reference. Each sheet includes sections for recording individual item responses, responses to the Overall items, and follow-up decisions, as well as a scoring grid that graphically displays the child's total scores in the developmental areas in relation to established cutoff scores that indicate whether further assessment or monitoring is warranted. The scoring grid is designed to be used primarily by service providers. Program staff can choose to use the entire Information Summary sheet or only the scoring grid section, or they may choose not to use this form at all.

ASQ-3 Support Materials

In addition to this *User's Guide,* which contains complete instructions for each of the phases of the ASQ-3 screening/monitoring system, numerous support materials accompany the ASQ-3. Several of these materials are included in this guide and include:

- Sample forms and letters to help establish a screening/monitoring program (e.g., letters to parents, letters to physicians, demographic sheets, evaluation forms; see Appendix D)
- Guidelines for choosing referral criteria
- Parent–child activity sheets that correspond to the ASQ-3 age intervals (see Appendix F)
- Suggested readings and a glossary (see Appendix A and Appendix B)

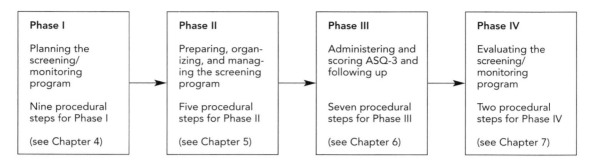

Figure 3.2. An overview of the four interrelated phases of the ASQ-3 system. Each phase includes a number of steps to be performed before the phase is completed.

- ASQ-3 technical report information that summarizes psychometric studies on the questionnaires (e.g., sample descriptions, analyses of reliability and validity, procedures for establishing cutoff points, comparisons of risk and nonrisk groups of children; see Appendix C)

Additional Support Materials

In addition to the support materials contained in this *User's Guide,* other resources are available to assist programs using ASQ-3 and ASQ:SE. These materials include the laminated *ASQ-3 Quick Start Guide* in English (Squires & Bricker, 2009e) and Spanish (Squires & Bricker, 2011) with ASQ-3 basics, designed as a handy reference for professionals on the go, and the *ASQ-3™ Learning Activities* (Twombly & Fink, 2013a; 2013b) intended to enhance child development and promote parent–child interaction. Some support materials can be used to assist with training, including DVDs: *Ages & Stages Questionnaires® on a Home Visit* (Farrell & Potter, 1995) describes procedures for completing the ASQ with parents while on a home visit, cultural adaptations, techniques for assisting parents to complete questionnaires, and suggestions for working in the home environment are enacted; *ASQ-3 Scoring & Referral* (Twombly et al., 2009) describes procedures for scoring and using the questionnaires; and *ASQ:SE in Practice* (Squires et al., 2004) introduces how to appropriately use ASQ:SE. The *ASQ-3 Materials Kit* contains most materials and toys needed for ASQ-3 completion. Finally, ASQ Pro and ASQ Enterprise support programs with online management, whereas ASQ Family Access enables programs to have parents complete questionnaires online. These materials are sold separately from the *User's Guide* and questionnaires, and more information can be found at www.agesandstages.com.

FOUR PHASES OF THE ASQ-3 SYSTEM

The ASQ-3 system is composed of four phases, each of which is outlined next. Figure 3.2 provides an overview and relationship of the phases.

Phase I: Planning the Screening/Monitoring Program

The first phase in the ASQ-3 system is planning the screening/monitoring program, which involves the following nine steps.

1. Communicate with community partners.
2. Include parental perspectives.
3. Involve health care providers.

4. Determine target population.
5. Finalize goals and objectives.
6. Determine program resources.
7. Determine administration methods and settings.
8. Determine depth and breadth of program.
9. Select referral criteria.

These steps, each of which is discussed in detail in Chapter 4, are suggested areas to consider before beginning to use the questionnaires. Some programs may not need to devote planning time to all of the steps because agency policies may already address them. For example, program goals and objectives may already be delineated and administration methods may already be defined by state guidelines. Completing the planning phase helps to ensure that the screening/monitoring system will run smoothly and efficiently once it is begun.

Phase II: Preparing, Organizing, and Managing the Screening Program

The second phase of the ASQ-3 system focuses on system management—paper or electronic tickler programs, record keeping, forms, policies, and procedures for determining follow up for children who are identified as needing further assessment and providing staff training. This phase, which contains the details for organizing the daily operation of the screening/monitoring program, includes the following steps:

10. Create a management system.
11. Prepare questionnaires.
12. Develop forms, letters, and a referral guide.
13. Articulate screening policies and procedures.
14. Provide staff training and support.

Chapter 5 outlines each of these steps and includes suggestions for maintaining child and family records and for establishing management systems. This chapter also includes brief information about managing the ASQ screening process online through ASQ Pro and ASQ Enterprise. Suggestions for developing forms and letters are given, as well as sample letters (blank samples appear in Appendix D). Staff training and ongoing support, an essential element of an effective screening/monitoring program, are also discussed in Chapter 5.

Phase III: Administering and Scoring ASQ-3 and Following Up

The third phase of the ASQ-3 system includes steps needed for administering and scoring questionnaires and establishing referral guidelines for families. Chapter 6 includes step-by-step directions for this phase. The steps for Phase III include the following:

15. Select the appropriate ASQ-3 age interval.
16. Assemble ASQ-3 materials.
17. Support parents' completion of ASQ-3.
18. Score the ASQ-3 and review the Overall section.
19. Interpret ASQ-3 scores.
20. Determine type of follow-up.
21. Communicate results with families.

Chapter 6 outlines the seven preceding steps, illustrating how to administer, score, and interpret ASQ-3. The chapter provides guidelines for follow up, including how to communicate with families. Chapter 6 explains how to select an ASQ-3 questionnaire based on a child's age or adjusted age, how to prepare the ASQ-3 materials prior to the screening, how to support parents' completion of the questionnaires, and how to determine the type of follow up a child may need.

Phase IV: Evaluating the Screening/Monitoring Program

The final phase of the ASQ-3 system, evaluating the screening/monitoring program, has two steps.

22. Assess progress in establishing and maintaining the screening/monitoring program.
23. Evaluate the program's effectiveness.

Chapter 7 describes this final phase and includes a worksheet to guide evaluation of progress. Information helpful in measuring effectiveness, including how to calculate over- and underidentification rates and how to survey parents for feedback, is given. Completing evaluation activities on an ongoing basis helps to ensure that program procedures are efficient and that the screening/monitoring system is effective—that is, that children in need of further diagnostic assessment are being identified.

ASQ-3 IN PRACTICE

Section III of the *User's Guide* provides practical information on the various ways in which ASQ-3 can be implemented. Chapter 8 illustrates options for ASQ-3 administration methods, and Chapter 9 describes how ASQ-3 can be used across a variety of settings. Chapter 10 presents scenarios to show different applications and methods for using the ASQ-3 with families. These case examples may be helpful for understanding different methods of use with families and specific strengths and limitations of these applications.

CONCLUSION

This chapter describes the components of the ASQ-3 system—the questionnaires, the procedures for using and scoring the questionnaires, and the support materials. The heart of the ASQ-3 system is the 21 child development questionnaires administered at regular intervals from 1 month to 66 months (5½ years) of age. Support materials assist with starting and maintaining the ASQ-3 system.

The four phases of establishing the ASQ-3 system are also outlined in this chapter. Planning the screening/monitoring program involves steps that are crucial to effectively using the ASQ-3 system. The nine planning steps are described in detail in Chapter 4. Determining a management system for the ASQ-3 is included in the second phase. This phase focuses on implementation and includes system creation, policies and procedures, using the questionnaires, and providing staff training and support, as well as procedures for determining follow up for identified children. These steps are described in detail in Chapter 5. Chapter 6 summarizes the steps for using and scoring the ASQ-3. Steps for the fourth phase, evaluating the screening/monitoring program, are discussed in Chapter 7. A description of these two steps—assessing progress in establishing and maintaining the monitoring program and evaluating the system's effectiveness—are included. Finally, Chapters 8–10 contain guidelines on administration methods and settings and family scenarios illustrating applications for using the ASQ-3.

II

Implementation of ASQ-3

4

Phase I: Planning the Screening / Monitoring Program

ASQ·3

A number of critical factors should be considered when initiating a screening and monitoring program such as the ASQ-3 system. This chapter describes each of the steps involved in the planning phase.

IMPORTANCE OF THE PLANNING PHASE

The planning phase contains important steps toward establishing a successful screening/monitoring program. Unless careful thought is given to each step of the planning phase, serious difficulties may arise later when the system is in operation. For example, if community health care providers are not consulted during this planning phase, then they may not refer children to participate in the screening/monitoring program. In addition, by involving health care providers early in the program, more appropriate criteria for participation in the program and enhanced cooperation for completing health and developmental assessments may result. If adequate time is spent during the planning phase, it is likely that time and energy will be saved during the implementation phase of the program. It is important to note that health care providers may be the ones driving screening/monitoring initiatives; however, the majority of ASQ users are community programs, so in many ways the planning process described in this chapter is approached from their perspective. See Chapters 8 and 9 for more detailed information about varying options for methods and settings used by ASQ screening programs.

STEPS IN THE PLANNING PHASE

Figure 4.1 provides a schematic of the steps necessary to begin screening/monitoring a designated population of children using the ASQ-3 system. Although the figure shows a linear, one-step-at-a-time approach to planning, it is possible to work on more than one step simultaneously or to rearrange the order of the steps.

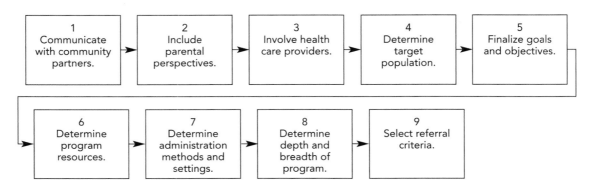

Figure 4.1. The planning phase of the ASQ-3 system includes nine important steps. These steps can be performed one at a time, or some may be undertaken simultaneously. Sometimes program staff will choose to complete the steps in a different order from the one shown here.

1. Communicate with Community Partners

Given the general lack of resources available to young children and their families, it is important to use resources efficiently and avoid duplicating services. Making agreements regarding which agencies will screen children and how information will be shared between service providers is an important step in using limited resources wisely. Many community agencies that provide services to young children and their families include developmental screening as part of their services. Some programs, such as Early Head Start and Head Start, are mandated in their performance standards to screen all children within a certain period of time after entry into the program. Other agencies, such as child welfare, operate under federal mandates that require personnel to refer children for developmental screening. For example, children under the age of 3 with documented abuse or neglect must be referred for developmental screening under the Keeping Children and Families Safe Act of 2003 (PL108-36), which amends the Child Abuse Prevention and Treatment Act (CAPTA) of 1974 (PL 93-247), as well as under the Individuals with Disabilities Education Act (IDEA) of 1990 (PL 101-476) and its amendments. Thus, a broad range of personnel from early education and care, health care, child welfare, public health, and parent education programs should be convened to discuss community screening efforts.

It is important to meet with agency representatives and stakeholders, including physicians and parent representatives, prior to implementing a screening/monitoring program. The community representatives should consider the following:

- What screening/monitoring efforts are currently underway in the community? Does the medical community provide developmental screening services? What other community agencies (e.g., school district, Head Start, child welfare, public health) provide screening?
- What populations are being screened/monitored, and are there gaps? Do certain geographic regions of the community have better identification rates than other regions? What different cultural groups are there in the community? Do these groups have access to developmental screening? Can diverse members of the community be reached in culturally appropriate ways?
- How can duplication of screening/monitoring efforts be avoided? Can agreements be reached regarding which agency will take the primary role in screening and then share developmental screening information among agencies? Should using a common child identification number to share information be considered?
- What types of screening tests are being used, and are these tests valid and reliable? Can community agencies agree on the use of common screening tests? Are tests being used to screen social-emotional development or for early autism detection?

- What types of resources are available in the community, and how can these resources be maximized? Do agencies need to prioritize which children are most vulnerable for developmental delay? Are physicians aware of reimbursements for developmental screening? Are current methods of screening costly?
- Is a comprehensive inventory of community resources available? What types of community resources are available for referral (e.g., early intervention/early childhood special education services, parenting education programs, mental health services, family support services)? Are community agencies ready to receive referrals?

Steps-Ahead of Eugene, Oregon, is funded to provide developmental screening and monitoring of children who are at risk for developmental delays. Steps-Ahead was created to deliver screening and monitoring services to all children in Lane County. Steps-Ahead has links with other agencies in the county serving young children and their families: Early Intervention Program of Lane County; Lane County Mental Health; Kids-Kan Head Start; Child Care Resource and Referral; Butler House Alcohol and Drug Treatment Program; White Bird Homeless Shelter; Sacred Mary Hospital Newborn Intensive Care Unit; Centro-Latino; and a number of community pediatricians. Representatives from these agencies, as well as several parent representatives, serve on an advisory board that provides ongoing advice and direction for the screening/monitoring program.

2. Include Parental Perspectives

Most communities are home to a variety of families with different backgrounds, experiences, and cultural values. Providing screening/monitoring services to families is important to consider during the planning process. Increasingly important is the issue of how to provide services in a culturally appropriate and respectful manner. Inviting family members with diverse backgrounds, including those who can serve as "cultural ambassadors," to participate in a planning group can assist in coming to know and understand parental perspectives on screening and monitoring. Family members can advise agencies on how to involve families with young children, as well as what types of follow-up services are needed in communities. Family members who represent different cultural groups can help review proposed screening protocols and provide feedback regarding the cultural appropriateness of items.

Parents may be able to provide information and insights about screening that are not readily available to most service providers. For example, a large community of ethnic Hmong families in Minnesota created the impetus for an audio version of the ASQ:SE. This was a helpful change because the Hmong culture has a strong oral tradition, and parents are less comfortable with written information. Although the ASQ is available in languages other than English (see www.agesandstages.com for more information), parent and other caregiver input may be essential to devising plans to best accommodate families with cultural experiences that may differ significantly in terms of practice and values. A discussion of factors to consider when translating ASQ-3 appears later in this chapter.

3. Involve Health Care Providers

Health care providers often have valuable medical information about their specific patients, as well as young children in general, that augments screening and monitoring outcomes. The American Academy of Pediatrics (AAP) has issued policy statements that make clear the importance of developmental screening and the critical role pediatricians should play in the early identification of children at risk for developmental delays, including autism. AAP's (2006) policy statement on screening recommended that pediatricians and other primary care providers screen all infants and young children for developmental delays during preventive care visits and be prepared to refer families to community-based resources. Recent recommendations on screening for autism (Johnson et al., 2007) are that pediatricians and other primary care providers should screen for autism and related disorders at 18 and 24 months. At the very least, physicians in most communities should be informed when their young patients are participating in screening and monitoring programs (after written consent to share results has been obtained from parents). In some cases, health care providers and their offices will be the ones conducting the ASQ-3 screening. See Chapter 9 for additional information on different screening providers and locations.

It is important to determine the medically sponsored and/or operated screening activities during the planning phase and to support these screening efforts by augmenting or complementing these services rather than trying to replace them. In addition, screening/monitoring programs should develop strategies to communicate screening results to the physicians of children being screened. Figure 4.2 shows a sample letter designed to explain to health care providers a family's participation in the monitoring program when an office other than that of the health care provider is conducting the screening. Figure 4.3 shows a sample letter designed to assist health care providers to understand the ASQ-3 screening results of their young patients. (Blank versions of these letters appear in Appendix D.)

4. Determine Target Population

Although some community programs and health care providers target universal screening as a goal, most community programs will need to prioritize and develop objective criteria for selecting whom to monitor. During the planning phase, advisory groups or program personnel may

---

Dear Dr. Goldenberg:
The parents or guardian of your patient, Sophia Martinez, have agreed to complete the Ages & Stages Questionnaires®, Third Edition (ASQ-3™), as part of Steps-Ahead developmental screening/monitoring program.

The ASQ-3 is a developmental screening and monitoring system designed for children from birth through age 5. More information on use of ASQ-3 in a medical setting can be found at www.agesandstages.com.

Parents or guardians are asked to respond to questions on the ASQ-3 about their child's development at 2-, 4-, or 6-month intervals from birth to 5 years. They answer items about activities their child can or cannot do. If the child obtains a score below the established cutoff on a questionnaire, the parent or guardian and the child's physician are notified so that further developmental support or assessment can be scheduled.

If you would like more information about our program, please contact Jennifer Davis at 541-555-0112.

Sincerely,

Katherine Kephart
Steps-Ahead

Figure 4.2.   A sample Physician Information Letter to health care providers. Appendix D contains a blank, photocopiable version of this letter.

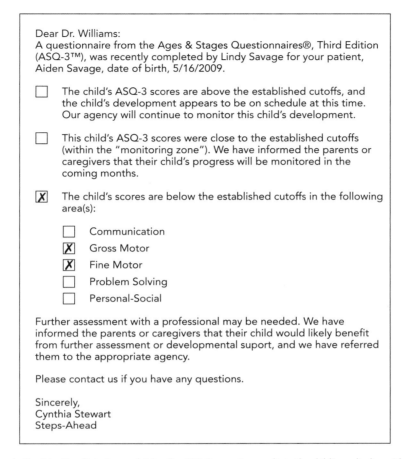

Dear Dr. Williams:

A questionnaire from the Ages & Stages Questionnaires®, Third Edition (ASQ-3™), was recently completed by Lindy Savage for your patient, Aiden Savage, date of birth, 5/16/2009.

☐ The child's ASQ-3 scores are above the established cutoffs, and the child's development appears to be on schedule at this time. Our agency will continue to monitor this child's development.

☐ This child's ASQ-3 scores were close to the established cutoffs (within the "monitoring zone"). We have informed the parents or caregivers that their child's progress will be monitored in the coming months.

☒ The child's scores are below the established cutoffs in the following area(s):

   ☐ Communication
   ☒ Gross Motor
   ☒ Fine Motor
   ☐ Problem Solving
   ☐ Personal-Social

Further assessment with a professional may be needed. We have informed the parents or caregivers that their child would likely benefit from further assessment or developmental suport, and we have referred them to the appropriate agency.

Please contact us if you have any questions.

Sincerely,
Cynthia Stewart
Steps-Ahead

Figure 4.3. A sample Physician Results Letter explaining the ASQ-3 screening results to the child's medical provider. Appendix D contains a blank, photocopiable version of this letter.

want to consider targeting certain geographical regions that are underserved, specific minority groups that may be high risk, or an age range that may maximize screening efforts (e.g., 36 months). Screening advisory groups can help determine where gaps exist in community services.

Several studies have found that although biological factors play a major role in predicting severe cognitive delays, these factors play only a minor role in predicting mild delays. Research findings have consistently reported that cumulative social and psychological risk factors are predictive of future cognitive delays. Children who have multiple risk factors in their lives are most compromised in terms of future development. Consequently, to maximize impact, screening/monitoring programs should not focus on selecting particular risk factors to determine their population but rather target children who have multiple risk factors in their lives.

Program resources and goals must be consistent with the risk factors chosen by the screening program personnel. Programs with limited resources may wish to target only children with multiple risk factors because they are more likely to experience developmental delays. If program resources are sparse, then targeting children who are experiencing multiple risk factors may be an especially compelling recommendation. Table 4.1 lists potential medical and environmental/social risk factors.

When identifying risk factors for a screening/monitoring program, it is important to review federal and state mandates as well as to examine selection criteria used by existing programs that may be serving the same community:

Table 4.1.   Possible risk factors for determining a screening/monitoring population

Medical	Environmental/social
Gestational and perinatal	Maternal age of 19 or younger
Intracranial hemorrhage (e.g., subdural, subarachnoid, intracerebral, or intraventricular hemorrhage; periventricular cystic leukomalacia)	Caregiver or infant interaction that is considered at risk
Neonatal seizures	Parents with disabilities or limited resources (e.g., history of mental illness or disability, mental retardation, sensory impairment, incapacitating physical disability, lack of knowledge about or ability to provide basic infant care)
Perinatal asphyxia (e.g., one or more of the following: 5-minute Apgar score of 4 or less, no spontaneous respiration until 10 minutes of age, hypotonia persisting to 2 hours of age, renal failure and other medical complications of asphyxia)	No or limited prenatal care
Small for gestational age (i.e., birth weight 2 standard deviations or more below the mean for gestational age)	Income below poverty level
Birth weight of 1,500 grams or less	No high school diploma
Mechanical ventilation for 72 hours or more	Atypical or recurrent accidents involving the child
Hyperbilirubinemia	Family interaction that is chronically disturbed
Central nervous system infection (including bacterial meningitis, herpes, or viral encephalitis/meningitis)	Family with inadequate or no health care
Congenital infection (e.g., TORCH)	Lack of stable residence, homelessness, or dangerous living conditions
Congenital defect involving the central nervous system (e.g., microcephaly, meningomyelocele)	Maternal prenatal alcohol or other substance abuse/use
Hydrocephalus	Parent with four or more preschool-age children
Multiple minor physical anomalies or a combination of major and minor anomalies (excluding infants with known syndromes or chromosome defects)	Parent with a developmental history of loss and/or abuse (e.g., perinatal loss; miscarriages; sexual or physical abuse; death of parent, spouse, or child)
Abnormal neuromotor examination results at time of nursery discharge (e.g., brachial plexus injury)	Parent with alcohol or other drug dependence
Gestational age of 34 weeks or less	Parent with severe chronic illness
Aspiration pneumonia	Parent–child separation
Maternal phenylketonuria or AIDS	Physical or social isolation and/or lack of adequate social support
Maternal prenatal alcohol or other substance abuse	
Family history of hearing loss	
Postnatal	
Head injury with loss of consciousness	
Central nervous system infection (e.g., bacterial meningitis, herpes, or viral encephalitis/meningitis)	
Nonfebrile seizures—single, prolonged, or multiple	
Failure to thrive or pediatric undernutrition (i.e., persistently slow rate of growth not associated with illness; weight/length at the third percentile or less)	
Recurrent apnea	
Chronic illness	
Chronic otitis media (middle-ear infections)	

Source: Benn (1993).

- *Federal and state guidelines for determining eligibility for Part C services:* Under IDEA and its amendments, each state is required to identify criteria for determining eligibility for intervention services. These criteria should be reviewed to ensure compatibility between the screening/ monitoring program and evaluation procedures used to determine eligibility for services.
- *Amendments to Child Abuse Prevention and Treatment Act (CAPTA):* The Keeping Children and Families Safe Act of 2003 requires that each state develop "provisions and procedures for referral of a child under the age of 3 who is involved in a substantiated case of child abuse or neglect to early intervention services funded under Part C of the Individuals with Disabilities Education Act." Most of these children have experienced a range of risk conditions and likely should be screened periodically, thus requiring the inclusion of abuse/neglect as a risk factor.

- *Risk factors used by other national, state, and local programs:* Reviewing the populations served by other programs available in the community can help ensure effective use of resources in targeting population needs. These programs might include those established to serve homeless children under the McKinney-Vento Homeless Assistance Act, as well as local Early Head Start, Healthy Start, Healthy Families America, Nurse-Family Partnership, and Parents as Teachers programs.
- *Risk factors used by existing community programs:* Reviewing the risk factors addressed by existing state or local screening/monitoring programs may permit the legitimate elimination of those factors from a new program. For example, if a state medical program is providing follow-up monitoring of low birth weight infants, then low birth weight can be eliminated as a risk factor for a new screening/monitoring program.

 The Steps-Ahead staff acknowledged their limited resources by modifying their original goal of screening and monitoring all children from birth to 5 years of age who were identified as having at least one risk factor. After consulting with the advisory board, Steps-Ahead staff decided they would need to reduce the number of children to be screened. To do this, the selection factors for participation in the program were changed. Instead of one risk factor, three risk factors were required to qualify an infant or young child for participation.

Given the change in risk criteria, staff recognized that fewer families in the community would be served. Steps-Ahead staff prepared to refer families they were unable to serve to other community resources and programs.

---

5. Finalize Goals and Objectives

During the planning phase, careful delineation of the program's goals and objectives by the major stakeholders (e.g., program staff, cooperating professionals, parents, community agencies) should be undertaken. Developing appropriate goals and objectives should help to ensure that the program is initiated efficiently and that day-to-day operations are effective. In addition, developing sound goals should assist in using available resources in the most cost-effective way. Several meetings of participating professionals may be required to develop a set of goals that reflect the purpose and intent of the program. As the amount of productive time spent during this step increases, so too does the likelihood that the program will operate satisfactorily for all involved. Although reasonable variation will occur across geographic sites, agencies, and personnel, the following goals are offered as guidelines. All, some, or none of these sample goals may be appropriate for particular programs.

- Increase the number of community partners that participate in developmental screening.
- Increase identification rates of children eligible for Part C (early intervention) and/or Part B Section 619 (early childhood special education) services under IDEA.
- Initiate screening efforts for children with identified risk factors that put them at risk for potential developmental delays (e.g., infants born prematurely).
- Develop a screening system within a community setting such as primary health care or child care.
- Increase involvement of parents in assessing their child's development.
- Increase collaboration and coordination among community agencies related to screening and referral through use of a common screening tool.
- Provide universal screening for all children within an age range (e.g., birth to 1 year, birth to 3 years, birth to 5 years) through a state- or communitywide initiative.

The primary goal of Steps-Ahead is to screen and monitor the development of children from birth to 5 years of age living within Lane County who have at least three documented risk factors. Screening and monitoring will be accomplished by having parents complete the ASQ-3 questionnaire for each age interval. Children are identified at 2 months and followed until their fifth birthday. Children are referred for further assessment if their performance on ASQ-3 indicates a possible developmental delay. Staff identified the following objectives for Steps-Ahead's use of the ASQ-3 system.

1. Educate referral sources about Steps-Ahead.
2. Inform participating families about the services of Steps-Ahead.
3. Identify, screen, and monitor referred children.
4. Refer children identified as having suspected delays to assessment sources.
5. Provide Child Find and public awareness information to the community.
6. Evaluate the efforts of Steps-Ahead.

6. Determine Program Resources

The success of any screening/monitoring program, no matter how economical, is dependent on matching its goals to available resources. The flexibility of the ASQ-3 system may provide additional opportunities for communities to utilize resources efficiently and expand screening efforts. All screening programs require resources to operate and support families when concerns arise; however, having parents observing and gathering information on their child's development may permit the use of limited resources for other purposes.

The ASQ-3 system was designed to be used by parents or other caregivers with minimal support from program personnel. Completing a questionnaire independently requires reading skills at a fourth- to sixth-grade reading level. Independent completion requires that parents are able to read and observe and report on their children's behaviors without assistance.

Clearly, not all parents will be able to complete questionnaires independently for a variety of reasons (e.g., cognitive disability, substance abuse, limited reading skills). Thus, many families may require support from program staff to successfully complete a questionnaire. Some parents may need minimal assistance such as item clarification or assistance reading some items. Other parents may need more in-depth assistance. For example, a parent with a cognitive disability may require someone to read and demonstrate all items. Also, a parent who speaks a language or dialect unfamiliar to program personnel may require an interpreter. Finally, a parent may need assistance with siblings in order to focus on the target child and complete the questionnaire. Even if parents require assistance initially, over time (and given the opportunity) they may become more independent and confident about their ability to report on their child's developmental status.

Determining resources may require some modification of the chosen goals and objectives in at least three ways. First, limited resources may require changes in program goals and objectives. For example, a program may have set a goal to monitor all infants discharged from the local hospital neonatal intensive care unit for a period of 3 years. An examination of resources may indicate that the necessary personnel and funds are not available to conduct such a large project; however, support may be available to monitor a small subgroup of infants at extremely high risk for developmental delays (e.g., babies weighing less than 1,000 grams at birth).

Second, limited resources may require changes in the means by which a goal is accomplished. Monitoring a group of infants may not be possible through home visits to every family, but it may be possible to monitor some children by using parents to follow their infants' development through a mail-out method, freeing up resources for weekly home visits to a family with more intensive needs.

Third, modifying goals may be necessary when a specific resource is unavailable. For example, the goal may have been for public health nurses to assess the development of a group of infants living in low-income housing. Upon learning that the area's public health nurses are unable to take on such a responsibility, the goal must be modified by utilizing paraprofessionals to support families in completing ASQ-3 and including the public health nurses in interpreting the results. As needed, the public health nurses can provide follow-up with families.

As soon as goals are selected and necessary resources are identified to meet those goals, agency personnel can begin to address the specific settings and methods needed to start a screening and monitoring program using ASQ-3.

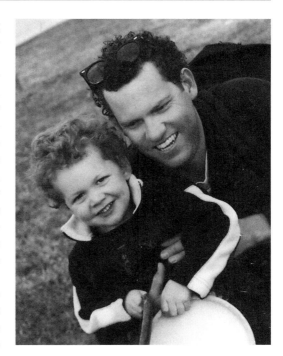

Case Study

In the planning phase, Steps-Ahead began by targeting one primary goal—to identify, screen, and monitor all of Lane County's children who have at least one risk factor for developmental problems. Risk factors were identified by the staff and advisory board at the inception of Steps-Ahead. Because the goals and objectives of Steps-Ahead are fairly broad, it was crucial that program resources be determined to see whether these goals could be met. The first step was to assess program resources, including personnel. The program was funded for one full-time program administrator, one full-time social worker, one half-time social worker, and one full-time secretary. Other resources, including supplies, equipment, and office space, were assessed and found to be adequate. The resources provided by the advisory board were then identified and included the following: follow-up assessment, professional consultation when needed, fundraising, and other in-kind support.

The next step was to evaluate these resources in terms of meeting program goals and objectives. As mentioned previously, when program staff considered the number of births in the county and the predicted percentage of participants in the program, they decided that some modification of the goal was necessary. After several meetings of the Steps-Ahead staff and the advisory board, the program's goals and objectives were amended to reflect the availability of resources. Thus, the goal was changed to screen and monitor only children with three or more risk factors.

7. Determine Administration Methods and Settings

The ASQ-3 system is flexible in that it can be used in different settings with a range of administration methods and differing levels of support to caregivers who are completing questionnaires. Most programs use a combination of settings or administration methods, depending on the varying needs of families. (See Chapter 8 for a more detailed discussion of methods for using

Table 4.2.   Completion methods for the ASQ-3

Completion method	Procedure	Considerations	Potential agencies, settings, or uses
Mail-out	Staff mail questionnaires to parents. Parents complete independently and mail back to a central location for scoring and feedback. An automatic reply (e.g., letter) is sent to parents whose children are not identified as at risk. Children who are identified as at risk or whose parents indicate concerns require a personalized response (e.g., telephone call, face-to-face contact with parent).	Mail-out is a cost-effective strategy for screening large numbers of children. Return rates for questionnaires can be increased with a variety of strategies.	Statewide and universal screening initiatives Community-based programs with limited resources Child welfare screening under the Child Abuse Prevention and Treatment Act (CAPTA) of 1974 (PL 93-247) and its amendments (e.g., PL 108-36)
Online	Staff invite parents of young children to complete questionnaires, and parents independently complete questionnaires online (e.g., through ASQ Family Access, a secure online questionnaire completion system). The online system scores and generates a report for professional review. A reply (e.g., letter) can be generated through the ASQ online management system (e.g., ASQ Pro, ASQ Enterprise) for parents whose children are not identified as at risk. Children who are identified as at risk or whose parents indicate concerns require a personalized response (e.g., telephone call, face-to-face contact).	Online questionnaire completion is a cost-effective strategy for screening large numbers of children It is important to know if parents tried items with their children.	Statewide and universal screening initiatives Primary health care screening
Telephone interview	Staff mail questionnaires to parents. Staff make a follow-up telephone call. Parents can complete questionnaires independently or with help from staff to read or understand items. Staff score and discuss results with parents.	This is a cost-effective strategy for screening large numbers of children. Parents need a copy of the questionnaires either mailed, dropped off, or accessed online so that they can see illustrations of items.	Early intervention and early childhood special education (EI/ECSE) assessment and eligibility Child welfare screening under CAPTA and its amendments
Home visit	Staff provide questionnaires in advance for parents to review and complete independently and the staff follow up with a home visit, or staff provide the support necessary during a home visit for parents to complete the questionnaires. Staff score questionnaires and discuss results with parents during the visit.	Only the support necessary for parents to complete the questionnaires should be provided. Materials available in the home or kit (available through Brookes Publishing) can be used. Adequate time is necessary for parents to try and/or observe items with the child.	Public health Early Head Start Parent education Child abuse prevention home visiting programs Child welfare screening under CAPTA and its amendments

ASQ-3.) In each setting, however, specific issues should be considered prior to implementing a screening program. Careful planning will ensure that the administration method chosen will provide accurate screening results as well as continue to maintain the underlying principle of ASQ—the meaningful inclusion of parents in their child's screening.

    Method of administration, setting, procedure, considerations, and potential uses for the ASQ-3 system are described in Tables 4.2 and 4.3. Families may receive a questionnaire through a mail-out system; complete the ASQ-3 online; or complete the questionnaire with the help of a professional or other staff member over the telephone or in the family's home. Settings for ques-

Table 4.3.   Completion settings for the ASQ-3

Completion setting	Procedure	Considerations	Potential agencies settings, or uses
Screening clinics	Staff ask parents to complete questionnaires using a paper version or a computer kiosk connected to an online system. Staff score and interpret results for parents.	Only the support necessary for parents to complete questionnaires should be provided. Adequate time, space, and materials need to be provided for parents to try items with the child.	Screening clinics EI/ECSE eligibility screening
Education and child care settings	Staff give parents questionnaires to complete and return, or parents and staff work together to complete questionnaires through a combination of classroom-based and home observations. Staff score and interpret results, discussing referral options with parents.	Parents should be included in the process and should receive only the support necessary to complete the questionnaires. Children may be performing more advanced skills in the home environment.	Head Start Preschools Child care programs Family child care
Primary health care office	Staff mail or direct parents to online questionnaires prior to appointment. Parents bring completed questionnaires to visit. Or, parents complete questionnaires at the office using a paper version or a computer kiosk connected to an online system. Staff or the online system scores the questionnaires, and staff review results with parents.	Children can be monitored through questionnaire screenings at regular intervals that correspond with well-child visits. Only the support necessary for parents to complete questionnaire should be given. If the questionnaires are completed at the office, adequate time, space, and materials need to be provided for parents to try items with the child.	Primary health care office Public health screening

tionnaire administration can include screening clinics, education and child care facilities, and a doctor's office or clinic. Support can be provided for any of these administration methods and settings (e.g., support can be provided in a mail-out system by calling parents and helping them complete the ASQ-3 over the telephone). An important consideration is to only provide as much assistance as is needed by each individual. Chapters 8 and 9 describe administration methods and settings in greater detail.

The following four factors may affect the distribution method and settings chosen.

1. Type of program (e.g., early intervention or special education, child care, child welfare, primary health care)
2. Available resources (e.g., financial resources; logistical resources such as space for completing ASQ-3, personnel and clerical support, and computer and online access)
3. Characteristics of parents (e.g., language and cultural diversity, literacy levels)
4. Program goals (e.g., identifying eligible children for special education services, increasing parental knowledge of child development, preventing child abuse)

Case Study   The Steps-Ahead staff decided their initial contact with parents would be within 1 month of the infant's birth. Based on information on the birth certificate completed in the hospital, the social worker determined whether the family met the required risk criteria. The social worker then called the family, explained the purpose of the screening program, and asked if the family was interested in participating. If the family expressed an interest in participating, then an introductory home visit was scheduled. During this visit, the Steps-Ahead social worker obtained the parents' consent to participate, enrolled the family in the program, provided an introduction to ASQ-3, and explained how this information would be used to support their child's development. The social worker answered any questions or concerns the parents had and provided several options for how the family would receive the questionnaires, either during home visits, on site, or by mail.

8. Determine Depth and Breadth of Program

During the planning phase, advisory groups and program personnel need to make decisions about the comprehensiveness of the screening program. These decisions will be influenced by the goals and objectives of the program, available resources, and recommendations from the field regarding best practice. In particular, three recommended practices should be considered: frequency of screening, breadth of screening, and type of screening measure.

Frequency of Screening

It is ideal to screen children at regular intervals, from 2 months to 5½ years, if possible. Again, ideally, children should be screened initially at 2 and 4 months; then at 4-month intervals until they are 24 months old; and at 6-month intervals until they reach 5 years. We do not recommend screening children more frequently than every 4–6 months (except at the 2- and 4-month age intervals) unless some reasons suggest more frequent screening would be useful (e.g., the child has suffered a serious illness, parents feel their child has changed markedly). More frequent screenings may result in inaccurate or incomplete filling out of forms in addition to no change in child status at short intervals. Children who are referred and found eligible for EI/ECSE services should *not* receive further screening. Children who score below the cutoffs and are referred for a more comprehensive assessment but do not qualify for services *should continue to be screened regularly*. These children have a higher likelihood of exhibiting a developmental problem later on (Glascoe, 2001).

Breadth of Screening

Developmental screening should address the major areas of development (i.e., motor, communication, cognitive, personal-social). In addition, recommended practice suggests that the social-emotional area of development should be screened annually. If parents or others have concerns about a child's behavior or if the child has experienced risk factors such as neglect and extreme poverty, then social-emotional screening should be conducted more frequently, preferably every 6 months.

Type of Screening Measure

The AAP (2006) recommended using a standardized developmental screening tool such as the ASQ-3 for children who appear to be at low risk for developmental problems at 9, 18, and 24 and/or 30 months. Children with suspected developmental problems should be screened with standardized tests more frequently. Screening for autism is recommended to begin at 18 months (Johnson et al. 2007). In addition to using formal screening measures, the AAP recommended that health care professionals perform *developmental surveillance* (informal assessments) at every well-child preventative visit, including asking for parent concerns, obtaining a developmental history, and identifying risk and protective factors. The ASQ-3 has been revised to be more sensitive to autism with the addition of questions about behavioral concerns as well as revisions to questions about early communication skills.

9. Select Referral Criteria

The final step of the planning phase focuses on discussing and selecting the criteria that program personnel will use to refer children for more extensive assessment. Examining children's performances on the ASQ-3 offers a straightforward way to determine those children who should be referred, those who should be monitored carefully, and those whose development appears to be proceeding without problem. The ASQ-3 generally identifies children who require further assessment and may be eligible for services and generally does not identify children who are not eligible for services. Scoring the questionnaires permits identifying those children who need further assessment and those who do not by comparing a child's score with the ASQ-3 cutoff scores. ASQ-3 cutoff scores provide the markers that separate children who require referral and assessment or monitoring from those who do not. (Chapter 6 provides detailed guidelines on scoring the ASQ-3.)

ASQ-3 Cutoff Scores

Cutoff scores for the five areas of development across each questionnaire age interval have been determined statistically. Using data from more than 18,000 questionnaires, the mean and standard deviation for each area of development were calculated. The cutoff points were derived by subtracting 2 standard deviations from the mean for each area of development on each questionnaire. (A detailed discussion of how cutoff points were determined is contained in Appendix C.)

Using the ASQ-3 cutoff scores, the following referral criteria are recommended.

- *Refer* a child whose score in one or more areas is on or below the established cutoff score (i.e., 2 standard deviations below the mean) for further assessment.
- *Monitor* a child whose scores fall close to the cutoff score (i.e., ≥ 1 and < 2 standard deviations below the mean). Some programs may choose to provide developmental activities for children whose scores fall in the monitoring zone and rescreen in a short period of time or refer the family to a community agency such as Head Start if appropriate.
- *Follow up* on a child whose scores are above the cutoff scores for each area but whose parent has indicated a concern in the Overall section of the questionnaire. Concerns may trigger a potential referral to any number of community agencies, from primary health care to parenting support groups.

After a child's area scores have been calculated for a specific questionnaire, they can be compared with the established cutoff points. The cutoff scores for each area are contained in Table 4.4. These cutoff scores were empirically derived using a large number of questionnaires, and the empirically derived cutoff points were chosen to minimize under- and overidentification; however, it should be emphasized that all screening measures make errors. Program staff may adjust their referral criteria or cutoff points so that children who are identified as having problems do, in fact, require further assessment.

Case Study

Steps-Ahead decided to use the referral criteria listed in the *ASQ-3 User's Guide*. Children with one or more areas below the cutoff scores were referred to the early intervention program of Lane County for a developmental assessment. If these children did not qualify for the early intervention program, then Steps-Ahead continued to monitor them using the ASQ-3 system. When a child's score was in the monitoring zone, parents were given ideas for activities that would help build the child's skills in that area. The child was rescreened in 4–6 months. When a child had one or more questionnaires with parent concerns marked in the Overall section, the social worker contacted the parent and discussed the concerns. Based on the discussion, the child continued to be monitored by Steps-Ahead or was referred for developmental assessment, or the family was linked with other needed services.

Table 4.4. ASQ-3 cutoff scores and monitoring zones as illustrated on the ASQ-3 Information Summary sheets

Questionnaire interval	Communication		Gross Motor		Fine Motor		Problem Solving		Personal-Social	
	Monitoring zone[a]	Referral cutoff[b]	Monitoring zone[a]	Referral cutoff[b]	Monitoring zone[a]	Referral cutoff[b]	Monitoring zone[a]	Referral cutoff[b]	Monitoring zone[a]	Referral cutoff[b]
2	35.19–22.77	22.77	48.58–41.84	41.84	39.98–30.16	30.16	36.55–24.62	24.62	42.14–33.71	33.71
4	43.44–34.60	34.60	46.52–38.41	38.41	40.60–29.62	29.62	44.38–34.98	34.98	42.54–33.16	33.16
6	39.27–29.65	29.65	33.95–22.25	22.25	37.04–25.14	25.14	39.06–27.72	27.72	36.83–25.34	25.34
8	42.73–33.06	33.06	41.35–30.61	30.61	47.95–40.15	40.15	45.05–36.17	36.17	44.60–35.84	35.84
9	30.00–13.97[c]	13.97	32.27–17.82	17.82	41.82–31.32	31.32	39.11–28.72	28.72	30.69–18.91	18.91
10	35.52–22.87	22.87	41.54–30.07	30.07	46.36–37.97	37.97	42.35–32.51	32.51	38.37–27.25	27.25
12	30.00–15.64[c]	15.64	35.71–21.49	21.49	43.36–34.50	34.50	38.16–27.32	27.32	33.73–21.73	21.73
14	31.63–17.40	17.40	39.44–25.80	25.80	34.97–23.06	23.06	34.82–22.56	22.56	35.76–23.18	23.18
16	30.45–16.81	16.81	47.11–37.91	37.91	41.97–31.98	31.98	40.95–30.51	30.51	37.22–26.43	26.43
18	30.00–13.06[c]	13.06	46.42–37.38	37.38	43.38–34.32	34.32	35.86–25.74	25.74	37.55–27.19	27.19
20	34.32–20.50	20.50	47.85–39.89	39.89	44.39–36.05	36.05	38.54–28.84	28.84	42.70–33.36	33.36
22	30.00–13.04[c]	13.04	39.11–27.75	27.75	39.09–29.61	29.61	39.16–29.30	29.30	40.31–30.07	30.07
24	38.20–25.17	25.17	46.40–38.07	38.07	43.43–35.16	35.16	39.59–29.78	29.78	41.34–31.54	31.54
27	37.22–24.02	24.02	39.14–28.01	28.01	31.08–18.42	18.42	38.79–27.62	27.62	36.11–25.31	25.31
30	43.56–33.30	33.30	44.84–36.14	36.14	33.02–19.25	19.25	38.63–27.08	27.08	41.94–32.01	32.01
33	37.37–25.36	25.36	44.04–34.80	34.80	27.90–12.28	12.28	38.78–26.92	26.92	39.85–28.96	28.96
36	41.43–30.99	30.99	45.84–36.99	36.99	32.57–18.07	18.07	41.13–30.29	30.29	44.07–35.33	35.33
42	38.54–27.06	27.06	45.15–36.27	36.27	33.68–19.82	19.82	39.82–28.11	28.11	41.25–31.12	31.12
48	41.82–30.72	30.72	42.74–32.78	32.78	30.58–15.81	15.81	42.04–31.30	31.30	38.47–26.60	26.60
54	42.82–31.85	31.85	44.58–35.18	35.18	31.72–17.32	17.32	39.68–28.12	28.12	42.55–32.33	32.33
60	42.80–33.19	33.19	41.72–31.28	31.28	39.05–26.54	26.54	41.29–29.99	29.99	46.96–39.07	39.07

[a]Scores higher than monitoring zone indicate typical development. Scores in monitoring zone may need further investigation.
[b]Scores at or below referral cutoff indicate a possible delay in development (further assessment with a professional is recommended).
[c]These four Communication area monitoring zones were adjusted slightly at 1.0 standard deviation below the mean.

TRANSLATING ASQ-3 FOR FAMILIES IN THE COMMUNITY

As the ASQ has become accepted and established in the early childhood field, there has been an increasing demand in the United States and abroad for translated versions. A Spanish translation of ASQ-3, as well as French and Korean translations of previous editions of the ASQ are available through Brookes Publishing. Translations of the ASQ-3 are in development in a number of languages. Brookes Publishing considers requests to translate questionnaires as needed for successful implementation within the community. For consideration and further information, please visit www.agesandstages.com.

Translating, or *adapting,* the ASQ-3 into other languages brings up several concerns and considerations, both linguistic and cultural. Linguistic issues include proper translation of items so that the words impart the same meaning while still being accessible to caregivers who may have minimal levels of education. For example, in one of the first Spanish adaptations, the term *stuffed animal* was translated as "an animal that is stuffed." This translation was too literal and might easily evoke different responses from caregivers of children with similar abilities. Another important issue is the cultural adaptability of items for cultures associated with other languages. Specific skills asked about on the ASQ-3 may not be practiced by children or may be developed at different developmental stages or ages. For example, the item that addresses the child's ability to feed him- or herself with a spoon may not be relevant in cultures in which chopsticks or tortillas are used as a primary eating utensil. An obvious substitution for some Asian families may be chopsticks; however, children may not master this skill until later than eating with a spoon. There may be several reasons for this: 1) Families may not encourage children to feed themselves until they are older, and 2) eating with chopsticks may require more advanced fine motor and cognitive skills than eating with a spoon. Certain items in the Communication domain that refer to English grammar or syntax may also present a challenge, especially in the older ASQ-3 intervals. For these items, programs must work with a speech-language pathologist or a linguist who is knowledgeable about the linguistic development of children in the target language. Similarly, careful attention must be paid to items that rely on references to environmental objects or materials. Certain items that may be commonplace in many North American environments may not be prevalent in other countries or cultures and may be unfamiliar to children and their caregivers. For example, an item on the 60-month questionnaire examines a child's ability to use comparative words: "A car is big, but a bus is _____ (bigger)." This would not be a valid comparison for children who live in rural communities or areas where there are no cars or buses. Whenever possible, these potential discrepancies must be taken into consideration and adaptations made.

A third issue arises when using a translated version of the ASQ-3 outside the United States, as the ASQ norms were developed on samples of American children. Children in other countries may develop at different rates. For example, although most mean scores across items did not differ between the American and Korean samples, at certain ages, Korean children's scores were significantly higher in the Fine Motor domain, whereas American children scored significantly higher in the Gross Motor domain (Heo, Squires, & Yovanoff, 2008). This issue brings into question the use of established ASQ-3 cutoffs with non-American populations.

Based on research and recommendations for adapting educational and psychological assessments into other languages (Beaton, Bombardier, Guillemin, & Ferraz, 2000; Hambleton, Merenda, & Spielberger, 2005), we have established guidelines for programs that are interested in adapting the ASQ-3 for use with speakers of non-English languages. Translating an assessment tool requires a series of translation and validation steps. Before beginning the translation process, however, we encourage programs to contact the publisher to find out what, if any, work has been done toward adapting the ASQ-3 into the target language. As previously mentioned, there is much demand for translations of the ASQ-3, both within and outside of the United States. Although not available commercially, unpublished adaptations of some or all of the ASQ question-naires exist in many languages. Programs interested in learning more about translations should see www.agesandstages.com.

Recommended Translation Process

Step 1: Translate Forward

Identify a native speaker who has an excellent grasp of American English and who is familiar with the early childhood field and child development. This native speaker translates the ASQ-3 from English into the target language.

Step 2: Translate Back

A different translator who is proficient in both languages and unfamiliar with the ASQ-3 trans-lates ASQ-3 back into English, without referencing or exposure to the original English version of ASQ-3.

Step 3: Compare the Back Translation with the Original ASQ-3

A native English speaker with strong familiarity with ASQ-3 (in some cases this may be one of the ASQ-3 developers) compares the back translation from Step 2 with the original ASQ-3 and identifies items in which discrepancies occur. Notes are made regarding discrepant items.

Step 4: Modify the Forward Translation

Based on discrepancies identified in Step 3, items in the initial translation are modified accord-ing to notes made by the ASQ-3 expert. Ideally, this step is done with the translator from Step 1 or at least with a native speaker who is familiar with child development.

Step 5: Pilot the Translated Version

Using the latest version of the adapted ASQ-3 developed in Step 4, the ASQ-3 translation is pilot tested with caregivers who are native speakers of the target language. Caregivers are asked to pro-vide feedback on any items that were difficult to understand or observe due to linguistic uncer-tainties or references to items that are culturally inappropriate.

Step 6: Modify the Pilot Version

Modifications are made to the pilot tested version after considering the feedback from caregivers in Step 5. This final version of the ASQ-3 translation is now ready for general use and can be used to establish local norms and develop cutoff scores for the intended population.

CONCLUSION

As previously noted, time devoted to the planning steps described in this chapter will likely be well spent in terms of ensuring the long-term success of a screening and monitoring program. The steps in Phase I provide a foundation on which the day-to-day activities of using the ASQ-3 system with young children and their families can take place. In the next chapter, pre-paring, organizing, and managing your screening system are described, including systems for managing data, preparing questionnaires, and developing strategies to train and support staff. Forms to assist with organizing and maintaining the monitoring system are included.

5

Phase II: Preparing, Organizing, and Managing the Screening Program

ASQ-3

Once the planning phase is complete, program personnel need to allocate sufficient time to prepare, organize, and develop strategies for managing all aspects of the screening/monitoring system.

STEPS IN THE PREPARING, ORGANIZING, AND MANAGING PHASE

This chapter discusses the five steps shown in Figure 5.1 that compose Phase II, including creating a management system; preparing questionnaires; developing forms, letters, and a referral guide; articulating screening policies and procedures; and providing staff training and support.

10. Create a Management System

This first step describes a series of strategies that permits the efficient operation of a screening/monitoring program, beginning with managing paperwork and ending with discussing systems to manage the timely sending and retrieving of questionnaires. This system may be enhanced through use of the ASQ online management system (ASQ Pro and ASQ Enterprise), which supports programs in effectively organizing and managing child and family data.

Assemble a Paper or Electronic File

Developing a process for assembling individual paper or electronic files for each child ensures that all questionnaires and forms concerning the child and family will be kept in a single location. All of the information in the paper or electronic file should be updated periodically. Developing a paper or electronic file entails several important steps.

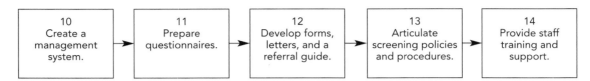

Figure 5.1. The five steps of Phase II of ASQ-3 implementation.

1. Assign the child an identification (ID) number. The first child to join the program might be assigned the number 001, the second 002, and so forth. ID numbers should be assigned for two reasons. First, children with the same or similar last names are less likely to be confused if ID numbers are assigned. Second, the use of ID numbers can help ensure confidentiality when necessary. The ASQ online system generates a unique ID number for each child and also allows previously assigned numbers to be recorded if desired by the user or program.
2. Place the Demographic Information Sheet in the child's paper or electronic file for easy access. The Demographic Information Sheet is discussed in detail later in this chapter and is shown later in this chapter as Figure 5.8.
3. Label the paper file with the child's name or other information that program personnel may find essential to locate the child's file, or input basic information into the electronic file in order to create a child's profile.

Create a Master List

Having a master list of participating children and targeted activities is essential to the smooth and efficient operation of a screening and monitoring program. The master list assists program personnel in ensuring that necessary information is collected and questionnaires are completed for each child participating in a monitoring program in a given agency. Figure 5.2 shows a master list format that can be used effectively for tracking on paper (a full-size photocopiable version appears in Appendix D). The ASQ online management system has various features that show listings of participating children.

Create a System to Manage ASQ-3 Implementation

The integrity of the ASQ-3 screening/monitoring program is dependent on adherence to a preset schedule. The schedule ensures that the parent who will complete the questionnaire receives it 1 or 2 weeks before the child reaches the indicated age interval (i.e., 2, 4, 6, 8, 9, 10, 12, 14, 16, 18, 20, 22, 24, 27, 30, 33, 36, 42, 48, 54, and 60 months). For infants born 3 or more weeks prematurely, the adjusted age should be used when completing the questionnaires until the infant's chronological age is 24 months (see Chapter 6 for details on how to calculate adjusted age). Completed questionnaires need to be responded to in a systematic and timely fashion, and a system needs to be developed to record screening results, make referrals, and monitor children over time. It is important to identify which staff will be responsible for each of the tasks involved in the ASQ-3 system.

Select a Questionnaire Distribution System

The method of use selected by the program or agency (e.g., mail-out format, online completion, home visit) will affect the way in which questionnaires are distributed and completed; however, some guidelines generally apply. Questionnaire distribution and receipt can be overseen through use of a variety of systems, including 1) computer-based systems to notify agency staff that a questionnaire should be distributed to a child at designated age intervals, 2) less technical strate-

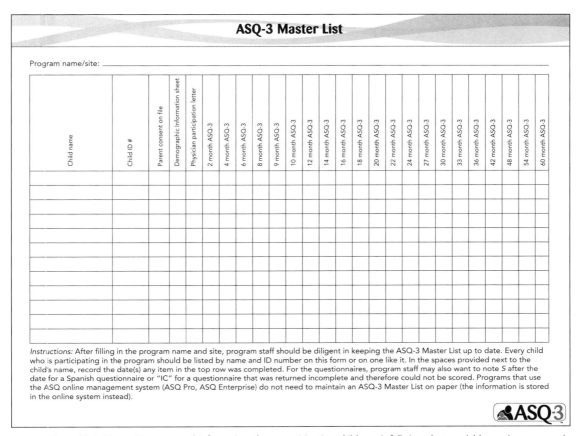

Figure 5.2. ASQ-3 Master List to record information about participating children. A full-size photocopiable version appears in Appendix D.

gies such as a card file tickler system that are adaptable to a mail-back system, or 3) other systems, such as personal calendars (paper or electronic) to keep track of when children should be screened. The following sections provide general information on computer-based systems, the card file tickler system, and other ASQ-3 tracking systems.

Computer-Based System   Agencies that have technical expertise in computer-based management systems may decide to create their own system for managing ASQ administration provided that they do not infringe on copyright and other intellectual property rights of the ASQ product line. (Programs with questions may contact rights@brookespublishing.com.) Or, agencies may prefer to use the online management system for ASQ available through Paul H. Brookes Publishing Co. (see www.agesandstages.com for detailed information). ASQ Pro is designed for single-site programs, and ASQ Enterprise is designed for multisite programs. Subscribers can manage their demographic and questionnaire data—for ASQ-3 and ASQ:SE—and organize their screening and monitoring programs. Subscribers can create user records for all staff at their program and profiles for the children they serve, generate questionnaire mailings and other communications, and record completed screening/monitoring activities as well as plan follow-up.

Tickler System   A second method of questionnaire distribution and receipt can be accomplished by using a card file tickler system that is adaptable to a mail-out system and other uses of the questionnaires. The tickler system uses index cards to keep track of the steps involved in mailing out ASQ-3 (although the tickler could be adapted for use with other methods of

ASQ-3 administration). A file box is sorted by weeks or months in a year, and as cards get pulled and refiled, they alert agency staff as to when certain activities need to occur. Detailed instructions for how to create a card file tickler system can be found in Appendix A at the end of Chapter 8 (the chapter that describes mail-out and other methods of administering the ASQ-3). The instructions for the tickler system also include critical information on completing questionnaires within the age administration range and on reminding parents before the due date to complete the ASQ-3 if they have not returned it in a timely manner.

Other Systems   A third method is developing a system that helps keep track of tasks related to ASQ-3. For example, a home visitor could take the birth dates of children on her caseload and project when the ASQ-3 would need to be administered in the upcoming year. She could use a day planner to make note of these dates. Agencies could post a master calendar with all children's projected ASQ-3 monitoring dates. Any number of systems can work to keep track of ASQ-3 activities, the important point being that a system *is created.*

11. Prepare Questionnaires

ASQ-3 questionnaires are designed to be reproduced from paper or PDF masters as needed by program staff (please see the conditions of the Photocopying Release on p. xxi and the End User License Agreement on the CD-ROM). Each questionnaire is clearly labeled at the top with the age interval and age administration range for ease of use by the staff in charge of photocopying, printing, and/or distributing the questionnaires.

ASQ Pro or ASQ Enterprise users may assemble and print individual or group questionnaire mailings with the system's communications feature. This enables users to select the appropriate questionnaire(s), customize parent letters or forms, and put the materials together for efficient mailing preparation. ASQ Family Access users may organize contact so that parents may complete ASQ-3 questionnaires online.

Family Information Sheet

The family information sheet for each questionnaire asks for identifying information about the child and family, and the answers to these questions will aid staff by indicating who is filling out the questionnaire at each interval, whether the correct interval has been completed (by comparing the date the questionnaire is completed with the child's date of birth or adjusted age), as well as whether any assistance was required completing the questionnaires.

There are two versions of each family information sheet available; users should select the appropriate version based on family and program needs. The standard family information sheets are included with the questionnaire paper masters. These are designed to be clear and accessible to parents who may be uncomfortable filling out forms or wary of being part of a "system." These family information sheets as well as a second, alternate set (data template version) designed to facilitate accurate data collection are included as PDF masters on the ASQ-3 CD-ROM. See Figure 5.3 for a sample of both family information sheets. In the ASQ-3 Spanish, the data template version of the family information sheets show the child's date of birth in day/month/year format (DDMMAAAA), which is often used in Spanish-speaking countries, instead of month/day/year (MMDDYYYY) format.

At the top right of each family information sheet is an illustration of a mother and infant. Programs may use this space to place their program logo or contact information if desired. As shown in Figure 5.3, the family information sheet provides space to insert, stamp, type, or write essential identifying information for the program. Once the monitoring system is operational, staff may wish to enter this information on all of the master family information sheets; this in-

Standard version (above left)

ASQ-3 Ages & Stages Questionnaires®

12 Month Questionnaire

11 months 0 days through 12 months 30 days

Please provide the following information. Use black or blue ink only and print legibly when completing this form.

Date ASQ completed: June 22, 2009

Baby's Information

Baby's first name: Carmen Middle initial: P. Baby's last name: Angelle

Baby's date of birth: June 30, 2008 If baby was born 3 or more weeks prematurely, # of weeks premature: _____ Baby's gender: ○ Male ● Female

Person filling out questionnaire

First name: Carol Middle initial: ___ Last name: Ankara

Relationship to baby: ○ Parent ○ Guardian ○ Teacher ○ Child care provider ○ Grandparent or other relative ● Foster parent ○ Other:

Street address: 4012 Star Dr.

City: Smith Rock State/Province: OR ZIP/Postal code: 97422

Home telephone number: 541-555-0122 Other telephone number: 541-555-0143

Country:

E-mail address: none

Names of people assisting in questionnaire completion: Liz Dawn, home visitor

Program Information

Baby ID #: 02189 Age at administration in months and days: 11-22

Program ID #: 303 If premature, adjusted age in months and days:

Program name: Steps-Ahead

P101120100

Second version (above right)

ASQ-3 Ages & Stages Questionnaires®

12 Month Questionnaire

11 months 0 days through 12 months 30 days

Please provide the following information. Use black or blue ink only and print legibly when completing this form.

Date ASQ completed: 0 6 2 2 2 0 0 9 M M D D Y Y Y Y

Baby's Information

Baby's first name: C A R M E N Middle initial: P Baby's last name: A N G E L L E

Baby's date of birth: 0 6 3 0 2 0 0 8 M M D D Y Y Y Y If baby was born 3 or more weeks prematurely, # of weeks premature: ___ Baby's gender: ○ Male ● Female

Person filling out questionnaire

First name: C A R O L Middle initial: ___ Last name: A N K A R A

Relationship to baby: ○ Parent ○ Grandparent or other relative ● Foster parent ○ Guardian ○ Teacher ○ Child care provider ○ Other:

Street address: 4 0 1 2 S T A R D R

City: S M I T H R O C K State/Province: O R ZIP/Postal code: 9 7 4 2 2

Home telephone number: 5 4 1 5 5 5 0 1 2 2 Other telephone number: 5 4 1 5 5 5 0 1 4 3

Country:

E-mail address: n o n e

Names of people assisting in questionnaire completion: Liz Dawn, home visitor

PROGRAM INFORMATION

Baby ID #: 0 2 1 8 9 Age at administration, in months and days: 1 1 2 2 M M D D

Program ID #: 3 0 3 If premature, adjusted age in months and days: ___ M M D D

Program name: S T E P S - A H E A D

E101120100

Figure 5.3. Samples of the family information sheet. The standard version (above left) is designed to be clear and accessible to parents (blank masters appear in print and PDF format in the ASQ-3 questionnaires box). The second version (above right) is designed to ensure accurate data collection (blank masters appear on the CD-ROM included with the ASQ-3 questionnaires box).

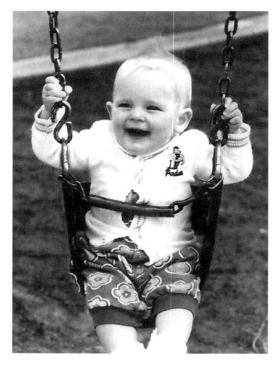

formation will need to be updated if any of the program's identifying information changes over time. Identifying information is vital when mail-out procedures are used. The name and telephone number of a contact person should be indicated to ensure that parents have access to a resource who can answer their questions or address their concerns. For online management system users, a logo can be uploaded and other program information can be updated as needed. The bottom of each version of the family information sheet has a section for information important to the program, which includes the child and program identification numbers as well as the child's age at administration and adjusted age as appropriate.

Questionnaire

The first page of each questionnaire contains a brief introduction for the parent and a summary of important points to remember; this list reminds parents to try to make questionnaire completion a game for the family to enjoy and provides space for staff to indicate when the questionnaire should be returned (see Figure 5.4). Programs may use the notes area on this page to include information as desired for the family. The questionnaire items immediately follow.

The next few pages of each questionnaire contain the 30 items that are arranged from easiest to most difficult behavior in five areas: Communication, Gross Motor, Fine Motor, Problem Solving, and Personal-Social. Each item is intended to be answered by filling in a circle in the columns labeled *yes, sometimes,* or *not yet.* A few items include space for the parent to write an example of the child's behavior. The final section of the questionnaire contains the Overall items, which are answered by marking *yes* or *no.* Depending on the response, an explanation may be requested, and space is provided for the parent to respond.

ASQ-3 Information Summary Sheet

The ASQ-3 Information Summary sheet provides a summary of the questionnaire. The top of the sheet indicates the age interval and has space to include brief identifying information about the child. The middle of the sheet has basic instructions for scoring and a bar graph to record scores for each area and indicate where the score falls in relation to the cutoff scores for referral and monitoring. There is an abbreviated Overall section to record responses and a guide for score interpretation and follow-up. At the bottom of the sheet, the program can record follow-up decisions made and use the optional item response grid to record item-level responses.

If agencies have an established agreement to share information about clients, and parents have provided written consent authorizing the sharing of their child's screening results with outside parties such as medical providers or preschool teachers, then sending this final page—the ASQ-3 Information Summary sheet—provides a complete summary of a child's ASQ-3 screening results. The receiving agencies, however, need to understand the ASQ-3 and how cutoff scores were derived in order to accurately interpret children's results. Figure 5.5 shows an ASQ-3 Information Summary sheet. Program personnel rather than parents complete the Information Summary sheet. (See Chapter 6 for details on completing the Information Summary sheet and interpreting results.)

ASQ-3   **12** Month Questionnaire   11 months 0 days
through 12 months 30 days

On the following pages are questions about activities babies may do. Your baby may have already done some of the activities described here, and there may be some your baby has not begun doing yet. For each item, please fill in the circle that indicates whether your baby is doing the activity regularly, sometimes, or not yet.

Important Points to Remember: **Notes:**

☑ Try each activity with your baby before marking a response.

☑ Make completing this questionnaire a game that is fun for you and your baby.

☑ Make sure your baby is rested and fed.

☑ Please return this questionnaire by _6/30/09_ .

COMMUNICATION   YES   SOMETIMES   NOT YET

1. Does your baby make two similar sounds, such as "ba-ba," "da-da," or "ga-ga"? *(The sounds do not need to mean anything.)*   ○   ○   ○   ——

2. If you ask your baby to, does he play at least one nursery game even if you don't show him the activity yourself (such as "bye-bye," "Peeka-boo," "clap your hands," "So Big")?   ○   ○   ○   ——

3. Does your baby follow one simple command, such as "Come here," "Give it to me," or "Put it back," *without* your using gestures?   ○   ○   ○   ——

4. Does your baby say three words, such as "Mama," "Dada," and "Baba"? *(A "word" is a sound or sounds your baby says consistently to mean someone or something.)*   ○   ○   ○   ——

5. When you ask, "Where is the ball (hat, shoe, etc.)?" does your baby look at the object? *(Make sure the object is present. Mark "yes" if she knows one object.)*   ○   ○   ○   ——

6. When your baby wants something, does he tell you by *pointing* to it?   ○   ○   ○   ——

COMMUNICATION TOTAL   ——

GROSS MOTOR   YES   SOMETIMES   NOT YET

1. While holding onto furniture, does your baby bend down and pick up a toy from the floor and then return to a standing position?   ○   ○   ○   ——

2. While holding onto furniture, does your baby lower herself with control (without falling or flopping down)?   ○   ○   ○   ——

3. Does your baby walk beside furniture while holding on with only one hand?   ○   ○   ○   ——

page 2 of 6

E101120200   Ages & Stages Questionnaires®, Third Edition (ASQ-3™), Squires & Bricker
© 2009 Paul H. Brookes Publishing Co. All rights reserved.

Figure 5.4. Sample of first page of an ASQ-3 questionnaire, showing "Important Points to Remember" and space for notes.

Cultural and Family Adjustments

Items on the ASQ-3 have been carefully selected, and, when possible, materials needed to complete the questionnaires are suggested. Although most parents will find the questionnaires easy to understand and use, there may be items that are not appropriate for a given family, culture, or geographic area. For example, on the 8 month questionnaire, parents are asked whether their child pats a mirror. In some cultures, opportunities for mirror play are not provided and, therefore, this item may not be appropriate for these families.

There also may be times when families do not have access to certain materials and/or are not familiar with certain objects or toys needed to complete items. In most of these situations, alternative materials may be substituted. It is important to examine the intent of the item, however, to ensure that the substituted materials adequately assess the targeted skill. For example, in Hawaii, home visitors found that children rarely used zippered coats or jackets, making items requiring the use of zippers difficult to observe. In order to assess these items, home visitors provided a large purse with a zipper that could be substituted for the zippered coat.

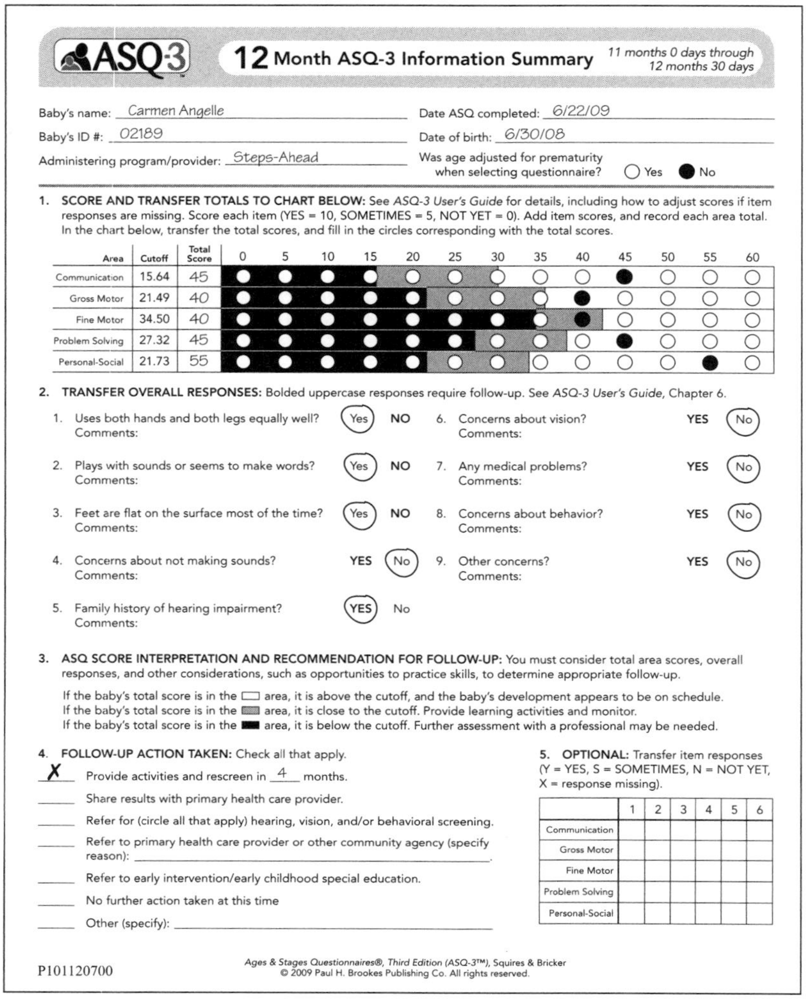

ASQ-3 **12 Month ASQ-3 Information Summary** *11 months 0 days through 12 months 30 days*

Baby's name: Carmen Angelle Date ASQ completed: 6/22/09

Baby's ID #: 02189 Date of birth: 6/30/08

Administering program/provider: Steps-Ahead Was age adjusted for prematurity when selecting questionnaire? ○ Yes ● No

1. **SCORE AND TRANSFER TOTALS TO CHART BELOW:** See *ASQ-3 User's Guide* for details, including how to adjust scores if item responses are missing. Score each item (YES = 10, SOMETIMES = 5, NOT YET = 0). Add item scores, and record each area total. In the chart below, transfer the total scores, and fill in the circles corresponding with the total scores.

Area	Cutoff	Total Score	0	5	10	15	20	25	30	35	40	45	50	55	60
Communication	15.64	45													
Gross Motor	21.49	40													
Fine Motor	34.50	40													
Problem Solving	27.32	45													
Personal-Social	21.73	55													

2. **TRANSFER OVERALL RESPONSES:** Bolded uppercase responses require follow-up. See *ASQ-3 User's Guide*, Chapter 6.

1. Uses both hands and both legs equally well? (Yes) **NO**
Comments:
2. Plays with sounds or seems to make words? (Yes) **NO**
Comments:
3. Feet are flat on the surface most of the time? (Yes) **NO**
Comments:
4. Concerns about not making sounds? **YES** (No)
Comments:
5. Family history of hearing impairment? (**YES**) No
Comments:
6. Concerns about vision? **YES** (No)
Comments:
7. Any medical problems? **YES** (No)
Comments:
8. Concerns about behavior? **YES** (No)
Comments:
9. Other concerns? **YES** (No)
Comments:

3. **ASQ SCORE INTERPRETATION AND RECOMMENDATION FOR FOLLOW-UP:** You must consider total area scores, overall responses, and other considerations, such as opportunities to practice skills, to determine appropriate follow-up.

If the baby's total score is in the ☐ area, it is above the cutoff, and the baby's development appears to be on schedule.
If the baby's total score is in the ▒ area, it is close to the cutoff. Provide learning activities and monitor.
If the baby's total score is in the ■ area, it is below the cutoff. Further assessment with a professional may be needed.

4. **FOLLOW-UP ACTION TAKEN:** Check all that apply.

_X_ Provide activities and rescreen in _4_ months.
___ Share results with primary health care provider.
___ Refer for (circle all that apply) hearing, vision, and/or behavioral screening.
___ Refer to primary health care provider or other community agency (specify reason): ________.
___ Refer to early intervention/early childhood special education.
___ No further action taken at this time
___ Other (specify): ________

5. **OPTIONAL:** Transfer item responses (Y = YES, S = SOMETIMES, N = NOT YET, X = response missing).

	1	2	3	4	5	6
Communication						
Gross Motor						
Fine Motor						
Problem Solving						
Personal-Social						

P101120700

Ages & Stages Questionnaires®, Third Edition (ASQ-3™), Squires & Bricker

Figure 5.5. An example of an ASQ-3 Information Summary sheet. (Blank masters of the ASQ-3 Information Summary sheets appear as hard copies in the ASQ-3 questionnaires box and in PDF format on the CD-ROM included with the ASQ-3 box.)

Determining when to make cultural adaptations may be difficult. As mentioned previously, there are times when items will need to be omitted because they are not culturally appropriate. Before the questionnaires are given to some families, it may be best to consult someone from a specific cultural background who has experience working with children and families from this culture; this is especially relevant when an interpreter is needed.

Another option when materials and equipment are not available is to encourage parents to look for objects outside the home. Many parks, child care centers, and schoolyards may have the needed objects. For example, in the southwestern United States, many homes are built without stairs. To complete Gross Motor items involving stairs, parents may use playground equipment in a local park or building. If appropriate substitutions cannot be made, then the item may need to be omitted and the questionnaire scored using the directions provided for missing responses (see Chapter 6).

Several families who have recently immigrated to the United States have been referred to the Steps-Ahead program. For the most part, these families share common values concerning child development. For a few families, however, strong beliefs against putting children on the floor to play until a certain age preclude the completion of many of the Gross Motor items on the ASQ-3. The Steps-Ahead social worker asked these parents if they could try some of the items on a table or bed. This adaptation seemed to work. The values of the families were respected, and at the same time information about the child's developmental progress was obtained.

12. Develop Forms, Letters, and a Referral Guide

This step covers a range of information associated with developing forms and letters essential for the smooth and efficient operation of a screening/monitoring program. The forms and letters described in this step of Phase II are offered as models or templates and will likely need to be modified by program personnel who choose to use them. Appendix D includes blank samples of forms and letters along with Spanish translations. The ASQ online management system contains customizable letter templates for use in a screening/monitoring program.

Information and Agreement Letter

Obtaining consent or agreement from a child's parent or guardian is an important prerequisite for participation in a screening/monitoring program. Personnel have four options for obtaining agreement to participate in the program: 1) telephone the parent or guardian to obtain initial consent, then include a written consent form with the first questionnaire; 2) send a letter to the parent or guardian soliciting written consent; 3) obtain consent online; or 4) obtain written consent in person. The way in which the initial approach to parents or guardians is made depends on the program's goals and resources. It is important to provide parents with as much information as possible about the screening and monitoring program when obtaining their consent to participate.

Figure 5.6 presents an example of a welcome letter that could be sent to a parent or other caregiver. It contains a brief description of the importance of early development and of the screening/monitoring program. The letter also explains the amount of parent participation expected and the activities of the program personnel. A blank version of this letter appears in Appendix D.

Most programs will want to ask parents to complete a consent form before beginning the screening process. Figure 5.7 offers an example of a form to be completed and signed by parents or guardians indicating their willingness to participate in the screening and monitoring program (a blank version appears in Appendix D). The form also gives parents and guardians the option of refusing to participate. Like the letter contained in Figure 5.6, this form should be modified as necessary to meet the specific needs of the program.

Demographic Information Sheet

After parents or guardians have signed a form indicating their wish to participate in the screening and monitoring program, a staff member should describe in more detail the procedures used in the program. At this time, parents should be asked to provide demographic information about their child and family. This information may help programs with interpretation of screening results. For example, language delays may be more common in children living in families where multiple languages are spoken; children who were born prematurely may have more medical

Dear Parent/Caregiver:

Welcome to our screening and monitoring program. Because your child's first 5 years of life are so important, we want to help you provide the best start for your child. As part of this service, we provide the Ages & Stages Questionnaires, Third Edition (ASQ-3), to help you keep track of your child's development. A questionnaire will be provided every 2-, 4-, or 6-month period. You will be asked to answer questions about some things your child can and cannot do. The questionnaire includes questions about your child's communication, gross motor, fine motor, problem solving, and personal-social skills.

If the questionnaire shows that your child is developing without concerns, we will provide some activities designed for use with ASQ-3 to encourage your child's development and will provide the next questionnaire at the appropriate time.

If the questionnaire shows some possible concerns, we will contact you about getting a more involved assessment for your child. Information will only be shared with other agencies with your written consent.

We look forward to your participation in our program!

Sincerely,

Katherine Kephart
Steps-Ahead

ASQ-3

Figure 5.6. A sample Parent Welcome Letter for parents or guardians (blank versions in English and Spanish appear in Appendix D).

problems in their preschool years. Ideally, this information is obtained in person, but it also can be gathered over the telephone or through the mail. Figure 5.8 shows an example of a Demographic Information Sheet (a full-size photocopiable version appears in Appendix D). Programs may use this sheet to gather demographic information when beginning to serve a particular child/family. The Demographic Information Sheet can be used to update demographic information annually or at greater or smaller intervals, depending on the program's needs. The program can indicate to parents which items to fill out and which sections will be completed by program staff (e.g., the Program Information section).

Before using any demographic form, staff should review it carefully to ensure it meets the program's specific information needs and any confidentiality and information-sharing guidelines that may affect the program. For programs using or planning to use the ASQ online management system (ASQ Pro and ASQ Enterprise), staff should be sure to gather the demographic data required to create child profiles in the online system. Information needed for the ASQ online management system include the child's name, date of birth, number of weeks premature (if applicable), gender, and address, as well as the parent's or caregiver's name, relationship to the child, telephone number, address, and primary and secondary home languages.

Consent Form

The first 5 years of life are very important for your child because this time sets the stage for success in school and later life. During infancy and early childhood, your child will gain many experiences and learn many skills. It is important to ensure that each child's development proceeds well during this period.

Please read the text below and mark the desired space to indicate whether you will participate in the screening/monitoring program.

(X) I have read the information provided about the Ages & Stages Questionnaires®, Third Edition (ASQ-3™), and I wish to have my child participate in the screening/monitoring program. I will fill out questionnaires about my child's development and will promptly return the completed questionnaires.

○ I do not wish to participate in the screening/monitoring program. I have read the provided information about the Ages & Stages Questionnaires®, Third Edition (ASQ-3™), and understand the purpose of this program.

Anne MacConnell
Parent's or guardian's signature

May 1, 2009
Date

Child's name: Emily MacConnell

Child's date of birth: May 26, 2008

If child was born 3 or more weeks prematurely, # of weeks premature: _____

Child's primary physician: Dr. Greene

ASQ-3

Figure 5.7. A Parent Consent Form to be signed by a child's parent or guardian, regarding participation in a screening/monitoring program (blank versions in English and Spanish appear in Appendix D).

Program Description Letters

Once parents have indicated their willingness to participate in the screening/monitoring program, staff should provide parents with an expanded verbal or written description of the monitoring program. It is important that parents' questions and concerns be addressed. It is equally important to ensure that parents understand the program and the options available to them. Parents' willingness to be (and remain) involved in the program may hinge on understanding expectations for their involvement. If the program is mailing the questionnaires, then a program description letter may accompany the first one (ideally, the 2 month interval). If another option is being used (e.g., home visits, one-time screening, primary health care provider monitoring), then the letter may accompany an appointment card. In any case, the letter should indicate that the parent or guardian may speak to a staff member to ask specific questions. A sample program description letter is contained in Figure 5.9. The reproducible document called "What Is ASQ-3™?" (see Figure 5.10) can be shared with parents at this point if desired. This handout, which appears in PDF format on the CD-ROM included with the ASQ-3 questionnaires box, offers a simple introduc-

Demographic Information Sheet

Today's date: _6/22/09_

Child's name (first /middle/last): _Carmen Angelle_

Child's date of birth (MM/DD/YYYY): __06__ / __30__ / _2009_

If child was born prematurely, # of weeks premature: _____

Child's gender: ○ Male ● Female

Child's ethnicity: _Mixed_

Child's birth weight (pounds/ounces): _4/16_

Parent/primary caregiver's name (first/middle/last): _Carol Ankara_

Relationship to child: _Foster parent_

Street address: _4012 Star Dr._

City: _Smith Rock_

State/Province: _OR_   ZIP/Postal code: _97422_

Home telephone: _541-555-0122_   Work telephone: _541-555-0143_

Cell/other telephone: _none_

E-mail address: _none_

Child's primary language: _English_

Language(s) spoken in the home: _English/Spanish_

Child's primary care physician: _Dr. Ford_

Clinic/location/practice name: _Bend, OR_

Clinic/practice mailing address: _Box 3590_

City: _Bend_

State/Province: _OR_   ZIP/Postal code: _97506_

Telephone: _541-555-0167_   Fax: _541-555-0198_

E-mail address: _____

Please list any medical conditions that your child has: _____

Please list any other agencies that are involved with your child/family: _WIC_

Program Information

Child ID #: _02189_

Date of admission to program: _6/22/09_

Child's adjusted age in months and days (if applicable): _303_

Program ID #: _____

Program name: _Steps-Ahead_

ASQ-3

Figure 5.8 A sample of a Demographic Information Sheet (blank versions in English and Spanish appear in Appendix D).

tion to developmental screening and the ASQ-3 and is designed to facilitate family participation in the screening/monitoring program. It does *not* describe how to complete the questionnaire.

Once parents have a general understanding of the program, the next step is to familiarize them with the questionnaires and the specific procedures used to complete them.

The Steps-Ahead staff decided that their initial contact with parents would be within 1 month of the infant's birth. Based on information on birth certificates completed in the hospital, the social worker determined whether each family met the required risk criteria. The social worker then sent a letter to the parents that explained the program. Within 1 week, she telephoned the parents to answer any questions they might have and to schedule a home visit. During the home visit, the Steps-Ahead social worker obtained the parents' consent to participate, enrolled the family, and described how to complete the questionnaires. The social worker also had parents choose whether they wanted to receive the questionnaires during home visits, while on site, or by mail.

Dear Mr. and Mrs. Gershenson:

Thank you for participating in the Steps-Ahead child screening/monitoring program. The enclosed questionnaire from the Ages & Stages Questionnaires®, Third Edition (ASQ-3™), is a screening tool that will provide a quick check of your daughter Maya's development. The information you supply will help reveal your child's strengths, uncover any areas of concern, and determine if there are community resources or services that may be useful for your child or your family.

We'd like to ask you first to fill out the enclosed family information sheet, which helps us be sure we have the most up-to-date information possible. Then, please try the activities on the questionnaire with your child and record what you see and any concerns you'd like to share.

Section 1: The first section of ASQ-3 includes five developmental areas. Each area has six questions that go from easier to more difficult skills. Your child may be able to do some but not all of the items. Read each question and mark

Yes if your child is performing the skill

Sometimes if your child is performing the skill but doesn't yet do it consistently

Not yet if your child does not perform the skill yet

Here is a brief description of the five developmental areas screened with ASQ-3:

Communication: Your child's language skills, both what your child understands and what he or she can say

Gross motor: How your child uses his or her arms and legs and other large muscles for sitting, crawling, walking, running, and other activities

Fine motor: Your child's hand and finger movement and coordination

Problem solving: How your child plays with toys and solves problems

Personal-social: Your child's self-help skills and interactions with others

Section 2: The Overall section asks important questions about your child's development and any concerns you may have about your child's development. Answer questions by marking **yes** or **no,** and if indicated, please explain your response.

Have fun completing this questionnaire with your child, and make sure he or she is rested, fed, and ready to play before you try the activities! Please be sure to send back the questionnaire within 2 weeks. If you have any questions or concerns, please contact Jennifer Davis at Steps-Ahead.

Sincerely,
Katherine Kephart
Steps-Ahead

Figure 5.9. Sample Parent ASQ-3 Questionnaire Cover Letter (blank versions in English and Spanish appear in Appendix D).

Letter to Primary Health Care Providers

Primary health care providers in most communities will appreciate receiving information about their young patients' participation in screening and monitoring programs if they are not conducting the screening themselves. Refer back to Figure 4.2 in Chapter 4 for a sample letter to a health care provider explaining the family's participation in a screening/monitoring program. Refer back to Figure 4.3 in Chapter 4 for a sample letter containing a brief description of the ASQ-3 and how to interpret the cutoff scores. This brief description can be attached when sending ASQ-3 results to primary health care providers. (Blank versions of these physician letters appear in Appendix D.) Health care providers who are administering the ASQ-3 to a child may find it helpful to ask the child's parents if the family is receiving any community services. If so, the health care provider may want to contact this agency (with the parents' written consent); this agency will likely appreciate receiving information about the child's screening and monitoring results.

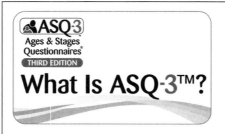

ASQ-3 is a set of questionnaires about children's development. It has been used for more than 20 years to make sure children are developing well. It is called a *screener* because it looks at how children are doing in important areas, such as speech, physical ability, social skills, and problem-solving skills. ASQ-3 can help identify your child's strengths as well as any areas where your child may need support.

As a parent or caregiver, you are the best source of information about your child. That's why ASQ-3 questionnaires are designed to be filled out by you. You will only need 10–15 minutes. It's that quick and easy. Here's how ASQ-3 works:

• You will answer each question "yes," "sometimes," or "not yet," based on what your child is able to do now. Your answers help show your child's strengths and areas where he or she may need practice.
• To answer each question, you can try fun and simple activities with your child. These activities encourage your child to play, move around, and practice day-to-day skills.
• After you complete the questionnaire, a professional will share the results with you.

If your child is developing without concerns, there is nothing more you will need to do. You may try the next ASQ-3 age level as your child grows and learns new skills. There are 21 questionnaires that you can use with children from 1 month to 5½ years old. If your child has trouble with some skills, your program will help you with next steps. Finding delays or problems as early as possible supports young children's healthy development.

You are an active partner in your child's learning and development. By completing ASQ-3 questionnaires, you are making sure your child is off to the best possible start!

> **To find out more, please talk to your health care or education professional, or visit www.agesandstages.com.**

Ages & Stages Questionnaires®, Third Edition (ASQ-3™), Squires & Bricker.
Copyright © 2009 Paul H. Brookes Publishing Co. All rights reserved.
Ages & Stages Questionnaires® is a registered trademark and ASQ-3™ is a trademark of Paul H. Brookes Publishing Co.

Figure 5.10. "What Is ASQ-3™?" parent handout. (A printable PDF master appears on the CD-ROM included with the ASQ-3 questionnaires box. A Spanish version is provided on the CD-ROM included with the ASQ-3 Spanish questionnaire box.)

Case Study Steps-Ahead involved physicians both as participants on the advisory board and with individual families when needed. The two physicians serving on the advisory board wrote letters to other physicians in the community describing the Steps-Ahead program. To ensure physician participation, Steps-Ahead staff notified physicians when families who were their patients enrolled in the program. (Parents indicated their child's physician on the ASQ-3 Demographic Information Sheet.) Steps-Ahead staff also shared ASQ-3 results with the child's health care provider after parents had given their written consent.

Feedback Letters

Once completed questionnaires are returned, program personnel will want to consider offering at least three types of feedback for children who 1) score above the cutoffs, 2) score near the cutoffs in at least one area and/or whose parents indicate a concern, or 3) score below the cutoff in one or more areas.

Dear Mr. and Mrs. Francini:

Thank you for completing the recent questionnaire from the Ages & Stages Questionnaires®, Third Edition (ASQ-3™), for your child. Your responses on the questionnaire show that your child's development appears to be progressing well.

Enclosed are activities designed for use with ASQ that you may use to encourage your child's development.

You'll receive another questionnaire in 4 months. Please remember that it is very important to complete all items and return each questionnaire as soon as you finish it. Feel free to call us if you have any questions.

Sincerely,

Mark Harrison
Steps-Ahead

Figure 5.11 A sample Parent Feedback Letter: Typical, for parents or guardians whose child's questionnaire scores are above the cutoff (blank versions in English and Spanish appear in Appendix D).

When Scores Are Above the Cutoffs   Most children for whom a questionnaire is completed will score above the cutoff scores in each developmental area. For these children, a letter can be sent to parents explaining that their child's development appears to be on schedule at this time and also indicating when the next questionnaire will need to be completed. Figure 5.11 shows a sample feedback letter for parents of children whose scores indicate they are developing typically.

When Scores Are in the Monitoring Zone   For questionnaires on which a child's score is close to the cutoffs (i.e., in the monitoring zone), a letter may be sent to parents explaining that their child appears to be developing on schedule but might benefit from practicing skills in a specific area of development. The program may choose to provide learning activities to support parents, such as the parent–child intervention activity sheets (in Appendix F at the end of this book and also on the CD-ROM in the ASQ-3 questionnaires box) or the separate *Ages & Stages Learning Activities,* which are available in English and Spanish. Parents can also be informed when the next questionnaire will need to be completed. Figure 5.12 contains a sample feedback letter

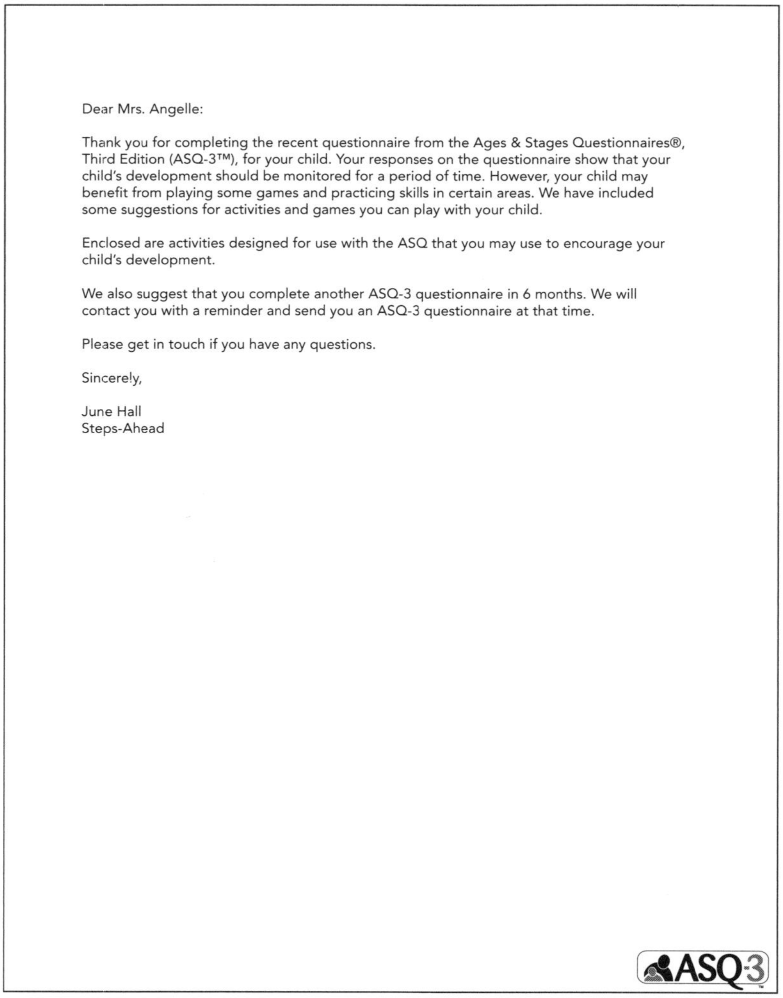

Dear Mrs. Angelle:

Thank you for completing the recent questionnaire from the Ages & Stages Questionnaires®, Third Edition (ASQ-3™), for your child. Your responses on the questionnaire show that your child's development should be monitored for a period of time. However, your child may benefit from playing some games and practicing skills in certain areas. We have included some suggestions for activities and games you can play with your child.

Enclosed are activities designed for use with the ASQ that you may use to encourage your child's development.

We also suggest that you complete another ASQ-3 questionnaire in 6 months. We will contact you with a reminder and send you an ASQ-3 questionnaire at that time.

Please get in touch if you have any questions.

Sincerely,

June Hall
Steps-Ahead

Figure 5.12. A sample Parent Feedback Letter: Monitoring, for parents or guardians, which indicates that the child's development needs monitoring (blank versions appear in English and Spanish in Appendix D).

for parents of children whose scores fall in the monitoring zone and who may benefit from practice in certain areas.

When Scores Are Below the Cutoffs or Parents Indicate Concerns   Parents should be contacted directly if they raise a concern on a questionnaire or if the child's score falls below the cutoff in one or more areas. The score or concern should be discussed and, if appropriate, further assessment options reviewed (see Chapter 6 for guidance on how to discuss results with families). In addition, the child's health care provider should receive a letter indicating further assessment is recommended (see Figure 5.13).

Create a Community Referral Guide

A comprehensive community inventory that lists services to parents of young children can be compiled during the planning phase or during the present phase to assist agencies when families request community resources and when a need for further assessment is indicated by ASQ-3 results. In addition, agencies involved in developmental screening need to keep an up-to-date list of local EI/ECSE agencies that provide developmental assessments and programs that provide

Dear Dr. Williams:

The ASQ-3 is a developmental screening and monitoring system designed for children from birth through age 5. More information on use of ASQ-3 in a medical setting can be found at www.agesandstages.com.

A questionnaire from the Ages & Stages Questionnaires®, Third Edition (ASQ-3™), was recently completed for your patient as follows:

Child's name: _Aiden Savage_____

Child's date of birth: _5/16/2008_____

Date completed: _5/20/2009_____

Questionnaire completed by: _Lindy Savage_____

○ The child's ASQ-3 scores are above the established cutoffs, and the child's development appears to be on schedule at this time. Our agency will continue to monitor this child's development.

○ This child's ASQ-3 scores were close to the established cutoffs (within the "monitoring zone"). We have informed the parents or caregivers that their child's progress will be monitored in the coming months.

Ⓧ The child's scores are below the established cutoffs in the following area(s):

   ○ Communication

   Ⓧ Gross Motor

   Ⓧ Fine Motor

   ○ Problem Solving

   ○ Personal-Social

   Further assessment with a professional may be needed. We have informed the parents or caregivers that their child would likely benefit from further assessment or developmental support, and we have referred them to the appropriate agency

Please contact us if you have any questions.

Sincerely,
Cynthia Stewart
Steps-Ahead

ASQ·3

Figure 5.13. A sample Physician Results Letter, for a child's health care provider, that indicates that the child's scores are below the cutoff in one or more areas of the ASQ-3 (a blank version appears in Appendix D).

intervention services to infants and young children. The list should include the following information for each entry.

- Agency name and address
- Contact person
- Telephone number
- Eligibility criteria for assessment and/or intervention
- Services provided

13. Articulate Screening Policies and Procedures

This step covers developing the necessary policies and procedures to ensure the effective and efficient operation of the screening/monitoring program. When planning a screening system, it is essential that policies and procedures be created to ensure that the process of screening is reliable and valid, as well as culturally appropriate and respectful of families. It can be a useful exercise

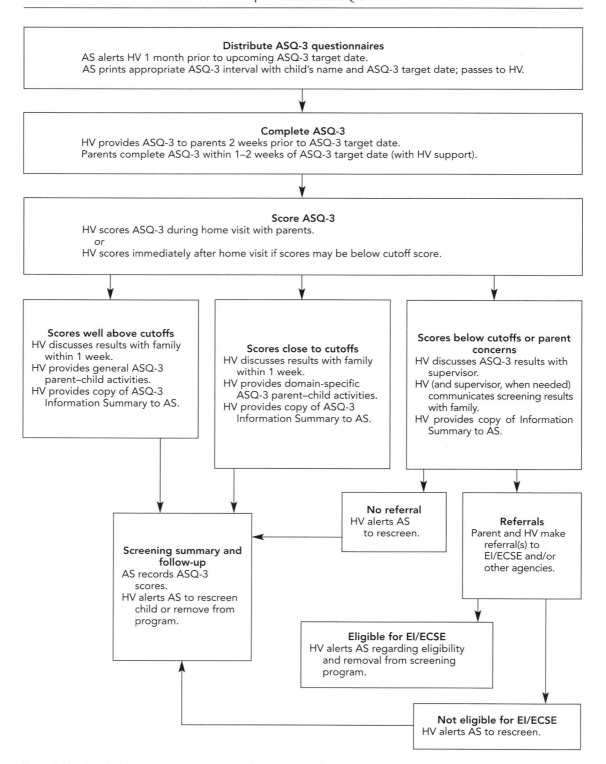

Figure 5.14.   Sample ASQ-3 system map. (*Key:* AS, administrative staff; EI/ECSE, early intervention/early childhood special education; HV, home visitor[s].)

Table 5.1. Procedures involved in an ASQ-3 screening/monitoring process and the competencies and skills necessary for their successful completion

Procedure	Necessary competencies and skills
Introduce the screening program, obtain consent, and gather demographic information	Communicate purpose of screening to families. Understand how ASQ-3 screening differs from other assessment processes. Describe features of ASQ-3 to families. Obtain consent to screen. Gather materials needed if not available in setting. Provide support only as needed for families to complete ASQ-3 items.
Distribute questionnaires in a timely manner	Calculate exact age of child, and choose appropriate interval to administer. Adjust for prematurity, if necessary. Use online, tickler, or informal management system.
Score ASQ-3	Score ASQ-3. Score domains with unanswered items. Enter item-level responses in online management system.
Interpret ASQ-3 results	Discuss factors with families that may affect a child's performance (e.g., biological, cultural). Understand cutoffs and interpret child's scores. Discuss concerns raised in Overall area.
Communicate screening results	Sensitively discuss results that fall in the monitoring zone or below cutoff area.
Conduct screening follow-up	Understand local early childhood/early special education providers and process for referring children to appropriate agencies. Identify resources for age-appropriate intervention strategies and activities to enhance development.

for an agency that is involved in screening children to create a "system map" that outlines and describes the steps involved in the screening program and who is responsible for which steps along the way. Supervisors, mentors, or senior staff play an important role in any screening program and may be involved at different steps in the process to ensure the integrity of the screening program. For example, although a staff member may have the skills necessary to support a family in administering the ASQ-3, he or she may need guidance from a more experienced staff person if the ASQ-3 indicates a potential delay in development. A sample system map of ASQ-3 procedures is in Figure 5.14.

In general, the necessary actions involved in questionnaire use include the following.

1. *Introducing the screening program, obtaining consent, and gathering demographic information:* Providing a general introduction to the screening/monitoring program and its purpose may be either written or conducted face to face. Although there are a variety of ways that consent may be obtained, it is important to identify who is responsible for this step in the process. Finally, how the demographic information is collected and who is responsible for gathering this information should be specified.

2. *Distributing questionnaires in a timely manner:* The responsibility for identifying which children need to be screened in any week, determining the appropriate intervals, and preparing the questionnaires should be clear. It is important to identify not only how this will occur but also who is the person responsible for reproducing and distributing questionnaires to parents. Depending on the type of setting/method, completing the ASQ-3 may be entirely the parents' responsibility (e.g., parents complete questionnaires online) or may require a staff person to provide assistance during a home visit. Although it may be clear that a home visitor will assist parents in the home, it may be less clear who is responsible to support families in clinic settings. Within each agency or setting, it should be stipulated which staff

members will provide support to families. At a minimum, program staff should have an understanding of the purpose of screening, the ASQ-3, and the necessary skills to support families as needed to complete the ASQ-3 (e.g., fluency in other languages).

3. *Scoring and interpreting ASQ-3 results:* The ASQ-3 is not a complicated tool; however, it is important to know who is responsible for its scoring, when scoring will occur, and who will interpret results. With supervision, paraprofessionals or clerical staff can reliably score questionnaires or input data for scoring in the ASQ online management system; however, a supervisor or other professional needs to interpret ASQ-3 results that fall in the monitoring zone or below the cutoff ranges. Providing the necessary support for paraprofessionals or less experienced staff during this step will ensure that referrals are appropriate and that consideration is given to other factors such as a child's health, cultural context, and opportunity to practice skills that may be influencing screening results.

4. *Communicating screening results:* Screening results can be communicated through letters, e-mails, over the telephone, or in person. Any results that suggest a potential delay or problem or any responses to a parent's concerns should be communicated in person by an experienced professional.

5. *Conducting screening follow-up:* Programs should have a policy that specifies what happens following screening, how it is recorded, and who is responsible for the specified follow-up. For example, it should be clear who will identify appropriate activities and provide them to the family of children whose scores fall in the monitoring zone. For children whose scores fall below screening cutoff scores, responsibility for identifying appropriate community referrals and supporting families should also be specified.

In planning these processes, it is useful to consider each step in relation to staff available for the screening/monitoring program. Table 5.1 contains a list of the procedures involved in the screening/monitoring process and the competencies and skills necessary for their successful completion.

14. Provide Staff Training and Support

Screening and monitoring with the ASQ-3 (or any screening tool) is a potentially complicated process, requiring an understanding of the purposes and limitations of screening, effective communication skills (particularly when sharing sensitive and potentially difficult information with parents), the ability to consider what factors may be influencing a child's performance on ASQ-3 (including cultural factors), and knowledge of community resources for appropriate referral.

Users of ASQ-3 should read the *User's Guide* thoroughly prior to initiating the screening and monitoring program. It is ideal that at least one member of the program staff attend an Introductory session and a Train-the-Trainers session (these are often combined) through Brookes On Location professional development seminars. Participants who attend Train-the-Trainers sessions will receive in-depth guidance as well as supporting materials that will assist in training others within their agency. Trainers can also provide follow-up coaching and consultation with staff who are beginning to use the ASQ-3 as well as shadow newly trained staff during their first screening experiences with families. Users are encouraged to go to www.agesandstages.com for specific information about a variety of training materials as well as available training seminar options.

Phase III, administering and scoring ASQ-3 and following up, is described in the following chapter. That phase addresses information that staff will need for ASQ-3 scoring, interpreting results, and sharing these results with families.

6

Phase III: Administering and Scoring ASQ-3 and Following Up

ASQ·3

After the planning phase of the ASQ-3 process is completed, program personnel can initiate Phase III of the ASQ-3 system, which is focused on the actual screening of children, scoring of the questionnaires, and follow-up activities. Chapter 8 describes mail-out procedures for programs choosing to mail ASQ-3 to families.

STEPS IN THE ADMINISTRATION, SCORING, AND FOLLOW-UP PHASE

As shown in Figure 6.1, Phase III is composed of seven steps: selecting the appropriate ASQ-3 interval to administer, assembling ASQ-3 materials, supporting parental completion, scoring ASQ-3 and reviewing the Overall section, interpreting ASQ-3 scores, determining appropriate follow-up, and communicating results.

15. Select the Appropriate ASQ-3 Age Interval

To obtain accurate outcomes, children must be screened using the correct age interval questionnaires (e.g., a 6-month-old child should be screened using the 6 month questionnaire). To begin, it is essential to determine a child's exact age in years, months, and days. Calculating a child's exact age can be done in at least two ways, which are shown in Figures 6.2 and 6.3. In Figure 6.2, a child's exact age can be calculated by subtracting the date of birth from the current date. Figure 6.3 shows how to calculate a child's exact age when it is necessary to borrow in subtraction.

Adjusting for Prematurity

Adjusting age for prematurity is necessary if a child was born 3 or more weeks before his or her due date and is chronologically under 2 years of age. This adjustment is essential to ensure that the correct age interval questionnaires are used with children born prematurely. The ASQ-3 system uses two methods for adjusting age for prematurity.

65

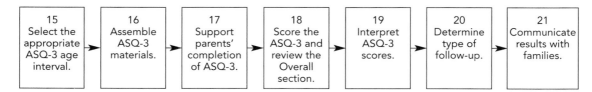

Figure 6.1. Phase III of ASQ-3 implementation and associated steps.

Adjusted Age   The first method for adjusting age for prematurity is calculating *adjusted age*. The adjusted age is calculated by subtracting the number of weeks of prematurity from the child's age. The resulting adjusted age is used to determine the appropriate ASQ-3 interval to administer on any given day.

Corrected Date of Birth   The second method for adjusting age for prematurity is termed *corrected date of birth* (CDOB). The CDOB is calculated by adding the number of weeks the infant was born premature to the child's date of birth (the CDOB is essentially the same date as the child's original due date). The target date for administering the ASQ-3 is then determined by adding the desired number of months (e.g., 16 months for the 16 month ASQ-3) to the child's CDOB.

After determining the child's CDOB or adjusted age, Table 6.1 should be used to determine which ASQ-3 interval should be used.

16. Assemble ASQ-3 Materials

The ASQ-3 can be used in a range of settings including homes, child care facilities, primary care offices, and clinics. To assess a child's behavioral competence, many of the items require the use of toys or other materials (e.g., blocks, stairs). Ideally, items can be assessed using familiar toys or objects; however, sometimes the required materials may not be present, even in a child's home. For example, some homes and clinics do not have stairs. Whatever the reason, it is helpful to plan ahead and consider which materials may be necessary to successfully complete a questionnaire.

Appendix E contains a chart listing the materials needed for each interval of the ASQ-3. It may be helpful for program personnel to create toy kits to ensure that materials are on hand when screening children. Programs also may purchase the *ASQ-3 Materials Kit*, which is available through Paul H. Brookes Publishing Co. If a toy kit is used, children should be given opportunities to become familiar with the toys and materials before an item is scored.

	Year	Month	Day
Administration date	2009	7	15
Date of birth	2005	3	10
Age of child	**4 years**	**4 months**	**5 days**

Figure 6.2. Calculating age. This example shows simple subtraction to calculate an exact age of 4 years, 4 months, 5 days. The 54 month questionnaire will be used.

	Year	Month	Day
Administration date	2008 ~~2009~~	18 (6 + 12 months) ~~6~~ 7	45 (15 + 30 days) ~~15~~
Date of birth	2007	10	28
Age of child	**1 year**	**8 months**	**17 days**

Figure 6.3. This example shows how to calculate exact age when it is necessary to borrow in sub-traction—30 days can be borrowed from the month column, and 12 months can be borrowed from the year column. Starting in the right column and moving left, begin with the day. Since 28 days cannot be subtracted from 15, subtract 1 month from the month column and add 30 days to the day column, making 45 days in the day column and leaving 6 months in the month column. Subtract 28 days from 45 days to get 17 days. Next, since 10 months cannot be subtracted from 6, subtract 1 year from the year column and add 12 months to the month column, making 18 months and leaving 2008 in the year column. Then subtract 10 months from 18 months to get 8 months. Finally, subtract 2007 from 2008 to get 1 year in the year column. This child is 1 year, 8 months, 17 days (or 20 months, 17 days) old at the time of administration, so the 20 month questionnaire will be used.

17. Support Parents' Completion of ASQ-3

To support parental completion of the ASQ-3, program personnel should begin by offering information and explanations about the screening process and monitoring system. Regardless of the setting and administration methods chosen, it is important to explain the purpose of screening and to describe the ASQ-3 system to parents. This explanation may occur in person, over the telephone, as a printed document shared with the parent, or in a letter mailed to a parent or caregiver completing the ASQ-3 for the first time. Following is the suggested content that should be addressed when explaining the ASQ-3 and how the screening process works to parents.

Table 6.1.   ASQ-3 age administration chart

Child's age	Use this ASQ-3
1 month 0 days *through* 2 months 30 days	2 month
3 months 0 days *through* 4 months 30 days	4 month
5 months 0 days *through* 6 months 30 days	6 month
7 months 0 days *through* 8 months 30 days	8 month
9 months 0 days *through* 9 months 30 days	9 *or* 10 month[a]
10 months 0 days *through* 10 months 30 days	10 month
11 months 0 days *through* 12 months 30 days	12 month
13 months 0 days *through* 14 months 30 days	14 month
15 months 0 days *through* 16 months 30 days	16 month
17 months 0 days *through* 18 months 30 days	18 month
19 months 0 days *through* 20 months 30 days	20 month
21 months 0 days *through* 22 months 30 days	22 month
23 months 0 days *through* 25 months 15 days	24 month
25 months 16 days *through* 28 months 15 days	27 month
28 months 16 days *through* 31 months 15 days	30 month
31 months 16 days *through* 34 months 15 days	33 month
34 months 16 days *through* 38 months 30 days	36 month
39 months 0 days *through* 44 months 30 days	42 month
45 months 0 days *through* 50 months 30 days	48 month
51 months 0 days *through* 56 months 30 days	54 month
57 months 0 days *through* 66 months 0 days	60 month

[a]May use the 9 or 10 month ASQ-3 with children in this age range.

Allay Fears About Screening

An important distinction between the ASQ-3 and other screeners is that the ASQ-3 is designed to illustrate what a child can do—not what he or she cannot do. ASQ-3 can and should be a positive experience that parents can share with their children because the ASQ-3 allows parents to be active participants in their children's development. However, many parents may feel uncomfortable about participating in a screening program for many different reasons, such as fear that their child will be labeled *below normal*. When discussing the purpose of screening with parents, consider using the following language:

- "The ASQ-3 is a screening tool that provides a quick check of your child's development."
- "Your answers will show your child's strengths and any areas in which your child may need more help or practice."
- "The information you provide will be helpful in determining whether your child needs further assessment."

Review "Important Points to Remember"

It is also important to give parents guidance and make them feel prepared to successfully complete a screening. Go over the items listed under "Important Points to Remember" on the front page of the ASQ-3:

- "Try each activity with your child before marking a response."
- "Make completing this questionnaire a game that is fun for you and your child."
- "Make sure your child is rested and fed."

Review the Structure of Items and the Developmental Areas

It may be helpful to describe briefly to parents the five developmental areas of the ASQ-3, the questionnaire items within these areas, and the Overall section:

- "The questions in each area go from easier to more difficult."
- "Your child may be able to do some, but not all, of the items."
- "There are five areas of development on the ASQ-3":
    1. *Communication*: "This refers to children's language skills and includes what they can say and what they can understand."
    2. *Gross Motor*: "This refers to children's use and coordination of their arms and legs when they move and play."
    3. *Fine Motor*: "This refers to children's movement and coordination of their hands and fingers."
    4. *Problem Solving*: "This refers to children's problem-solving skills and how they play with toys."
    5. *Personal-Social*: "This refers to children's self-help skills and their interactions with others."
- "The Overall section asks questions about your child's overall development and about any concerns you may have about your child's development."

Tell Parents About the Possible Responses

It also may be helpful to explain to parents the options for scoring items:

- "*Yes* indicates that your child is performing the skill."

- "*Sometimes* indicates that your child is just beginning to perform the behavior (i.e., emerging skill) or performs the skill on occasion, but not all the time"
- "*Not yet* indicates that your child is not yet performing the behavior."

Because the ASQ-3 is used in a range of settings and with different populations, it may be necessary to offer expanded information or additional support to some parents or other caregivers. Support provided may range from being available to answer questions, to reading the items, to assisting parents in eliciting and interpreting their children's responses.

18. Score the ASQ-3 and Review the Overall Section

Each questionnaire contains 30 items that cover five developmental areas and an additional set of questions about the child's overall health and development. This step explains the scoring procedure for the 30 questions on each questionnaire and how to address a parent's responses to the Overall questions. This step also explains how to use the scoring bar graph with cutoffs and the monitoring zone on the ASQ-3 Information Summary sheet. The *ASQ-3 Scoring & Referral* DVD (Twombly et al., 2009), available from Paul H. Brookes Publishing Co., Inc., is also discussed.

After a parent or other caregiver has answered the items on a questionnaire, a professional should use the scoring procedure outlined below:

1. *Review the questionnaire for omitted items.* If all items are answered, proceed to Step 2. If any questions were omitted, try to determine why; if appropriate, gather the necessary information to score the unanswered questions, then go to Step 2. If it is not possible (e.g., parent cannot be contacted) or appropriate (e.g., for cultural reasons) for the parent to answer the item, see the procedures outlined in the following section, Scoring Questionnaires with Omitted Items.

2. *Correct items marked "not yet" or "sometimes" if more advanced items are scored "yes or sometimes."* On a few of the questionnaires, there are items that ask about behaviors the child may have performed at one time but no longer does because he or she has acquired more advanced skills (e.g., sitting without using hands for support versus sitting while leaning on his or her hands for support). On these questions, parents are instructed to answer *yes* to items their child performed earlier but no longer does. If parents mistakenly answer *not yet* or *sometimes* to an easier item (e.g., pertaining to sitting while leaning on hands for support) but *yes* to a more advanced item (e.g., sitting without using hands for support), the response for the earlier item should be changed to *yes* before the area score is computed. Refer to the asterisked scoring instructions on the questionnaires for details.

3. *Score each item on the questionnaire.* For each questionnaire item, parents may mark *yes, sometimes,* or *not yet* by filling in a bubble for each item response. A scoring line is provided to the right of the response bubbles, as shown in Figure 6.4. The scoring system assigns 10 points for each *yes,* 5 points for each *sometimes,* and 0 points for each *not yet* response. In the ASQ online management system, scores are generated once a questionnaire is marked complete. For programs scoring questionnaires by hand, these scores may be hand recorded on the scoring lines.

   a. *Yes* = 10 points
   b. *Sometimes* = 5 points
   c. *Not yet* = 0 points

4. *Total the points in each of the five developmental areas.* Obtain area total scores for Communication, Gross Motor, Fine Motor, Problem Solving, and Personal-Social. This is done when you finalize a questionnaire within the ASQ online management system. If a program is working on paper, the total area score can be recorded on the line at the end of each

COMMUNICATION

| | YES | SOMETIMES | NOT YET |

1. Does your baby chuckle softly?

2. After you have been out of sight, does your baby smile or get excited when he sees you?

3. Does your baby stop crying when she hears a voice other than yours?

4. Does your baby make high-pitched squeals?

5. Does your baby laugh?

6. Does your baby make sounds when looking at toys or people?

COMMUNICATION TOTAL

Figure 6.4. An illustration of the section of the questionnaire for scoring each item and for calculating the area score. (In this illustration, items from the 4 month questionnaire are shown.)

area on the questionnaire (see Figure 6.4). If any items were omitted, go to the next section, Scoring Questionnaires with Omitted Items. After adjusting the total area score, go to Step 5.

5. *Transfer the total area scores to the ASQ-3 Information Summary sheet.* There are two ways to indicate scores on the ASQ-3 Information Summary sheet on which scores can be recorded. Each area total score can be filled in next to the cutoff score in the scoring grid. The total area scores also can be bubbled in on the bar graph portion of the scoring grid (see Figure 6.5). A total area score may be *above* cutoffs, *close to* cutoffs (in the monitoring zone), or *below* cutoffs. On the scoring grid, the dark shading indicates the empirically derived 2 standard deviations below the mean cutoff score in each developmental area. The lightly shaded *monitoring zone* was developed to address concerns about careful monitoring of a child whose performance falls close to the cutoff score. The monitoring zone spans the range from 1 to 2 standard deviations below the mean. If a child scores in the monitoring zone, then program staff may refer a child for further assessment, provide learning activities in that area of development, or monitor development in that area in the upcoming months. In addition, program personnel may either reduce or expand the monitoring zone to adjust for available community resources. Total area scores that fall below the cutoff indicate a need for further assessment in these areas. These area scores are automatically generated, and the Information Summary sheet can be printed using the ASQ online management system.

6. *Record individual item responses.* The grid at the bottom right of the ASQ-3 Information Summary sheet provides space to record responses to individual questionnaire items (see Figure 6.6). If program staff wish to return completed questionnaires to parents, the ASQ-3 Information Summary sheet can be used as a 1-page summary of all questionnaire

Area	Cutoff	Total Score	0	5	10	15	20	25	30	35	40	45	50	55	60
Communication	34.60														
Gross Motor	38.41														
Fine Motor	29.62														
Problem Solving	34.98														
Personal-Social	33.16														

Figure 6.5. The section of the ASQ-3 Information Summary sheet designed to record area scores. (In this illustration, the 4 month summary sheet is shown. For each ASQ-3 interval, the Cutoff column on the summary sheet shows the cutoff scores for that particular interval.)

information, including individual questionnaire item responses. This may be valuable at a later time if a staff person must determine whether a child needs a more in-depth developmental assessment. Programs that plan to use the ASQ online management system and that wish to return completed questionnaires to parents should use the item response grid. The individual item responses will be needed when program staff enter screening data in the online system.

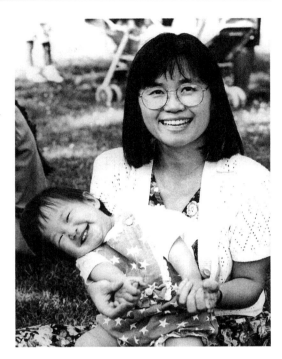

7. *Read the responses in the Overall section carefully.* When reading through the Overall section, note any parent concerns. In most cases, these concerns should be discussed to identify potential problems. Transfer the *yes* and *no* responses in the Overall section to the middle portion of the ASQ-3 Information Summary sheet, along with any relevant comments.

The Overall section questions focus on health and developmental issues such as hearing, vision, behavior, quality of a child's skills, and general parent concerns that may require follow-up. The Overall section, which contains questions such as "Do you think your child hears well?" and "Does anything about your child worry you?" is not scored, but it should serve as a general indicator of parental concerns.

Parents answer these questions by selecting *yes* or *no* and, when appropriate, explaining their responses. For example, a child may pass many of the expressive items in the communication area on the 30 month questionnaire and receive scores that are above the cutoff point. However, the child's parents may have noted *no* in response to the questions, "Do you think your child talks like other toddlers his [or her] age?" or "Do other people understand most of what your child says?" In such a case, a child may be able to put together the words in a sentence, but

5. OPTIONAL: Transfer item responses (Y = YES, S = SOMETIMES, N = NOT YET, X = response missing).						
	1	2	3	4	5	6
Communication						
Gross Motor						
Fine Motor						
Problem Solving						
Personal-Social						

Figure 6.6. Illustration of the grid at the bottom right of the ASQ-3 Information Summary sheet for recording responses to individual questionnaire items.

the child's poor articulation interferes with his or her ability to communicate effectively. Many children are eligible for services on the basis of their articulation (particularly preschool-age children), and, therefore, a referral for further assessment should be discussed with the child's caregiver. A detailed discussion of interpreting parents' answers on the Overall section appears later in this chapter in Reviewing the Overall Section of the ASQ-3.

Scoring Questionnaires with Omitted Items

When a parent does not provide answers to all of the items on a questionnaire, attempts should be made to contact the parent as soon as possible to obtain his or her response(s) to the missing item(s). If the missing responses are provided, the person scoring the questionnaire should follow the steps outlined in the previous section. *Please note that an area should **not** be scored when more than 2 items are left unanswered.*

Sometimes, parents omit items because they are unsure of how to respond or because they have concerns about their children's performance on those items. For whatever reason, it is important to reach parents when items are left unanswered to obtain an answer. If contacting the parent is not possible, or if it is inappropriate to complete the item, then an adjusted total area score can be computed. Adjusted total area scores do not penalize children for unanswered items. An adjusted total area score is computed by dividing the total area score by the number of items answered in that area.

total area score ÷ number of items answered in that area = average total score for that area

This formula will yield a number between 0 and 10. The adjusted item score is then added to the other item scores, producing a total area score that can be compared against the cutoff points on the ASQ-3 Information Summary sheet. If two items were omitted, then the adjusted item score is added twice to the other item scores.

average total score + scores for other items = adjusted total area score

Another method to determine adjusted total area scores is to use the information provided in Table 6.2; this information is also available in the *ASQ-3 Quick Start Guide*. After calculating the total area score (with omitted items), find that score on the left-hand column and follow across to determine the adjusted total area score. This adjusted total area score can be compared against the cutoff points on the ASQ-3 Information Summary sheet.

Table 6.2. Score adjustment chart for the ASQ-3 when item responses have been omitted

Area score (for the items that have responses)	Adjusted total area score (one omitted item)	Adjusted total area score (two omitted items)
50	60	—
45	54	—
40	48	60
35	42	52.5
30	36	45
25	30	37.5
20	24	30
15	18	22.5
10	12	15
5	6	7.5
0	0	0

Reviewing the Overall Section of the ASQ-3

Regardless of a child's scores, when a parent records a concern in the Overall section of the questionnaire, program staff should respond. Important concerns that parents indicate may call for a follow-up assessment or referral for services. Autism, cerebral palsy, articulation difficulties, and hearing impairment are examples of these important concerns that may be indicated on the Overall section.

Table 6.3 contains a list of Overall section questions and the intent behind each one. In general, a "red flag" answer to an Overall question (shown on the ASQ-3 Information Summary sheets in the Overall section as boldface, uppercase **YES** and **NO** responses, indicates that a follow-up telephone call or visit is necessary. Any concern about development noted by parents in the Overall section should be discussed with the parents, and a referral should be made if appropriate. Keep in mind that these questions are not diagnostic; they can only serve as a guide for discussion and the potential need for further assessment.

19. Interpret ASQ-3 Scores

Once a questionnaire is complete and has been reviewed and scored, an interpretation of the results should be performed by a professional. After scoring the questionnaire, there are several options that visually indicate whether a child may need further assessment. The professional should

Table 6.3. ASQ-3 Overall questions by age interval and possible problem indicators

ASQ-3 intervals	Overall question	Possible problem indicator of	Examples of referrals
2–14	Does your baby use both hands/legs equally well?	Cerebral palsy	Health care provider; motor specialist
2–14	When you help your baby stand, are his/her feet flat on the surface most of the time?	Cerebral palsy	Health care provider; motor specialist
16–60	Do you think your child talks like other toddlers/children his/her age?	Articulation delay; speech-language disorder	Early intervention/early childhood special educator (EI/ECSE); speech-language pathologist (SLP)
16–60	Can you understand most of what your child says?	Articulation delay; speech-language disorder	EI/ECSE; SLP
30–60	Can other people understand most of what your child says?	Articulation delay; speech-language disorder	EI/ECSE; SLP
16–60	Do you think your child walks, runs, and climbs like other toddlers/children his/her age?	Neurological conditions; cerebral palsy	EI/ECSE; health care provider; motor specialist
All	Do you think your baby/child hears well?	Hearing impairment	EI/ECSE; audiologist
All	Does either parent have a family history of childhood deafness or hearing impairment?	Hearing impairment	EI/ECSE; audiologist
All	Do you have concerns about your baby's/child's vision?	Visual impairment; strabismus	Primary health care provider
All	Has your baby/child had any medical problems in the last several months?	If ear infections, possible hearing impairment; other medical problems could indicate a very long list of issues	Primary health care provider; audiologist for hearing evaluation
All	Do you have any concerns about your baby's/child's behavior?	Regulatory disorder; autism; attention-deficit/hyperactivity disorder; oppositional defiant disorder; anxiety disorder; depression	EI/ECSE; health care provider; infant mental health or behavioral specialist
All	Does anything about your baby/child worry you?		

be able to interpret the results of the ASQ-3 by viewing the area totals. If the area total for any given developmental area falls within the darkest shaded section of the bar graph on the ASQ-3 Information Summary sheet scoring grid (see Figure 6.5), it is recommended that the child be referred for further assessment. If the area total for any given developmental area falls within the lightly shaded section of the bar graph (a monitoring zone between 1 and 2 standard deviations below the mean), the professional should decide either to continue monitoring the child or to refer the child for further assessment. If the area total falls within the white portion of the bar graph, the child is doing well in that developmental area and should continue to be monitored as appropriate.

Each developmental area contains six items that address skills in that area. Each item has an approximate developmental quotient range between 75 and 100. An item that has a developmental quotient of 100 is a skill that most children should be able to perform at a given age. The rationale for selecting this restricted range is that children who are performing above 100 are probably developing without problems, whereas children scoring below 75 may have significant problems. Most typically developing children will have area scores well above the cutoff points, indicating no apparent problems.

Cutoff Scores

The ASQ-3 system uses cutoff scores to determine whether a child's score on a questionnaire indicates that the child is developing typically or whether he or she should be referred for a more comprehensive assessment. The cutoff scores have been generated for each area of development on each questionnaire based on more than 18,000 questionnaires completed by parents of children between 1 and 66 months of age. The cutoff points were derived by subtracting 2 standard deviations from the mean (average score) for each area of development (e.g., Fine Motor). Therefore, the mean for each area represents the average performance of a large number of children. The standard deviation represents the amount of variance for each mean score (i.e., how many scores are likely to vary in a particular area). Means and standard deviations by ASQ-3 questionnaire for each age interval are listed in Table 6.4.

The cutoff scores listed in Table 6.5 were selected to minimize the percentages of children overidentified and underidentified. The cutoff scores vary by area of development and by questionnaire age interval. The technical report in Appendix C provides a more thorough discussion of the analyses conducted on the ASQ-3.

Table 16 in Appendix C provides data that can be used to make possible changes in cutoff scores (e.g., 1 standard deviation below the mean rather than 2 standard deviations). The sensitivity, specificity, false negative, false positive, underidentification, and overidentification rates when these cutoff points are adjusted are given.

20. Determine Type of Follow-Up

After the child's questionnaire has been scored and the Overall section has been reviewed, several follow-up options should be considered on the basis of the child's screening results. The ASQ-3 Information Summary sheet provides a list of potential actions that may follow administration of the ASQ-3, based on the child's scores and the parent's responses to the Overall questions. These different types of follow-up options and procedures are explained in the following sections.

Children Whose Scores Indicate Typical Development

Children whose scores are well above the cutoff points are considered typically developing and do not require further assessment. Children can be rescreened at 4- to 6-month intervals, and parents can be provided with developmental activities when appropriate, such as the intervention activities in Appendix F. Parents should be informed in person, over the telephone, or

Table 6.4. ASQ-3 means and standard deviations (*SD*) by questionnaire interval

Questionnaire interval	Communication		Gross Motor		Fine Motor		Problem Solving		Personal-Social	
	Mean	SD	Mean	SD	Mean	SD	Mean	SD	Mean	SD
2	47.62	12.42	55.32	6.74	49.80	9.82	48.48	11.93	50.57	8.43
4	52.28	8.84	54.63	8.11	51.58	10.98	53.79	9.41	51.92	9.38
6	48.90	9.63	45.64	11.69	48.93	11.90	50.41	11.35	48.31	11.48
8	52.40	9.67	52.09	10.74	55.75	7.80	53.92	8.87	53.35	8.75
9	38.55	12.29	46.72	14.45	52.31	10.49	49.51	10.39	42.47	11.78
10	48.17	12.65	53.02	11.47	54.72	8.38	52.19	9.84	49.49	11.12
12	43.22	13.79	49.92	14.22	52.22	8.86	48.99	10.84	45.73	12.00
14	45.85	14.23	53.09	13.64	46.87	11.91	47.08	12.26	48.34	12.58
16	44.08	13.64	56.31	9.20	51.96	9.99	51.39	10.44	48.01	10.79
18	42.30	14.62	55.46	9.04	52.44	9.06	45.99	10.13	47.90	10.35
20	48.14	13.82	55.82	7.96	52.73	8.34	48.24	9.70	52.04	9.34
22	44.94	15.95	50.48	11.37	48.58	9.49	49.02	9.86	50.54	10.24
24	51.23	13.03	54.73	8.33	51.70	8.27	49.40	9.81	51.14	9.80
27	50.43	13.21	50.27	11.13	43.74	12.66	49.95	11.16	46.92	10.82
30	53.81	10.25	53.54	8.70	46.78	13.76	50.18	11.55	51.87	9.93
33	49.38	12.01	53.28	9.24	43.52	15.62	50.65	11.86	50.74	10.89
36	51.88	10.44	54.68	8.84	47.07	14.50	51.97	10.84	52.82	8.74
42	50.02	11.48	54.03	8.88	47.55	13.87	51.54	11.72	51.39	10.13
48	52.92	11.10	52.71	9.97	45.35	14.77	52.78	10.74	50.34	11.87
54	53.79	10.97	53.98	9.40	46.12	14.40	51.25	11.56	52.77	10.22
60	52.42	9.62	52.17	10.44	51.57	12.52	52.59	11.30	54.84	7.89

Table 6.5. ASQ-3 referral cutoff scores as illustrated on the ASQ-3 Information Summary sheets

Questionnaire interval	Communication	Gross Motor	Fine Motor	Problem Solving	Personal-Social
2	22.77	41.84	30.16	24.62	33.71
4	34.60	38.41	29.62	34.98	33.16
6	29.65	22.25	25.14	27.72	25.34
8	33.06	30.61	40.15	36.17	35.84
9	13.97	17.82	31.32	28.72	18.91
10	22.87	30.07	37.97	32.51	27.25
12	15.64	21.49	34.50	27.32	21.73
14	17.40	25.80	23.06	22.56	23.18
16	16.81	37.91	31.98	30.51	26.43
18	13.06	37.38	34.32	25.74	27.19
20	20.50	39.89	36.05	28.84	33.36
22	13.04	27.75	29.61	29.30	30.07
24	25.17	38.07	35.16	29.78	31.54
27	24.02	28.01	18.42	27.62	25.31
30	33.30	36.14	19.25	27.08	32.01
33	25.36	34.80	12.28	26.92	28.96
36	30.99	36.99	18.07	30.29	35.33
42	27.06	36.27	19.82	28.11	31.12
48	30.72	32.78	15.81	31.30	26.60
54	31.85	35.18	17.32	28.12	32.33
60	33.19	31.28	26.54	29.99	39.07

Note: Scores at or below referral cutoff indicate a possible delay in development (further assessment with a professional is recommended). For monitoring zone score information, see Table 4.4 in Chapter 4.

through mail or e-mail that their child's development seems typical. An example of a feedback letter to parents of children whose scores indicate on-schedule development can be found in Figure 5.11 in Chapter 5 (blank versions in English and Spanish appear in Appendix D).

Children Whose Scores Indicate the Need for Monitoring

Program staff may choose an appropriate interval of follow-up screening for a child whose score falls in the lightly shaded monitoring zone, or they may decide to refer a child whose score falls in the monitoring zone. Chapter 5 provides a description of the monitoring zone and how it can be used.

Children Whose Scores Indicate the Need for Further Assessment

For children whose scores on the questionnaires fall below the cutoff scores, some level of action should be taken. If scores or overall responses indicate a concern, it is recommended that a conversation with the family occur either in person or over the telephone.

- *Follow-up:* Follow-up action should occur for any child whose score in a particular area is *close to* the cutoffs or falls within the monitoring zone. Children whose scores are close to the cutoffs in one or more areas may be provided developmental activities (e.g., intervention activities in Appendix F; *Ages & Stages Learning Activities,* Twombly & Fink, 2004, 2008, specific to the areas of concern and rescreened in 4–6 months. Rescreening in a shorter time frame (e.g., 1–2 months) also may be recommended. If a child receives scores that are low but not below the cutoff points in *several* areas of development, the child may need to be referred for further assessment.
- *Referral:* A referral should be made for any child whose scores in one or more developmental areas are below the established cutoff point (i.e., 2 standard deviations below the mean) for that questionnaire interval. Children whose scores fall *on or below* the cutoff scores are *identified* (i.e., considered to be in need of follow-up) and should be referred for further assessment.
- *Other follow-up:* Follow-up action should occur for any child whose family has indicated concern(s) on the Overall section of the questionnaires. Table 6.3 provides guidance on Overall section questions, the problems that may be indicated by the possible answers to these questions, and examples of potential referrals.

Follow-up actions may be recorded in the ASQ online management system so that programs can have records of decisions made and any actions taken. (For more details, see the user's guides available in the ASQ online management system.)

Activities to Encourage Development

Follow-up for children with typical results, as well as for children for whom monitoring and/or referral is indicated, can include giving parents and teachers ideas for games and fun events. Intervention activities in English and Spanish are included in this *User's Guide* in Appendix F, grouped according to age range. The *ASQ-3™ Learning Activities* also provide games and fun ideas for interactions, arranged by developmental domain and age range, and are available in English and Spanish (Twombly & Fink, 2013a, 2013b). The *ASQ-3™ Learning Activities* were originally developed as part of a preschool program in Hawaii that matched children's needs, as measured on the ASQ, with focused games and activities in the developmental areas targeted on the ASQ. The intervention activities and the *ASQ-3™ Learning Activities* use materials that most families and preschool programs have. Children with ASQ-3 scores close to the referral cutoff scores (i.e., children whose scores are within the monitoring zone) may benefit by practicing skills targeted in these activities.

21. Communicate Results with Families

Referral Considerations

Parents should inform and direct the referral process. Parents should decide specific next actions to be taken and a time line for taking these actions. Staff will need to individualize the assistance they give families based on family resources and needs. Before making a referral to a community agency or specialist, it is important to consider what factors may have affected a child's perform-ance on the ASQ-3. The Parent Conference Sheet (provided in the Supplemental Materials sec-tion of the ASQ-3 box and on the CD-ROM accompanying the ASQ-3 box) can be a useful tool for organizing conversations with parents about results and next steps.

- *Opportunity:* Did the child have the opportunity to try the items or the time to practice the skills? If not, it may be appropriate to provide the child further opportunity to try the items before making a referral.
- *Health/biological factors:* Does the child have a health condition or medical factors that may have affected his or her performance? For example, does the child have a hearing impairment? If so, a referral to the primary health care provider may be appropriate as part of a referral for further assessment.
- *Cultural factors:* Are there cultural reasons that the child's performance on the questionnaire was not optimal? For example, does the family feed the toddler (e.g., put food in his or her mouth), leaving the child with little opportunity to use a spoon or fork? The practice of feed-ing a young child may have benefits to the parent–child relationship that outweigh the ben-efits of the child's learning how to use utensils. It may be clear from looking at other skills in the Fine Motor area that the child's fine motor development is on target and that the utensil-use item should be omitted.
- *Environmental factors:* Are there environmental factors that may have affected the child's performance? For example, has there been a recent stressful event in the child's life that may have caused a developmental regression? Does the child have older siblings who talk for him or her?

Suggestions for Talking to Parents When Results Indicate the Need for Further Assessment

Sharing ASQ-3 results that identify a child as needing further assessment can be an extremely sensitive conversation. Program personnel need to prepare carefully for these discussions and should conduct them with compassion and empathy. Parents may react defensively or become angry at the person who is delivering the information. It may be helpful to role-play difficult conversations with a trusted peer or supervisor before communicating screening results with par-ents. The setting for the conversation should be private, and it should take place at a time that is convenient for the family. Consider cultural practices (e.g., Should other family members be invited to the meeting?) and language issues (e.g., Is an interpreter needed?). Delivering ASQ-3 results for a child whose scores are below the cutoffs should always be done in person or, alter-natively, over the telephone; parents should never receive results of this type by mail or e-mail. Keep in mind the following points when sharing results with parents:

- Provide screening information as quickly as possible.
- Assure parents that the conversation is confidential.
- Remind parents about the purpose of screening. Make sure they understand that screening only indicates the need for further assessment and does not diagnose a child.
- Review ASQ-3 results, emphasizing the child's strengths.
- Avoid terms such as *test, fail, normal,* or *abnormal.*
- Use language such as *well above cutoffs, close to cutoffs,* and *below cutoffs* when explaining cutoffs and a child's scores.
- Discuss information that may have affected scores (e.g., opportunity, health history, cultural or environmental factors).
- Listen to parents' perceptions of their child and be open to new ideas and viewpoints.
- Discuss parent concerns and provide specific, nonjudgmental examples of your concerns.
- Emphasize parents' current skills and resources.
- If parents are interested, provide information about community resources and referral options.
- Remember that you are there to help the parents take the next steps and to facilitate the process.

Community Referral Information

To assist in making appropriate, timely referrals, it is helpful to keep up-to-date lists of community agencies that provide developmental assessments and programs that provide intervention services to infants and young children. The list should include the following information for each entry:

- Agency name and address
- Contact person
- Telephone number
- Eligibility criteria for assessment and/or intervention
- Services provided

Case Study

FAMILY SCENARIOS

Sam was chronologically 5 months old when the 4 month ASQ-3 was completed by his parents, Joyce and Bill Fuller. Because Sam was born 4 weeks premature, Steps-Ahead adjusted his birth date for prematurity. Joyce and Bill adopted Sam when he was 2 weeks old; Sam's birth mother had received no prenatal care during the pregnancy. Sam's birth weight was low for his gestational age, and he tested positive for drug exposure. He was hospitalized for 2 weeks with newborn tremors, hypertonia, and respiratory distress. As shown in Figure 6.7, all of Sam's scores on the 4 month ASQ-3 were in the monitoring zone, with the Gross Motor total falling below the cutoff point. In the Overall section, Joyce and Bill commented that Sam stands on his toes (rather than flat on his feet), doesn't sleep at night, and cries a lot. Given the low scores and the concerns noted by Sam's parents, the Steps-Ahead social worker is recommending further assessment, with special attention to Sam's motor abilities.

    Delia was born 4 months ago to Janice Conley. There were no problems at birth, and Delia's birth weight and other medical characteristics were typical. Delia and her family qualified for participation in Steps-Ahead because Janice was 19 at the time of Delia's birth and she had not completed high school. Janice also has another child, Jamie, who is 2 years old. Delia's scores on the ASQ-3 (see Figure 6.8) are well above the cutoff points in all areas, and Janice did not list any concerns in the Overall section. Steps-Ahead will continue to monitor Delia's development and will mail the 8 month questionnaire to Janice in approximately 4 months.

Kinko is 30 months old. Kinko's mother, Choi-yu, received the 30 month ASQ-3 by mail. On the 30 month questionnaire, Kinko's scores are well above the cutoff points and indicate that she is developing typically. Choi-yu did not indicate any concerns about Kinko's development in the Overall section. Kinko originally was referred to Steps-Ahead because she was born 6 weeks prematurely and because Choi-yu was being treated for chronic depression. Steps-Ahead sent Choi-yu a copy of the completed 30 month ASQ-3, the intervention activities for 30- to 36-month-olds, and a letter similar to the Parent Feedback Letter: Typical shown in Appendix D. Steps-Ahead will continue to monitor Kinko's development and will send another questionnaire when Kinko is 33 months old.

Jake is 12 months old. His mother, Naomi, completed the 12 month ASQ-3 in her home with the assistance of a social worker from Steps-Ahead. Jake was referred to Steps-Ahead because his birth weight was extremely low and because Naomi was a teenager with a reported history of substance abuse and domestic violence. Jake's scores on the 12 month ASQ-3 were in the monitoring zone for most areas of development and were below the referral cutoff point for Problem Solving. Jake's 8 month ASQ-3 scores also had been in the monitoring zone, but none fell below the referral cutoff points. On the Overall section of the 12 month ASQ-3, Naomi indicated that she felt very stressed and was having trouble with Jake's newfound mobility. The Steps-Ahead social worker discussed the results of the questionnaire with Naomi and made a referral for further developmental testing. Naomi was linked with agencies that would help provide parenting support. She was given the completed ASQ-3, and the social worker kept the ASQ-3 Information Summary sheet for Steps-Ahead. After modeling some activities, the social worker also gave Naomi intervention activities for 12- to 16-month-olds. Naomi signed a release to notify Jake's pediatrician of the questionnaire results and Steps-Ahead's recommendation for further testing. Jake was tested by the early intervention services agency and was found to be eligible for services. Jake no longer will be monitored by Steps-Ahead. His records will be forwarded to the early intervention program after Naomi signs a release form.

Gabriella is 16 months old. Sylvia and Juan, Gabriella's parents, completed the 16 month ASQ-3 in their home with the assistance of a social worker from Steps-Ahead. Gabriella was referred to Steps-Ahead because of her pediatrician's concern about her development and history of chronic ear infections. Gabriella's scores on the questionnaire were well above the cutoff points in all areas except Communication and Problem Solving. In those areas, her scores were in the monitoring zone. Gabriella's parents expressed concern in the Overall section in response to the question, "Do you think your child talks like other toddlers his [or her] age?" Earlier, Gabriella's parents had completed questionnaires when she was 8 and 12 months old. Both of these questionnaires showed Gabriella's development to be well above the cutoff points in all areas. Given the results of Gabriella's 16 month questionnaire and the noted parental concerns, the Steps-Ahead social worker called Gabriella's parents to discuss the options. Sylvia and Juan decided to wait and watch Gabriella's development in the Communication and Problem Solving areas. The social worker gave Sylvia and Juan the 16 month questionnaire and intervention activities for 16- to 20-month-olds. The social worker also gave Gabriella's parents the 20 month ASQ-3 and the intervention activities for 20- to 24-month-olds to help them watch for skills that Gabriella should begin to develop in the coming months. Steps-Ahead will continue to monitor Gabriella's development with the ASQ-3. Special attention will be given to the Communication and Problem Solving areas on the 20 month ASQ-3.

Jeffrey is 20 months old. He lives with his grandmother and his brother and sister. Jeffrey's grandmother completes the questionnaires, which she receives by mail. Jeffrey was referred to Steps-Ahead because he was prenatally exposed to drugs and had a history of abuse by his biological mother. Jeffrey's grandmother has completed question-

4 Month Questionnaire

ASQ-3

3 months 0 days
through 4 months 30 days

On the following pages are questions about activities babies may do. Your baby may have already done some of the activities described here, and there may be some your baby has not begun doing yet. For each item, please fill in the circle that indicates whether your baby is doing the activity regularly, sometimes, or not yet.

Important Points to Remember:

☑ Try each activity with your baby before marking a response.
☑ Make completing this questionnaire a game that is fun for you and your baby.
☑ Make sure your baby is rested and fed.
☑ Please return this questionnaire by _____.

Notes:
_____
_____
_____

COMMUNICATION

	YES	SOMETIMES	NOT YET	
1. Does your baby chuckle softly?	○	⊗	○	5
2. After you have been out of sight, does your baby smile or get excited when he sees you?	○	○	⊗	0
3. Does your baby stop crying when she hears a voice other than yours?	○	⊗	○	5
4. Does your baby make high-pitched squeals?	⊗	○	○	10
5. Does your baby laugh?	○	⊗	○	5
6. Does your baby make sounds when looking at toys or people?	⊗	○	○	10
			COMMUNICATION TOTAL	35

GROSS MOTOR

	YES	SOMETIMES	NOT YET	
1. While your baby is on his back, does he move his head from side to side?	⊗	○	○	10
2. After holding her head up while on her tummy, does your baby lay her head back down on the floor, rather than let it drop or fall forward?	⊗	○	○	10
3. When your baby is on his tummy, does he hold his head up so that his chin is about 3 inches from the floor for at least 15 seconds?	○	⊗	○	5
4. When your baby is on her tummy, does she hold her head straight up, looking around? (She can rest on her arms while doing this.)	○	⊗	○	5

page 2 of 5

E101040200

ASQ-3

4 Month Questionnaire page 3 of 5

GROSS MOTOR (continued)

	YES	SOMETIMES	NOT YET	
5. When you hold him in a sitting position, does your baby hold his head steady?	○	⊗	○	5
6. While your baby is on her back, does your baby bring her hands together over her chest, touching her fingers?	○	○	⊗	0
			GROSS MOTOR TOTAL	35

FINE MOTOR

	YES	SOMETIMES	NOT YET	
1. Does your baby hold his hands open or partly open (rather than in fists, as they were when he was a newborn)?	○	○	⊗	0
2. When you put a toy in her hand, does your baby wave it about, at least briefly?	⊗	○	○	10
3. Does your baby grab or scratch at his clothes?	⊗	○	○	10
4. When you put a toy in her hand, does your baby hold onto it for about 1 minute while looking at it, waving it about, or trying to chew it?	⊗	○	○	10
5. Does your baby grab or scratch his fingers on a surface in front of him, either while being held in a sitting position or when he is on his tummy?	○	⊗	○	5
6. When you hold your baby in a sitting position, does she reach for a toy on a table close by, even though her hand may not touch it?	○	○	⊗	0
			FINE MOTOR TOTAL	35

PROBLEM SOLVING

	YES	SOMETIMES	NOT YET	
1. When you move a toy slowly from side to side in front of your baby's face (about 10 inches away), does your baby follow the toy with his eyes, sometimes turning his head?	⊗	○	○	10
2. When you move a small toy up and down slowly in front of your baby's face (about 10 inches away), does your baby follow the toy with her eyes?	⊗	○	○	10
3. When you hold your baby in a sitting position, does he look at a toy (about the size of a cup or rattle) that you place on the table or floor in front of him?	⊗	○	○	10
4. When you put a toy in her hand, does your baby look at it?	⊗	○	○	10
5. When you put a toy in his hand, does your baby put the toy in his mouth?	○	○	⊗	0

E101040300

Figure 6.7. The scoring sections of Sam Fuller's 4 month ASQ-3 revealed scores in the monitoring zone in four of the five developmental areas, with his Gross Motor score falling below the cutoff point. His parents also indicated concerns in the Overall section. On the basis of these results, the home visitor who scored the questionnaire is recommending further assessment.

Figure 6.7. (continued)

ASQ3   (continued)   **4 Month Questionnaire** page 5 of 5

OVERALL   (continued)

3. Do you have concerns that your baby is too quiet or does not make sounds like other babies? If yes, explain: ○ YES   ⊗ NO

4. Does either parent have a family history of childhood deafness or hearing impairment? If yes, explain: ○ YES   ⊗ NO

5. Do you have concerns about your baby's vision? If yes, explain: ○ YES   ⊗ NO

6. Has your baby had any medical problems in the last several months? If yes, explain: ○ YES   ⊗ NO

7. Do you have any concerns about your baby's behavior? If yes, explain: ○ YES   ⊗ NO

8. Does anything about your baby worry you? If yes, explain: ⊗ YES   ○ NO

He has problems sleeping, night walking, colic? He cries a lot. My older children are frustrated with his crying. It builds tension. I will try anything.

Ages & Stages Questionnaires®, Third Edition (ASQ-3™), Squires & Bricker
© 2009 Paul H. Brookes Publishing Co. All rights reserved.

E101040500

ASQ3

PROBLEM SOLVING   (continued)   **4 Month Questionnaire** page 4 of 5

	YES	SOMETIMES	NOT YET	
6. When you dangle a toy above your baby while she is lying on her back, does your baby wave her arms toward the toy?	○	○	⊗	0
			PROBLEM SOLVING TOTAL	40

PERSONAL-SOCIAL

	YES	SOMETIMES	NOT YET	
1. Does your baby watch his hands?	⊗	○	○	10
2. When your baby has her hands together, does she play with her fingers?	○	○	⊗	0
3. When your baby sees the breast or bottle, does he seem to know he is about to be fed?	⊗	○	○	10
4. Does your baby help hold the bottle with both hands at once, or when nursing, does she hold the breast with her free hand?	○	○	⊗	0
5. Before you smile or talk to your baby, does he smile when he sees you nearby?	⊗	○	○	10
6. When in front of a large mirror, does your baby smile or coo at herself?	○	⊗	○	5
			PERSONAL-SOCIAL TOTAL	35

OVERALL

Parents and providers may use the space below for additional comments.

1. Does your baby use both hands and both legs equally well? If no, explain: ⊗ YES   ○ NO

2. When you help your baby stand, are his feet flat on the surface most of the time? If no, explain: ○ YES   ⊗ NO

He is on his toes a lot.

Ages & Stages Questionnaires®, Third Edition (ASQ-3™), Squires & Bricker
© 2009 Paul H. Brookes Publishing Co. All rights reserved.

E101040400

ASQ-3 — 4 Month Questionnaire

3 months 0 days through 4 months 30 days

On the following pages are questions about activities babies may do. Your baby may have already done some of the activities described here, and there may be some your baby has not begun doing yet. For each item, please fill in the circle that indicates whether your baby is doing the activity regularly, sometimes, or not yet.

Important Points to Remember:

☑ Try each activity with your baby before marking a response.
☑ Make completing this questionnaire a game that is fun for you and your baby.
☑ Make sure your baby is rested and fed.
☑ Please return this questionnaire by _____.

Notes:

_____

COMMUNICATION

	YES	SOMETIMES	NOT YET	
1. Does your baby chuckle softly?	⊗	○	○	10
2. After you have been out of sight, does your baby smile or get excited when he sees you?	⊗	○	○	10
3. Does your baby stop crying when she hears a voice other than yours?	⊗	○	○	10
4. Does your baby make high-pitched squeals?	⊗	○	○	10
5. Does your baby laugh?	⊗	○	○	10
6. Does your baby make sounds when looking at toys or people?	○	⊗	○	5
		COMMUNICATION TOTAL		55

GROSS MOTOR

	YES	SOMETIMES	NOT YET	
1. While your baby is on his back, does he move his head from side to side?	⊗	○	○	10
2. After holding her head up while on her tummy, does your baby lay her head back down on the floor, rather than let it drop or fall forward?	⊗	○	○	10
3. When your baby is on his tummy, does he hold his head up so that his chin is about 3 inches from the floor for at least 15 seconds?	⊗	○	○	10
4. When your baby is on her tummy, does she hold her head straight up, looking around? (She can rest on her arms while doing this.)	⊗	○	○	10

E101040200

page 2 of 5

ASQ-3 — 4 Month Questionnaire

page 3 of 5

GROSS MOTOR *(continued)*

	YES	SOMETIMES	NOT YET	
5. When you hold him in a sitting position, does your baby hold his head steady?	⊗	○	○	10
6. While your baby is on her back, does your baby bring her hands together over her chest, touching her fingers?	⊗	○	○	10
		GROSS MOTOR TOTAL		60

FINE MOTOR

	YES	SOMETIMES	NOT YET	
1. Does your baby hold his hands open or partly open (rather than in fists, as they were when he was a newborn)?	⊗	○	○	10
2. When you put a toy in her hand, does your baby wave it about, at least briefly?	⊗	○	○	10
3. Does your baby grab or scratch at his clothes?	⊗	○	○	10
4. When you put a toy in her hand, does your baby hold onto it for about 1 minute while looking at it, waving it about, or trying to chew it?	⊗	○	○	10
5. Does your baby grab or scratch his fingers on a surface in front of him, either while being held in a sitting position or when he is on his tummy?	⊗	○	○	10
6. When you hold your baby in a sitting position, does she reach for a toy on a table close by, even though her hand may not touch it?	⊗	○	○	10
		FINE MOTOR TOTAL		60

PROBLEM SOLVING

	YES	SOMETIMES	NOT YET	
1. When you move a toy slowly from side to side in front of your baby's face (about 10 inches away), does your baby follow the toy with his eyes, sometimes turning his head?	⊗	○	○	10
2. When you move a small toy up and down slowly in front of your baby's face (about 10 inches away), does your baby follow the toy with her eyes?	○	⊗	○	5
3. When you hold your baby in a sitting position, does he look at a toy (about the size of a cup or rattle) that you place on the table or floor in front of him?	⊗	○	○	10
4. When you put a toy in her hand, does your baby look at it?	⊗	○	○	10
5. When you put a toy in his hand, does your baby put the toy in his mouth?	⊗	○	○	10

E101040300

Figure 6.8. Delia Conley's scores on the 4 month ASQ-3 indicated typical development, and her mother did not list any concerns in the Overall section. Steps-Ahead will continue to monitor Delia's developmental progress.

PROBLEM SOLVING (continued)

	YES	SOMETIMES	NOT YET	
6. When you dangle a toy above your baby while she is lying on her back, does your baby wave her arms toward the toy?	○	⊗	○	5

PROBLEM SOLVING TOTAL   50

PERSONAL-SOCIAL

	YES	SOMETIMES	NOT YET	
1. Does your baby watch his hands?	⊗	○	○	10
2. When your baby has her hands together, does she play with her fingers?	⊗	○	○	10
3. When your baby sees the breast or bottle, does he seem to know he is about to be fed?	⊗	○	○	10
4. Does your baby help hold the bottle with both hands at once, or when nursing, does she hold the breast with her free hand?	○	⊗	○	5
5. Before you smile or talk to your baby, does he smile when he sees you nearby?	⊗	○	○	10
6. When in front of a large mirror, does your baby smile or coo at herself?	⊗	○	○	10

PERSONAL-SOCIAL TOTAL   55

OVERALL

Parents and providers may use the space below for additional comments.

1. Does your baby use both hands and both legs equally well? If no, explain: ⊗ YES   ○ NO

2. When you help your baby stand, are his feet flat on the surface most of the time? If no, explain: ⊗ YES   ○ NO

E101040400

OVERALL (continued)

3. Do you have concerns that your baby is too quiet or does not make sounds like other babies? If yes, explain: ○ YES   ⊗ NO

4. Does either parent have a family history of childhood deafness or hearing impairment? If yes, explain: ○ YES   ⊗ NO

5. Do you have concerns about your baby's vision? If yes, explain: ○ YES   ⊗ NO

6. Has your baby had any medical problems in the last several months? If yes, explain: ○ YES   ⊗ NO

7. Do you have any concerns about your baby's behavior? If yes, explain: ○ YES   ⊗ NO

8. Does anything about your baby worry you? If yes, explain: ○ YES   ⊗ NO

E101040500

Figure 6.8. (continued)

naires since he was 8 months old. Results from these questionnaires indicate that Jeffrey's development is well above the cutoff points; however, Jeffrey's grandmother has noted that he is unable to sleep at night. She reported finding him asleep on their living room couch on some mornings. The Steps-Ahead social worker called Jeffrey's grandmother to discuss her concerns. On the basis of their discussion, the social worker recommended that Jeffrey be seen by his pediatrician to evaluate his sleeping problem. In the meantime, the social worker gave Jeffrey's grandmother the completed 20 month ASQ-3 and the intervention activities 20- to 24-month-olds. On examination, Jeffrey's pediatrician found that he had asthma and prescribed appropriate medication for him. Jeffrey's grandmother reported to Steps-Ahead that Jeffrey's sleeping habits have improved. Steps-Ahead will continue to monitor Jeffrey's development with the ASQ-3.

CONCLUSION

Phase III, administration and scoring procedures and follow-up, describes a series of steps necessary for using the questionnaires. The information on administration provides information on how to choose the correct ASQ-3 interval, what materials are needed, and how to support parents completing the ASQ-3. The information on scoring provides instructions for scoring and recording results of the ASQ-3. Although the scoring instructions may seem complicated on the first reading, a short practice session with two or three questionnaires should clarify most concerns. The sections that discuss ASQ-3 score interpretation provide detailed information on the structure of the questionnaires and on how the cutoffs were established. Recommended guidelines for follow-up based on a child's scores or overall concerns are provided. Finally, suggestions are given for talking to parents of children whose questionnaire scores fall below the cutoff points and/or when parental concerns are noted in the Overall section.

This *User's Guide* is intended to be a reference; there are many sections in this chapter that will need to be reviewed as monitoring program operations begin. Options, such as those for using questionnaires and ways to give parents feedback, may need to be exercised until a system is established that fits individual program needs. Chapter 7 describes the final phase of the ASQ-3 system: evaluating the screening/monitoring program.

7

Phase IV: Evaluating the Screening/ Monitoring Program

ASQ-3

Phase IV of implementing ASQ-3 screening/monitoring program focuses on evaluating the programs in terms of the program's implementation progress and the effectiveness of the screening tool. This phase has two steps, which are shown in the shaded portion of Figure 7.1. As with any screening program, each step in implementing an ASQ-3 screening/monitoring program should lead to the next one.

Evaluation is the systematic collection of data on screening activities so that the accuracy and overall success of the program can be measured. Evaluation data will assist in decision making about program operations as well as measure effectiveness in identifying children in need of intervention services. Funding sources, parents, boards of directors, lawmakers, community members and the medical community are examples of potential audiences for evaluation reports.

STEPS IN THE EVALUATION PHASE

As indicated in Figure 7.1, the evaluation of the ASQ-3 screening/monitoring program provides information about the attainment of program goals and may also suggest new goals. Ongoing evaluation may result in the modification of procedures and steps in all four phases of the program.

22. Assess Progress in Establishing and Maintaining the Screening/Monitoring Program

Contemplating the evaluation of the screening process should not begin at the end of Phase II. Rather, knowing the goals of the evaluation process facilitates the collection of necessary information as the program progresses.

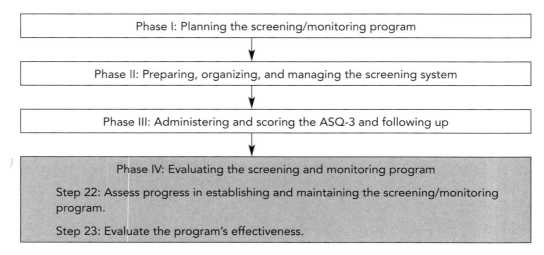

Figure 7.1.   The four phases of ASQ-3 implementation, including the two steps of Phase IV. (Phases I–III are discussed in Chapters 4–6.)

Setting up and maintaining a screening and monitoring program for a large number of children require a range of activities. The Implementation Progress Worksheet (see Figure 7.2; a full-size version of this worksheet appears in Appendix D) was developed to assist program personnel in efficiently monitoring the variety of required phases and steps necessary for initiation and maintenance of the program. The items on this worksheet mirror the 23 steps in the four phases of setting up an ASQ-3 screening/monitoring program. The worksheet is intended to be of assistance during the initiation and early stages of developing the monitoring program; however, staff may find it useful to refer back to the worksheet at designated intervals (e.g., quarterly) even after the program has been institutionalized.

Tasks

The left column of the Implementation Progress Worksheet lists each of the steps necessary to establish the ASQ-3 system (e.g., finalize goals and objectives, determine program resources) in the order in which they are described in this *User's Guide*.

Actions

To the right of the Tasks column are five "action" columns: Personnel Needs, Information Needs, Supplies and Equipment Needs, Person/Agency Responsible, and Projected Completion Date. In each column, personnel can enter the indicated information for the individual steps.

For the Include Parental Perspectives step, personnel from the Steps-Ahead program might enter the following information:

- *Personnel Needs:* Social workers to make individual contacts with parents of infants identified on birth certificates and clerical staff to prepare letters to parents and take telephone messages
- *Information Needs:* Current names, addresses, and telephone numbers (if available) of families
- *Supplies and Equipment Needs:* Office supplies, including stamps, computer and software for word processing, letterhead, and a telephone with two lines
- *Person/Agency Responsible:* Social workers will have responsibility for obtaining consent to participate from parents; thereafter, social workers will have responsibility for ongoing contact with participating parents for feedback and for altering the ASQ-3 method of use when requested.

Implementation Progress Worksheet

Use the following scale for progress rating(s): 0, not applicable; 1, not begun; 2, partially begun or implemented; 3, fully completed or implemented.

Tasks	Personnel needs	Information needs	Supplies and equipment needs	Person/agency responsible	Projected completion date	Progress rating 11/2	4/1	7/1	10/1
Phase I: Planning the screening/monitoring program									
1. Communicate with community partners.		Contacts	Database	L.A.	2/15	2			
2. Include parental perspectives.	Parents	Contact		S.G./L.A.	Ongoing	2			
3. Involve health care providers.	M.D. input	Contacts		P.K.	2/15	1			
4. Determine target population.				Board		3			
5. Finalize goals and objectives.				Board	3/1	2			
6. Determine program resources.	Accounting	Fiscal reports		Fiscal	12/31	3			
7. Determine administration methods and settings.				Board	12/31	3			
8. Determine depth and breadth of system.				Board	3/1	2			
9. Select referral criteria.		Dates		Board	12/31	3			
Phase II: Preparing, organizing, and managing the screening program									
10. Create a management system.	0.02 FTE		Database	R.G.	3/1	1			
11. Prepare questionnaires.			ASQ-3	N.P.	4/1	1			
12. Develop forms, letters, and a referral guide.			ASQ-3	L.A.	2/1	1			
13. Articulate screening policies and procedures.	Board			S.G./L.A.	3/1	1			
14. Provide staff training and support.	L.A.	Dates	Training matl.	L.A./L.T.	12/31, 3/1	1			

(continued)

ASQ-3

Implementation Progress Worksheet *(continued)*

Tasks	Personnel needs	Information needs	Supplies and equipment needs	Person/agency responsible	Projected completion date	Progress rating 11/2	4/1	7/1	10/1
Phase III: Administering and scoring ASQ-3 and following up									
15. Select the appropriate ASQ-3 age interval.	Clerical		ASQ-3	L.T.	Ongoing	1			
16. Assemble ASQ-3 materials.	Clerical		ASQ-3	L.T.	Ongoing	1			
17. Support parents' completion of ASQ-3.	Home visitor			S.G./Home visitor	Ongoing	1			
18. Score the ASQ-3 and review the Overall section.	Home visitor			Home visitor	Ongoing	1			
19. Interpret ASQ-3 scores.	Home visitor			Home visitor	Ongoing	1			
20. Determine type of follow-up.	Home visitor	Comm. resource	Resource guide	Home visitor	Ongoing	1			
21. Communicate results with families.	Home visitor	Comm. resource	Resource guide	Home visitor	Ongoing	1			
Phase IV: Evaluating the screening/monitoring program									
22. Assess progress in establishing and maintaining the screening/monitoring program.	Board	Board		L.A./Board	Quarterly	2			
23. Evaluate the program's effectiveness.	Evaluator	Reports		L.A./Board	Quarterly	1			

ASQ-3

Figure 7.2. Sample of an Implementation Progress Worksheet. The items on this worksheet mirror the steps in the four phases of the ASQ-3 system. (A blank version appears in Appendix D at the end of this book.)

- *Projected Completion Date*: Parents to be contacted for consent within 1 month after birth of child or within 1 month after child returns home from the hospital

Progress Rating

The final column provides four spaces to indicate the quantitative level of progress attained toward the specific step's completion. The rating scale includes the following numeric values:

0 = *Not applicable*
1 = *Not begun*
2 = *Partially begun or implemented*
3 = *Fully completed or implemented*

During initial start-up, program staff may want to evaluate their progress weekly using the Implementation Progress Worksheet. Later, monthly or quarterly evaluations of progress may be sufficient. Tasks to evaluate will change as a program matures and as more children are being monitored. As program objectives are modified, it may be necessary to begin a new worksheet reflecting these new objectives.

For example, for Step 2, Include Parental Perspective, which is analyzed in the case study in Chapter 4, the goal of garnering parents' support of the monitoring program 1 month after the birth of their child may not allow sufficient time. This task may need to be changed to contacting and mailing information to parents at 1 month and waiting until the infant is 2 months or older to make a home visit and explain the ASQ-3 system.

Although most programs will strive for ratings of 3 on targeted steps, there may be instances in which a rating of 2 is sufficient. Limited resources, lower priority, or modification of steps may be reasons for these lower ratings. If a modification occurs, steps should be rewritten and reevaluated.

23. Evaluate the ASQ-3 Program's Effectiveness

The final step shown in Figure 7.2 is to *evaluate the program's effectiveness.* Every monitoring program, even those with limited resources, should conduct some form of evaluation to determine the effectiveness of the program and the procedures being used. The following areas of evaluation are recommended:

- Parent feedback
- Effectiveness of questionnaires in accurately identifying children who need further assessment
- Feedback from personnel using the questionnaires

How extensively each of these areas can be evaluated will depend on the program's resources and staff expertise. The evaluation procedures described next are simple and straightforward; they represent the basic minimal amount of evaluation data that program personnel should collect.

Parent Feedback

Feedback from parents should be sought at least yearly. A simple, short survey can be included with a questionnaire once a year (e.g., 12, 24, 36, 48, 60 months). Figure 7.3 is an example of such a survey (blank versions in English and Spanish appear in Appendix D). This type of feedback will assist program personnel in making adjustments to procedures that will help ensure parental participation and satisfaction.

Dear Parent,

Would you please take a few minutes to evaluate our questionnaires? We appreciate your participation in our program and hope that our services have been helpful to you.

Please circle the number that best expresses your opinion.

1. Approximately how many minutes did it take you to fill out each questionnaire? __9__ minutes. Did you consider this amount of time:

very little time			too much time
1	(2)	3	4

Comments:

2. Did the questionnaires alert you to skills or activities your child could do that you were not sure about?

very few			very many
1	2	(3)	4

Comments:

3. After filling out the questionnaires, did you have any new ideas about how to interact or play with your child?

very few			very many
1	(2)	3	4

Comments:

4. Were any items unclear or difficult to understand?

very few			very many
(1)	2	3	4

Comments:

5. Did you enjoy participating in this program?

very little			very much
1	2	3	(4)

Comments:

If you have any further comments about the questionnaires, please write them on the back of this form.

ASQ-3

Figure 7.3. Sample of a Parent Feedback Survey. Feedback from parents should be sought at least yearly. (Blank versions appear in English and Spanish in Appendix D at the end of this book.)

Questionnaire Effectiveness

To examine the effectiveness of the questionnaires, it is imperative to keep records of the number of children identified as needing further assessment and the outcomes of their subsequent developmental assessments. By recording this information, it is possible to determine the percentages of children accurately identified by the questionnaires as having delays and those who were incorrectly recommended for further evaluation. These calculations provide information on the sensitivity and overidentification rates for the group of children being monitored. Providing information on the effectiveness of a screening program may help personnel in a variety of ways. First, data on the effectiveness of the screening program may be requested and appreciated by funding sources. Second, additional information may be provided about the monitoring of implementation goals. For example, a program may project a screening rate of 10%. If the program's goal of 10% is not realized (i.e., percent screened is significantly higher or lower), the criteria used to include children in the program may need to be modified.

		Follow-up assessment	
		Intervention needs	No intervention needs
Ages & Stages Questionnaires®	Identified by questionnaires as needing further assessment	True positives A	False positives (overidentification) B
	Not identified by questionnaires; developing typically	False negatives (underidentification) C	True negatives D

Percentage of children identified as needing further assessment:

$$\frac{A + B}{A + B + C + D}$$

Sensitivity   The proportion of children correctly identified by the questionnaires as needing further assessment:

$$\frac{A}{A + C}$$

Specificity   The proportion of children correctly identified by the questionnaires as developing typically:

$$\frac{D}{B + D}$$

Overidentification   The proportion of children (of the total number of children for whom a questionnaire was completed) incorrectly identified by the questionnaires as needing further assessment:

$$\frac{B}{A + B + C + D}$$

Underidentification   The proportion of children (of the total number of children for whom a questionnaire was completed) incorrectly excluded by the questionnaires:

$$\frac{C}{A + B + C + D}$$

Positive predictive value   The proportion of children identified by the questionnaires as needing further assessment who will, in fact, have intervention needs:

$$\frac{A}{A + B}$$

Figure 7.4.   Formulas for calculating the percentage of children appropriately identified as needing further assessment and the sensitivity, specificity, and over- and underidentification rates.

Figure 7.4 provides formulas for calculating the percentage of children appropriately identified as needing further assessment and the sensitivity, specificity, and overidentification and underidentification rates. Specificity and underidentification rates cannot be calculated unless a program conducts follow-up assessments with children who are not identified by the questionnaires as needing further assessment and also with children who are identified as needing further assessment.

Personnel Feedback

It is important to seek formal or informal feedback from personnel using the questionnaires, to learn which procedural steps work well and which ones do not. The ASQ-3 system is flexible, and program personnel can and should make adjustments in its use to ensure efficient, effective application.

Determining Next Steps

Once the evaluation of the screening/monitoring program has been completed, program staff should review and discuss results. Actions should be taken based on these results, such as adjusting screening cutoff points when greater (or fewer) numbers of children are being identified as needing further assessment. Other actions might include having staff review questionnaires to check that parent concerns in the Overall section of the ASQ-3 are being considered and that questionnaires are being scored accurately. Modifying program eligibility so that more (or fewer) children are referred for further assessment is a final example of actions to be taken based on evaluation results. At least once a year, staff should meet to examine ways to improve the activities associated with the screening/monitoring program. Parents should also be invited to review program evaluation results and suggest improvements and modifications in the system.

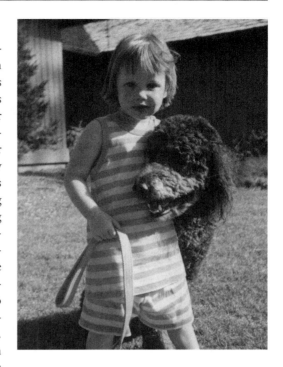

Screening Tests and Evaluation

Screening tests, as defined in Chapter 1, provide a brief snapshot of a child's current developmental skills. Screening tests are designed for use with large groups of children at relatively low cost. These brief tests contain few items and, thus, do not offer comprehensive assessments of children's development. These features, although appropriate for screening, make such brief tests inappropriate for most other evaluation purposes. Results of a screening test such as the ASQ-3 are not designed to measure a child's progress over time, just as individual developmental assessments are not designed for screening purposes.

Conducting the appropriate type of evaluation is highly dependent on using measures and/or procedures designed to fit or meet the purposes of the evaluation. The types of evaluation purposes and their associated assessments are shown in Table 7.1. Screening requires the use of a screening measure; determining eligibility usually requires a measure that provides in-depth developmental information and permits comparing children against established norms. To evaluate child progress, a curriculum-based assessment such as High/Scope (Weikart & Schweinhart, 2000) or the Assessment, Evaluation, and Programming System for Infants and Children (AEPS®; Bricker, 2002) should be used.

Table 7.1. Purposes and types of assessment

Type	Purpose	Examples
Screening test	Is the child in need of further testing?	ASQ-3, DIAL III
Eligibility test/diagnostic assessment	Is the child eligible for special services?	Battelle, Bayley
Programmatic/curriculum-based assessment	Is the child making progress?	AEPS®, Creative Curriculum

A formal curriculum such as High/Scope (Weikart & Schweinhart, 2000) or the Creative Curriculum (Dodge, Colker, & Heroman, 2002) needs to be used with goals and objectives against which child progress can be measured. Alternately, in-depth observations, child products such as drawings, and video recordings of a child's play and projects need to be gathered over time.

Curriculum-based measures such as the Carolina Curriculum (Johnson-Martin, Atter-meier, & Hacker, 2004) or the AEPS® (Bricker, 2002) are ideal for delineating step-by-step objectives that can be used for measuring child progress toward long-range goals, especially for children with delays in development. Screening tests are not sensitive enough to show progress toward outcomes; these tests are designed only to identify those children who need further assessment.

Therefore, the ASQ-3 should *not* be used to show whether a child or children in a class are making progress. ASQ-3 scores do not measure children's skills above the questionnaire level (i.e., no ASQ-3 age interval includes any items that are out of reach of the typically developing child of that age), so they will not measure the full range of a child's abilities. ASQ-3 scores indicate only whether a child's skills are above or below the screening cutoff scores in a specific developmental area.

As a developmental screening test, the results of the ASQ-3 were designed to identify children who need further developmental assessment. Some child care and early childhood programs have chosen to use the ASQ-3 to reflect general classroom status—percentages of children in each class scoring above and below the cutoff scores. This type of analysis does not reflect the purpose for which the ASQ was developed; it may be difficult to show improvements in child progress through this method.

Case Study

After 6 months, the Steps-Ahead staff reviewed their progress in completing targeted tasks (see Figure 7.2). For the planning phase, goals and objectives, program resources, and method of use steps were fully implemented and had met projected dates of completion. Criteria for participation, involving parent perspectives and physicians, and determining referral criteria were only partially implemented, receiving ratings of 2. Although criteria for participation and for referral had been determined, it was believed that more time was needed to evaluate how these guidelines were functioning within program parameters. Staff decided to continue to record the numbers of children served and numbers of children referred for further assessment; in 3 months, the staff would meet to evaluate how well these actual numbers corresponded with their projections.

In terms of involving physicians, more work was needed to inform physicians at private hospitals in the area and to garner support from the health maintenance organizations at these private hospitals. Advisory board staff and social workers were designated to work with the private hospitals.

In terms of including parental perspectives, staff felt positive about their relationships with families. However, they decided to add two parents to the advisory board so that parent input would be ongoing. Staff also undertook the development of a satisfaction questionnaire for parents to complete along with the 12 month questionnaire.

Regarding Phase II (Preparing, Organizing, and Managing Your Screening Program), all clerical and office tasks related to setting up and maintaining child files had been completed. Procedures for the tickler system, scoring, and recording questionnaire results appeared to be working well. For these clerical and office tasks, staff decided to reevaluate progress in 3 months, when there were larger numbers of children participating in the screening/monitoring system.

For the task of determining follow-up for children who were identified as needing further assessment, staff believed that, to date, there were insufficient numbers to rate progress. The early intervention program in the county had assessed 6 of the 10 children referred to date and had shared the results with Steps-Ahead. Parents of two of the identified children had requested further monitoring with the questionnaires before referral. Two children had been assessed by physicians at a health maintenance organization, but these results had not been received by Steps-Ahead.

For Phase III (Administering and Scoring ASQ-3 and Following Up), the Implementation Progress Worksheet was completed and all steps were rated (see Figure 7.2). Steps receiving ratings of 2 were targeted, and staff were assigned new tasks. Progress toward full implementation of these steps was to be evaluated during monthly staff meetings. The next program evaluation meeting was scheduled for 3 months later.

CONCLUSION

Phase IV, Evaluating the Screening and Monitoring Program, involves two major steps: assessing progress in the establishment and maintenance of the program and evaluating the system's effectiveness. Progress can be assessed by screening/monitoring project staff during monthly or quarterly staff meetings and should not require extensive information or data that go beyond the day-to-day operations of the program. The second step, evaluating the system's effectiveness, is also of prime importance. Information may be needed from outside referral agencies to determine child assessment outcomes. These data are necessary to determine whether the program is really working: Are the right children being identified for further assessment? Are they then referred for early intervention services? Evaluation of the monitoring program should be ongoing, and revision of steps and activities will be necessary as the program grows and changes.

Examples to illustrate different applications and settings in which the ASQ-3 can be used with children and families are described in Section III. These examples are meant to illustrate many of the opportunities and issues that may come up when using the ASQ-3 in the variety of settings illustrated in Table 4.3. These family scenarios may be useful when training staff in ASQ-3 administration, scoring, and referral.

III

ASQ-3 in Practice

8

ASQ-3 Completion Methods

This chapter expands on the methods for obtaining completed ASQ-3 questionnaires that are introduced in Chapter 4. Mail-out, online, telephone interview, home visit, and on-site completion options are discussed. The material in this chapter underlines the questionnaires' flexibility and adaptability—an important advantage of using ASQ-3 to monitor children's development. Accompanying the descriptions are examples of how different agencies and programs are using ASQ-3.

There are also two appendixes that follow this chapter. Appendix 8A contains procedures for using a card file tickler system. Appendix 8B details the steps and decisions involved in implementing ASQ-3 while on a home visit.

MEETING THE NEEDS OF DIVERSE PROGRAMS AND SETTINGS

A great strength of the ASQ-3 system is the flexibility it provides in terms of how it can be used (e.g., mail out, online, telephone interview, home visit, on site), when it can be used (i.e., with any child between 1 and 66 months of age), and where it can be used (e.g., at home, in a physician's office). Since publication of the first edition, ASQ has been used by pediatric and family care practices, well-infant clinics, health care programs, screening clinics, and educational intervention programs.

Communities in the United States that provide screening vary considerably in terms of which agencies and professionals have the responsibility to monitor the developmental status of young children. The physical facilities, personnel, and resources of these varied programs require flexibility in screening measures and procedures. For example, one countywide screening program has state dollars to monitor the development of all newborns deemed to be at risk in this rural area. This program operates from a small office with two staff members who track the developmental progress of 150 infants per year, whereas in a nearby metropolitan area, all developmental screening is conducted by primary care physicians using office staff. These practices only assess the developmental status of children if requested by parents. Such diversity requires using adaptable measures, such as the ASQ-3. Although initially developed as a mail-out system, the

ASQ has been used successfully in individual communities employing a wide range of other approaches to collecting questionnaires.

The mail-out approach is the first option for ASQ-3 questionnaire completion. The mail-out method requires that the ASQ-3 be mailed to parents who, in turn, complete the questionnaire and return it by mail to a central location, such as the office of the primary health care provider, a clinic, or a screening program.

The ASQ Family Access online questionnaire completion system is the second option for questionnaire completion. Through this online system, the professional can direct a caregiver to a secure web site to fill out a questionnaire. The system ensures that the correct ASQ-3 interval is selected and that the questionnaire is complete. Data are transmitted to the program's online management system account for verification, and the questionnaire is scored and screening results are saved to the child's electronic record. (Programs using the ASQ online management system can also enter data from paper questionnaires to be scored and stored in the online management system.)

A telephone interview is the third option for completing the ASQ-3. Prior to the telephone interview, the ASQ-3 is mailed to parents. Once the questionnaire is received, parents are given a few days to review and try items with their child, if possible. At a mutually agreed-on time, a telephone interview ensues, during which the questionnaire is completed.

Conducting a home visit is another option for completing the ASQ-3. While working with the family in the child's home, the home visitor assists caregivers in completing the questionnaire.

ASQ-3 can also be completed on site at a program's physical location, such as in a waiting room. When using this completion option, toys and objects (e.g., blocks, pencil and paper, mirror) must be available so that the parent may try all questionnaire items with the child.

Although these are the five primary options typically employed for completing questionnaires, these options may be combined or other variations may be used as necessary to meet the requirements and resources of programs and their personnel.

Mail Out

Mail-out methods generally entail using the questionnaires by mailing them to families at set intervals. Parents complete the questionnaires and usually return them by mail. Mailings can be prepared manually by program staff or through mailings generated through the online management system. Once returned, the questionnaire is scored, and the results are shared with parents. The mail-out option permits the dynamic monitoring of large populations of infants and children at low cost. The ASQ system was originally designed as a mail-out system and has been used this way consistently in hundreds of programs both nationally and internationally.

For optimal results when using the mail-out method in a primary health care practice, it is recommended that the ASQ-3 be mailed to parents *or* that parents be directed to the ASQ online questionnaire completion system 1–2 weeks prior to the well-child checkup. Parents can then complete the ASQ-3 at home, trying each item with the child as necessary, and send the completed questionnaire to the health care provider's office prior to the visit. As an alternative, parents can bring the completed questionnaire to the office at the time of the appointment.

Mail-Out Considerations

Mailing out the ASQ-3 for parents or other primary caregivers to complete is appropriate if parents or caregivers are capable of reading the items, observing the child's activities, and accurately scoring the items with little or no assistance. Prior to mailing a questionnaire, it is important to determine how the ASQ-3 will be introduced to parents or caregivers. An initial face-to-face meeting is the preferred way to introduce the screening and monitoring program and the

ASQ-3. This face-to-face introduction is reassuring and helpful for parental "buy-in," and it may help to maximize the ASQ-3 return rates. Chapter 6 offers guidance on introducing the ASQ-3 to parents and caregivers. If a face-to-face introduction is not possible, then a letter should be sent with the first ASQ-3 questionnaire to introduce the program. (See Chapter 5 for examples of letters; blank sample letters in English and Spanish are available in Appendix D at the end of this book.)

When completed questionnaires are returned, timely feedback should be given to parents. Sending a properly worded letter is appropriate when the results of the screening indicate a child is developing typically or may need monitoring only in one area. If the child's performance on ASQ-3 items is below the cutoff score in any area, or if parents indicate a concern, then it is important to follow up with a telephone call rather than sending a letter. In general, it is recommended that program personnel do not include the Information Summary sheet that shows scoring results when sending parents feedback. This sheet requires explanation by professional personnel about the scoring cutoffs and results.

Primary health care practices, screening clinics, educational programs, and other types of programs that are monitoring large numbers of children will need a system for keeping track of important dates that include when questionnaires are to be mailed and returned and when feedback needs to be provided. Timely tracking of questionnaire dissemination and feedback requires an electronic or paper-based system. See Appendix 8A at the end of this chapter for procedures for using a card file tickler system for tracking the mailing of ASQ-3 to families.

Mail-Out Procedures

In the ASQ-3 questionnaires, a master mailing sheet is provided. For programs that use the mail-out completion option, the name of the screening program and its address should be stamped, printed, or typed on a copy of the mailing sheet, and the parent's name and address also should be written or typed on that sheet (see Figure 8.1). A contact telephone number and name should be included in order that parents may obtain assistance if necessary. After the child's identifying information is specified on the mailing sheet and the questionnaire is ready to be mailed, the questionnaire and mailing sheet should be folded and taped at the ends and top, with the mailing sheet on the outside of the folded packet. Or, staff may prefer to use an envelope to mail each ASQ-3. In these cases, a self-addressed stamped envelope should be enclosed to encourage return of the completed questionnaire.

The return date is a common concern when using the ASQ-3 mail-out method. To increase return rates, the following steps are suggested.

1. Make a follow-up telephone call a few days after the questionnaire is mailed to ensure receipt and to answer any questions.
2. If a questionnaire is not returned within 2 weeks, then make a second telephone call to remind parents to return the questionnaire.

It is important to adhere to the time schedule for sending questionnaires and feedback. Parents should receive the appropriate questionnaire on time and should receive timely feedback in writing, by telephone, or in person. As mentioned previously, it may be important to include an introductory letter to parents in the first questionnaire that explains the screening program and purpose of the questionnaires (see Chapter 5, Figure 5.10).

Examples of Strategies to Improve Return Rates

*   Introduce parents to the screening program and the ASQ-3 prior to sending out the first questionnaire. Introductions can be done by letter or ideally through a telephone call or face-to-face contact with the family (see Chapter 6 for more information about introductions).

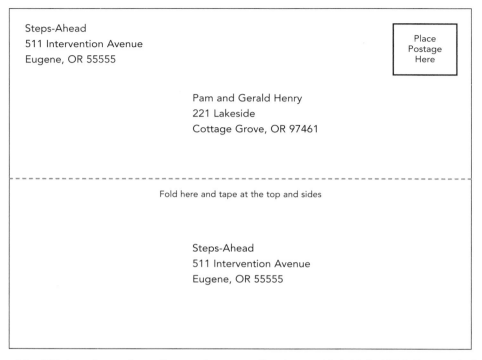

Steps-Ahead
511 Intervention Avenue
Eugene, OR 55555

Place
Postage
Here

Pam and Gerald Henry
221 Lakeside
Cottage Grove, OR 97461

Fold here and tape at the top and sides

Steps-Ahead
511 Intervention Avenue
Eugene, OR 55555

Figure 8.1.   With the mail-out option, staff can use the master mailing sheet provided with the ASQ-3. The example shown here is ready to be mailed to Joseph Henry's family for questionnaire completion.

- Provide a contact name and number in the notes section on the first page of the questionnaire.
- Send the ASQ-3 in an envelope that will catch a parent's attention or that is personalized in some way.
- Provide an intervention activity material (e.g., a pack of 4 crayons with the 16 month ASQ-3) with the questionnaire when it is mailed.
- Provide a birthday card with the questionnaire on the child's first, second, third, fourth, and fifth birthdays.

When you send feedback to the families, include the following:

- Local restaurant, toy, or book coupons with questionnaire results
- Activity ideas, such as those provided in Appendix F of this *User's Guide*
- A copy of the completed questionnaire for parents
- A copy of the next questionnaire so that parents can look for skills in the coming months

MAIL-OUT EXAMPLE

Several pediatricians serve on the board of directors for the Steps-Ahead program. In particular, Dr. Bram found the ASQ-3 useful as a screening tool for his patients. Initially, he decided to try the questionnaires with a small number of patients, with the goal of adopting the ASQ-3 system as his primary developmental screening test. Dr. Bram selected 50 families with children between the ages of 1 month and 24 months. He sent a letter that described the ASQ-3 system and the purpose of completing the questionnaires along with the handout "What Is ASQ-3™?" and asked parents to participate. Dr. Bram's office staff mailed the appropriate questionnaires using the mail-out procedures previously described. When parents brought their children to his office for well-child checkups, Dr. Bram reviewed the results of the questionnaires with the parents and answered questions as needed.

As part of his analysis of the ASQ-3 system, Dr. Bram computed return rates and percentages of children needing referral; he also asked how parents felt about completing the questionnaires. His return rate averaged 80%, and the percentage of children needing referral (based on scores in one or more areas of development below the cut-off point) was 12%. Parents' responses during the well-child checkups indicated they felt the questionnaires were informative and easy to complete. Dr. Bram also felt the questionnaires gave parents a springboard from which they could ask questions about their child's development.

Online

Online questionnaire completion refers to using ASQ Family Access via the Internet to enter and securely transmit information completed by parents or caregivers. The ASQ online questionnaire completion system enables programs to set up secure, personalized web sites for parents to access in order to enter appropriate demographic information, print the targeted questionnaire interval, and complete the ASQ-3 items. Results may be reviewed via the ASQ online management system (ASQ Pro or ASQ Enterprise).

By using the ASQ online management system, users can create and manage child records, screenings, and screening results. The online management system scores completed ASQ-3 (or ASQ:SE) questionnaires, organizes and manages communications with parents, and tracks follow-up and other activities.

Online Considerations

The ASQ online questionnaire completion system is cost effective and can enable programs to reach large numbers of families. Parents have the flexibility to complete a questionnaire online in their home or in another location, such as at a kiosk in a physician's office. Important considerations for online completion include parents' level of comfort with this electronic format and their access to the Internet. It is critical that the online method facilitate questionnaire completion without placing a barrier between parent and program, especially for parents who may be uncomfortable in the absence of direct contact with the professional. In addition, it is important to remind parents to try each activity and directly observe their children's skills. Often, parents of young children go online when their young children are asleep or are otherwise occupied, and some parents may try to complete the ASQ-3 from memory. Simple reminders to provide adequate opportunities for children to perform ASQ-3 (or ASQ:SE) items can help ensure accurate screening results. Using the ASQ Family Access online questionnaire completion system helps address or minimize important issues, such as incomplete questionnaire data, administration of an incorrect age interval or language, and the high cost of mailings.

In addition, the online management system has some significant advantages over a paper management system in terms of efficiency and accuracy. For instance, because scoring is automated, the time it takes professionals to score a questionnaire is reduced, and scoring errors are eliminated.

Online Procedures

The flexibility of using the ASQ online questionnaire completion and online management systems depends on how a user would like to reach children and their families and whether the user has access to ASQ Pro or ASQ Enterprise as well as ASQ Family Access. Parents who are invited to complete their child's questionnaire online through ASQ Family Access receive a URL to visit to set up a user name and password and begin screening. Users can direct parents to the web page in the form of a letter, e-mail, or telephone call. The program sets up preferences for the web site (e.g., inclusion of logo, welcome message to parents, follow-up note upon completion), and parents simply fill out demographic information and enter responses to the appropriate questionnaire items. When parents are finished completing the questionnaire, the user is alerted in the ASQ Pro or ASQ Enterprise online management system account and can accept the screening for scoring and inclusion in the online management system.

A typical ASQ online management system user will create and store child records, including results of screenings completed by hand after receiving the questionnaire in the mail as well as results collected through the online parent completion system. The online management system will score the questionnaire, store it, and generate reports and communications as desired by the user. Regardless of the questionnaire delivery and return options, users of the online management system can manage general follow-up, subsequent screenings, referrals, and additional communications with parents or caregivers. The online management system does not, however, replace key interaction with a knowledgeable staff person, who should discuss the screening results and next steps with the parents or caregivers, respond to questions or concerns, and offer information for appropriate referrals to local community services if necessary.

ONLINE EXAMPLES

Miss Hancock received a 36 month questionnaire in the mail from her daughter, Rain's, primary health care provider. Included with the questionnaire were instructions on completing the questionnaire and bringing it with her to Rain's next scheduled visit. When Miss Hancock arrived, the nurse collected the completed questionnaire and entered it into the computer, generating results that the nurse placed in Rain's file for the doctor to go over with Miss Hancock. Questionnaire data were added to the program's ASQ Pro records.

Ms. Perry took her twin boys, Joey and Jeff, to a primary health care practice that has kiosk-based computer access to the ASQ-3 through ASQ Family Access. While waiting in the office for a well-child visit, Ms. Perry was given directions by office staff on how to access the appropriate age ASQ-3 for her children. Following the directions, she completed a 36 month ASQ-3 for each of her boys. She received a reply indicating that the doctor would be discussing the screening results for both children with her shortly. Ms. Perry then discussed the results with her family physician during the boys' well-child checkup. The physician encouraged Ms. Perry to contact her local early intervention provider to obtain a more comprehensive assessment of Jeff, who scored below the cutoff in several areas.

Telephone Interview

The telephone interview method often combines the mail-out method with a personal interview over the telephone. This completion option usually requires mailing a questionnaire to a family, which is then followed up by a telephone interview to complete the questionnaire. This combination method is effective for families who may not be equipped to complete a questionnaire independently (e.g., parents with limited literacy); however, it is more costly to conduct and therefore most programs may use it only with families who cannot or will not complete the questionnaires without assistance. The telephone interview option can also be used when it is not possible to schedule a visit to a child's home.

Telephone Interview Considerations

Programs that have large numbers of children to screen may find that using the mail-out completion option in combination with the telephone interview option maximizes effectiveness and resources. The mail-out option was designed for use with parents who can independently complete the ASQ-3, whereas the telephone interview option can be reserved for the few families who require assistance to complete the questionnaires. The telephone interview option is possible if primary health care practices, screening clinics, or educational programs have personnel who can consistently conduct quality telephone interviews.

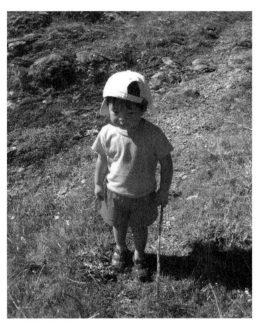

Photo by Ching-I Chen

Telephone Interview Procedures

A copy of the age-appropriate questionnaire is mailed to the parents prior to the interview (see previous section in this chapter on mail-out procedures). This allows parents the opportunity to try the items on the questionnaire and mark responses prior to the scheduled telephone interview. During the interview, program personnel can follow up with parents regarding questions or concerns and clarify items. If parents are unable to try an item before the telephone interview or are unsure how their child would perform a particular item(s), then the interviewer can call back or schedule a follow-up meeting so the parents have time to try the item(s) with the child. If possible, parents should try all items with their child before questionnaire results are finalized.

The procedures for implementing the telephone interview completion option closely follow those used for the mail-out system, with a few exceptions. First, the program must dedicate staff time to interview families, and the interviewer must be knowledgeable about child development, local resources, referral agencies, and procedures for completing the ASQ-3. Calling ahead to schedule the interview with the parent will serve to ensure that parents have received the ASQ-3 and will try the questionnaire items with their child before the interview. During the interview, either the interviewer or parents can read items. Parents and the interviewer can discuss questions and concerns as the items are read. The questionnaire can be scored by both the parent and interviewer. If parents are unsure of how their child will perform a particular item(s) and were unable to observe if the child has the skill, then the interviewer can offer to call back so the parents have time to observe or try that item(s) with the child. Parental concerns and needs can also be addressed during the follow-up telephone call.

Case Study

TELEPHONE INTERVIEW EXAMPLE

At times, Steps-Ahead personnel will assist parents in completing the ASQ-3 through a telephone interview. The Briggs family lives in a remote location, more than 2 hours by car from the Steps-Ahead office. The family indicated they prefer a home visit rather than receiving the questionnaire by mail, but the staff are unable to make home visits at every questionnaire age interval. When it is not possible for a home visitor to travel to the family, the questionnaire is mailed prior to a scheduled telephone interview. A home visitor then calls Mrs. Briggs and completes the questionnaire with Mrs. Briggs over the telephone. This approach gives the family some personal contact, and if questions arise, the home visitor can provide immediate feedback.

Home Visit

ASQ-3 can be used across a broad range of programs that have some form of home visitation by their staff. The advantages of using ASQ-3 on home visits are numerous. Parents can ask questions as they complete the questionnaire and can discuss concerns about their child's development with the home visitor. In addition, the questionnaires can be incorporated into more comprehensive curricula; for example, the ASQ-3 could be used in conjunction with an abuse and neglect prevention program to help parents understand their child's development over time. Of all of the ways to complete ASQ-3, the home visiting completion option is the most costly.

Home Visit Considerations

It is crucial for home visitors to receive training and guidance on explaining the purpose of developmental screening and on providing assistance for completing the questionnaire in a home setting. It is important that home visitors understand that ASQ-3 was designed to be completed by parents or other primary caregivers. Home visitors should be nondirective and only offer assistance when requested by parents. In addition to maintaining independent parent completion of the questionnaire to the extent possible, home visitors should also use materials familiar to the child. Although it may be helpful for home visitors to assemble a toy kit as backup, using materials familiar to children, when possible, usually provides a more accurate picture of their development.

Another important recommendation for home visits is to encourage parents or caregivers to try each item with their child. Parents or caregivers should take time to carefully answer each question as well as to discuss concerns and results. If the screening process is rushed, then unintended consequences may occur. Rushing ASQ-3 completion may result in over- or under-identification because the observations of children were insufficient to accurately score each item. Parents may become unnecessarily alarmed if results suggest a potential problem when the child's development is actually typical for his or her age group. Conversely, necessary services for a child may be withheld if questionnaire results erroneously find the child's development to be typical for his or her age group when, in fact, a significant delay exists.

Home Visit Procedures

Ideally, questionnaires should be mailed 1–2 weeks before the scheduled home visit to give parents the opportunity to observe their child's performance of items over time (see the mail-out options discussed earlier in this chapter). The home visitor should begin by explaining the screening process and describing what his or her role will be. It is important to explain the purpose of the questionnaires and instructions for their completion in language that is easy to understand.

After the questionnaire is completed and reviewed, the home visitor may choose to score the questionnaire with the parents, offering immediate information and feedback and making referrals as appropriate. The ASQ-3 Information Summary sheet, which shows scores and follow-up decisions, can also be completed with parents. This form allows parents to score and/or review the questionnaire with assistance from the home visitor.

There may be times when supervisors choose to have home visitors gather screening information from families but share questionnaire outcomes with supervisors prior to discussing the results with parents. This is particularly important if a home visitor is newly hired or inexperienced or when families have complex needs. When results of the ASQ-3 indicate the need for further assessment, it is important for home visitors to be prepared to explain the next steps. These conversations may be difficult and emotionally charged for family members and, consequentially, home visitors may need to have previous discussions with supervisors prior to presenting concerning results to parents. Reviewing the discussion in Chapter 6 about communicating results with the family may be helpful.

When discussing results, a home visitor may offer activities that support positive parent–child interactions and encourage development. The ASQ-3 intervention activities sheets, found in Appendix F, or the *Ages & Stages Learning Activities* (Twombly & Fink, 2004, 2008), which provides activities focused on different areas of development, can be left with parents. For specific steps on using the ASQ-3 on home visits, see Appendix 8B at the end of this chapter.

HOME VISIT EXAMPLE

Some of the families participating in Steps-Ahead have a home visitor who helps them complete the ASQ-3. Lonni and her infant, Amanda, were enrolled in Steps-Ahead 2 years ago when Amanda was born prematurely; Lonni was 16 years old at the time. Lonni qualified for other programs that assisted her in finding housing and a parent support group. Lonni and her service coordinator from Steps-Ahead have participated in several team meetings with other agency personnel to develop a comprehensive intervention plan.

When Lonni was first asked to complete the ASQ-3 with the home visitor, she said that observing her child and completing the ASQ-3 was a waste of time. While acknowledging Lonni's skepticism, the home visitor asked if they could work together to complete the ASQ-3 for Amanda. With Lonni's approval, the home visitor read each item and talked about observing Amanda's performance. The home visitor commented on how well Amanda was able to walk, run, and manipulate objects. The home visitor noted, however, that Amanda's performance in the language area seemed to lag a little behind what would be expected of most 2-year-olds. The home visitor asked Lonni if she would like some activities that might help her encourage Amanda's language development. Lonni agreed, and the home visitor spent time discussing the suggested activities and how Lonni might engage Amanda in more book reading. At the next questionnaire interval, Lonni showed more interest in completing the ASQ-3 and seemed pleased that Amanda's language development was now on target for her age. At the end of the visit, Lonni asked when they would complete the next ASQ-3.

On-Site Option

Questionnaires may be completed on site (e.g., in a doctor's waiting room) for parents who do not return the questionnaires and for parents with no permanent address. Completing the ASQ-3 on site has several drawbacks, however. First, toys and objects (e.g., blocks, pencil and paper, a mirror) must be available so that parents can try the questionnaire items with their child. Second, parents may not have the time necessary to accurately complete the questionnaires in an office or clinic environment, or the child may be uncooperative and/or may not have the time needed to demonstrate each targeted skill. These issues must be considered when interpreting results. Are the results an accurate reflection of the child's ability, or did any of the previous reasons influence the child's performance? Scores in the monitoring zone or below the referral cutoffs may require follow-up. For example, it may be appropriate to offer a second copy of the ASQ-3 for parents to complete at home and then return to the office.

CONCLUSION

ASQ-3 can be administered in many ways. The purpose of this chapter has been to describe five primary ways of completing the ASQ-3: using mail-out, online, telephone interview, home visit, and on-site completion options. Considerations and recommendations for using each option were offered as well as an example illustrating the method. The ways of administering the ASQ-3 described in this chapter can be used separately or can be combined. It is important for program personnel to examine their screening goals, survey their available resources, and then choose the option that best fits their needs.

8A

Procedures for Using the Card File Tickler System

The card file tickler system provides a simple, low-tech approach to tracking all of the activities involved in mailing out the ASQ-3. To begin, locate an index card file box. Place dividers for each month (e.g., January, February, March) in the file box. Include subdividers for each month and arrange them by day, week, biweekly interval, or month, depending on the number of children monitored. Complete an individual index card for each child monitored in the program. Figure 8A.1 shows a sample card for Joseph Henry; a blank sample card is provided as well for program staff to photocopy on an as-needed basis (see Figure 8A.2). The card contains space to record essential identifying information for the child and family, as well as a tracking grid to assist program staff.

The sample grid includes a column listing the program's planned activities in the order the activities are to be administered and columns for each age interval at which a questionnaire is to be completed. Upon completion of each activity in the first column, staff enters the date in the appropriate column. The activities column contains entries for follow-up, which may not be necessary if the questionnaire is completed and returned to the program on schedule. After a questionnaire is mailed or given to the parents, the card is refiled in chronological order under the month and week the questionnaire should be returned. All activities associated with tracking the child's progress are filed by date under the appropriate month and week.

For example, Joseph's card (see Figure 8A.1) is filed under the week of September 15 because that date is 1 week before Joseph will become 12 months old. When September 15 arrives, the card is reviewed, and Joseph's parents are sent a 12 month questionnaire. A notation is made on the card indicating that a reminder call should be made to the parents on September 19, approximately 4–5 days after the questionnaire was mailed, and that the questionnaire should be returned by September 22. The card is filed under the week of September 19 until the call is made and the questionnaire is returned.

If the questionnaire were to be returned before September 22, then this would be indicated on the card. In addition, other important information should be recorded on the card when possible (e.g., feedback sent, results of questionnaire, whether child was referred for services). A

Child's name __Joseph Henry__
Parent's or guardian's name __Pam & Gerald Henry__
Address __221 Lakeside, Cottage Grove, OR 97461__
Telephone __541-555-0149__ Message __None__

Corrected date of birth __None__
Child's gender __M__
Date of birth __Sept. 22, 2007__

ACTIVITIES	2 MO	4 MO	6 MO	8 MO	9 MO	10 MO	12 MO	14 MO	16 MO	18 MO	20 MO	22 MO	24 MO	27 MO	30 MO	33 MO	36 MO	42 MO	48 MO	54 MO	60 MO
Send questionnaire							9-15-08		1-15-09												
Sent questionnaire							9-15-08														
Call—instructions							9-19-08														
Called							9-19-08														
Expected return							9-22-08														
Returned							9-22-08														
If not, called																					
Results							OK														
Feedback sent							9-28-08														
Parent called with concern							—														
Physician notified							—														
Referral							—														
Refile card (y/n)							Y														

Comments:

Figures 8A.1. The card file tickler system includes a card for each child participating in the program. As shown on this sample card completed for Joseph Henry, essential identifying information is recorded, and staff uses the grid to track the distribution and return of questionnaires. Basic results are also recorded.

Child's name _____

Parent's or guardian's name _____

Address _____

Telephone _____ Message _____

Corrected date of birth _____

Child's gender _____

Date of birth _____

ACTIVITIES	2 MO	4 MO	6 MO	8 MO	9 MO	10 MO	12 MO	14 MO	16 MO	18 MO	20 MO	22 MO	24 MO	27 MO	30 MO	33 MO	36 MO	42 MO	48 MO	54 MO	60 MO
Send questionnaire																					
Sent questionnaire																					
Call—instructions																					
Called																					
Expected return																					
Returned																					
If not, called																					
Results																					
Feedback sent																					
Parent called with concern																					
Physician notified																					
Referral																					
Refile card (y/n)																					

Comments:

Figure 8A.2. This blank sample card for the card file tickler system may be photocopied for program use. (Please see the conditions of the Photocopying Release on p. xxi.)

space is also provided at the bottom of the card to record any additional comments or information relevant to the child. The date for mailing the next questionnaire is recorded, and the card is refiled under the appropriate month and day.

Joseph's parents returned the questionnaire on September 25; the results indicated typical development, and staff sent feedback to them on September 28. Joseph's parents are scheduled to receive a 16 month questionnaire next; thus, the card is refiled under the week of January 15, approximately 4 months after the last questionnaire was completed. If Joseph's parents had not returned the questionnaire by September 22, then they would have been called and a new return date would have been recorded with the card.

SPECIFIC STEPS FOR USING A TICKLER SYSTEM

Careful adherence to the following steps is the first guideline for ensuring a high return rate. In all steps, *target* refers to the assigned date for completing the questionnaire; for infants who were born 3 or more weeks prematurely and who are less than 24 months of age, this target date corresponds with the corrected age rather than the chronological date of birth.

1. Pull the child's card from the tickler file box.
2. Complete the identifying information on the first page of the appropriate ASQ-3 interval.
3. Record the questionnaire target date (e.g., the date the child will be 16 months) under *Expected return* on the tickler file card.
4. Prepare the questionnaire for mailing, either by stapling or taping the ends or by putting it in an envelope. If stapled or taped, then the program's return address and a stamp should be added to the mailing sheet. If mailed in an envelope, then a program-addressed, stamped envelope should be included.
5. Record the date the questionnaire is mailed on the child's tickler file card under *Sent questionnaire.*
6. Record a date 3 or 4 days after mailing in the *Call—instructions* column.
7. Refile the card under the date marked in the *Call—instructions* column.
8. Check the tickler file and call parents on the date marked for *Call—instructions* to ensure that the questionnaire was received and to answer any questions the parents may have about completing the questionnaire.
9. Record the date the parents were contacted in the *Called* column.
10. Refile the tickler file card in the file box under the date in the *Expected return* column.
11. If the questionnaire is returned before the expected return date, then record the date returned under the *Returned* column.
12. If the questionnaire is not returned by the expected return date, then call the child's parents and record the date in the *If not, called* column.
13. Score the questionnaire according to the instructions in Chapter 6 and record the results on the Information Summary sheet.
14. If the questionnaire results indicate the child is developing typically, then send a feedback letter (see Chapter 5 for examples of feedback letters; see Appendix D at the end of this book for blank sample letters as well as Spanish versions of the letters) and an intervention activities sheet (see Appendix F at the end of this book). If program resources permit, then send parents additional incentives that may increase return rate (see discussion in this chapter about mail-out incentives).
15. If the questionnaire results indicate that a child is identified as needing an in-depth assessment, then call the child's parents to discuss options. Refer the child for further assessment, if indicated.

16. Ask the parents if they want the questionnaire results sent to the child's physician. Obtain the parents' written consent to share questionnaire results with other agencies and the child's physician.

17. Determine whether the child will continue to be monitored using the questionnaires. Monitoring would be discontinued for three reasons: 1) at the parent's request, 2) if the child was older than 5 years, or 3) if developmental delays were identified on the follow-up assessment and the child then began receiving early intervention services.

18. Refile the child's tickler file card under the date that corresponds to 1 week before target date for the next questionnaire age interval.

8B

Using the ASQ-3 on Home Visits

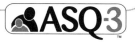

The following list details the steps and decisions involved in implementing the ASQ-3 system while on a home visit. In addition, a DVD, *The Ages & Stages Questionnaires® on a Home Visit* (Farrell & Potter, 1995), is also available from Paul H. Brookes Publishing Co.

- Obtain consent from the parent(s) to participate in the monitoring program.
- Telephone and schedule a home visit date and time.
- Photocopy the language-appropriate (English or Spanish) and age-appropriate questionnaire.
- Arrange for an interpreter if necessary.
- Mail the age-appropriate questionnaire to the child's home 2 weeks before the visit.
- Assemble appropriate toys and materials needed to complete the questionnaire.
- Determine whether the parents are capable of reading and comprehending the questionnaire.

For parents who are unable to read or are otherwise unable to complete the questionnaire (e.g., as a result of mental illness, developmental disability, or a language difference):

- The home visitor may read the items on the questionnaire.
- The home visitor may demonstrate for parents how to elicit the behavior required for questionnaire items.

For parents who are able to read and comprehend the questionnaire:

- Parents can read and administer the questionnaire with the home visitor's assistance.
- The home visitor may demonstrate how to elicit the behaviors required for questionnaire completion.

To describe the questionnaire, the home visitor can give the following information:

- Describe the ASQ-3 system as a tool parents can use to check their child's development.
- Clarify the home visitor's role (i.e., to read and demonstrate how to elicit desired behavior).
- Provide ideas for involving family members, including siblings, in eliciting behaviors described on the questionnaires.

After describing the questionnaire, the home visitor can do the following:

- Complete the family information sheet (i.e., demographic information) with the parent.
- Enter the parent's name in the section called "Person filling out questionnaire."
- Explain the scoring system.
    - *Yes* indicates the child is performing the behavior.
    - *Sometimes* indicates the child is just beginning to perform the behavior (i.e., it is an emerging skill).
    - *Not yet* indicates the child is not yet performing the behavior.
- Introduce each area of development on the questionnaire.
    - *Communication* items focus on language skills—both what the child understands and what he or she can say.
    - *Gross Motor* items focus on large muscle movement and coordination.
    - *Fine Motor* items focus on small muscle movement and coordination.
    - *Problem Solving* items focus on the child's play with toys.
    - *Personal-Social* items focus on the child's interactions with toys and other children.
- Administer the questionnaire.
    - If necessary, read each item.
    - Paraphrase items as needed for parents who seem to need clarification.
    - When appropriate, rephrase questions in terms of the family's values or cultural orientation.
    - Comment on the child's accomplishments whenever possible. Praise the child directly. Highlight the parents' strengths and reinforce positive parent–child interactions.
    - Adapt materials used for questionnaire items to the family's culture and values (e.g., some cultures do not use mirrors).
    - For items the parents cannot answer with certainty, have them try to elicit the behaviors while the home visitor is present.
    - If the child is uncooperative, and the parents are unsure whether the child can perform a behavior, then the home visitor can call parents in 1–2 weeks, thereby giving the parents more time to try the item(s).
    - Complete the Overall section, paying close attention to the parents' concerns.
    - Offer suggestions and resources when appropriate.
    - Encourage dialogue about the child's development and parenting issues.
- Score the questionnaire.
    - The home visitor can do the scoring or show the parents how to do the scoring.
    - Compare the child's area scores with the cutoff scores indicated on the Information Summary sheet.
    - Discuss the results with the parents.
    - Explain the area scores.

- Using the bar graph scoring grid on the Information Summary sheet, show the parents where the child's scores fall in relation to the cutoff scores.
- Encourage dialogue with the parents about the child's development.
- Discuss referral options if necessary.
- Offer intervention activity suggestions (see Appendix F at the end of this book) appropriate to the child's current and upcoming questionnaire age interval.
- Describe some of the activities with the parents.
- Encourage the parents to arrange the activities in an accessible place (e.g., on refrigerator door).
- Make arrangements for follow-up, referral, or the next home visit.

9

ASQ-3 Settings

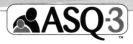

As indicated in Chapter 8, the mail-out, online, telephone interview, home visit, and on-site options for ASQ-3 questionnaire completion can be used across a variety of programs that may wish to conduct developmental screening. In addition, screening clinics, child care settings, center-based educational programs (e.g., preschools, Head Start programs), and primary care practices offer exceptional opportunities to engage parents in the developmental screening of their young children. The following sections offer information and recommendations for developmental screening in these settings.

Appendix 9A at the end of this chapter describes specific steps for using the ASQ-3 with teachers and parents. This appendix also describes how teachers and child care providers can work together with parents to administer the ASQ-3.

SCREENING CLINICS

Screening clinics (also known as "round ups") are usually joint community efforts held annually that provide developmental assessments for a large number of children that focus on general development, hearing, and vision, as well as medical and dental evaluations. Recommendations and referrals are made to EI/ECSE programs, hospitals, and other community resources as appropriate. Screening clinics are usually sponsored by a network of providers who combine their agencies' efforts to provide communitywide early childhood assessments.

The ASQ-3 has been the measure of choice for many screening clinics conducted throughout the United States for several reasons. First, the questionnaires are economical to use because they can be completed by parents rather than professional staff. Second, most parents and other caregivers find the questionnaires to be user friendly, easy to complete, and a reasonable time investment. Third, many parents comment on the value of completing an ASQ-3 because it gives them a better understanding of what their child should be doing developmentally. Finally, the extensive data based on the reliability and validity of the ASQ-3 permits professional staff to be confident that, in most cases, the ASQ-3 results will be accurate.

Screening clinics may be organized using a variety of formats. Often, each agency has its own space or room where parents and their children can complete the ASQ-3 with the appropriate toys and objects available to complete each interval. Parents can complete the ASQ-3 items independently with their children or with assistance from staff. Information on community resources and referrals can be given to families when necessary.

Prior to the screening, clinic staff will need to assemble the necessary toys and objects (e.g., clipboards, pencils) to complete questionnaire assessments. Staff will need to be on hand to assist parents, score questionnaires, and provide feedback. Some programs have used creative means for helping parents try items and score the questionnaires. For example, different stations or areas can be set up for each developmental area on the questionnaire (e.g., Communication, Fine Motor). Parents and children rotate through each station, completing items for that area.

Case Study

SCREENING CLINIC EXAMPLE

Three human services agencies in a small rural county offer an annual screening clinic to all interested parents of children birth to 5 years of age. Carla Jones is a single mother with an infant who participates in the county WIC program. WIC staff encouraged Carla to participate in the screening. Carla brought her infant to the screening clinic, where she was assigned a "helper" who assisted Carla in completing the 8 month questionnaire for her infant. Upon completion, Carla and the clinic helper scored the questionnaire, which indicated the infant's scores in the Gross Motor and Fine Motor areas were below the cutoff scores for her age. Without alarming Carla, the clinic helper suggested they talk to the staff person, Ms. Owens, from the county's evaluation program. Ms. Owens and Carla discussed the ASQ-3 results and together decided to have Carla bring her infant to the evaluation agency to complete a more comprehensive assessment.

CHILD CARE SETTINGS

Providing developmental screening in child care settings is often an efficient and effective strategy for screening large numbers of young children, especially when using a measure such as the ASQ-3. Many children are served by child care programs, and in many instances, child care providers may have enough contact with children to accurately complete the questionnaire. Child care providers, however, should first enlist parents to complete the ASQ-3 for their child whenever possible. Parents should be provided the opportunity to complete the questionnaire for two important reasons. First, many parents benefit by acquiring information about their child's development and what skills should be targeted for the future. Second, parents usually know more about their child than anyone else and acquiring that information should be part of developmental screening. Having a child care provider work in partnership with a parent and begin observations of ASQ-3 skills in the child care setting is an excellent strategy to consider. Meeting together to compare observations and discuss a child's development provides the opportunity to discuss the child's strengths and, if necessary, discuss any developmental or behavioral concerns.

Case Study

CHILD CARE SETTING EXAMPLE

Little Ducklings is a child care program for children ages 2–5 years whose parents are eligible for child care subsidies. The child care program is open from 7:30 A.M. to 5:30 P.M. Monday through Friday, and many of the children attend full time. During enrollment, parents are informed that the program provides developmental screening as part of its services. During parent orientation, Katie's mother was given the age-appropriate

ASQ-3 (36 months) for her daughter, introduced to its purpose and content, and provided time to complete the questionnaire and ask any questions that arose. A meeting was scheduled with Katie's mother and Katie's child care provider to review the results. The child care provider used the age-appropriate questionnaire to begin observing Katie's skills in the child care setting. She also planned activities to try to elicit some of the items for which direct direct observation is more necessary. A week before the scheduled meeting, a program secretary called to remind Katie's mother of the upcoming meeting. At the meeting, Katie's mother and child care provider compared their results on the ASQ-3. With two items, Katie's mother was able to provide examples of skills Katie mastered that the child care provider had not been able to observe. Katie's mother and the child care provider combined their observations to create one final ASQ-3. The child care provider was planning to focus on providing fine motor opportunities to Katie because her ASQ-3 scores fell in the monitoring zone in the Fine Motor area.

CENTER-BASED EDUCATIONAL PROGRAMS

Most communities offer center-based educational programs for young children. Many of these programs, such as Head Start, target preschool-age children, whereas other programs, such as Early Head Start, focus on infants and toddlers. Some programs offer developmental screening to their families as an additional service, whereas Head Start and Early Head Start programs are required to provide developmental screening to all children in their programs.

Enrollment in a center-based educational program is an excellent time to introduce the purpose of screening and ASQ-3 to parents. A second opportunity is during planned parent meetings. Including screening as one of the activities of a center-based program makes it a universal process and therefore does not stigmatize any child or family. Parents can be given the age-appropriate ASQ-3 interval for their child during enrollment and begin looking through it in anticipation of answering questions. Classroom teachers can also be given the age-appropriate questionnaire interval for the child and begin making observations of the child in the classroom. A meeting can be arranged between the parent and classroom teacher to review the results of the questionnaire, and differences in observations can be discussed. If the parent does not bring the questionnaire to the meeting, then teachers can review their observations carefully with the parents to see if there are any changes parents would like to make to the ASQ-3. Items marked *not yet* should be discussed carefully to determine if the parent has observed those skills in the home environment, and answers to questions in the Overall section should be finalized with parents.

Although there is some flexibility in ASQ-3 administration procedures, teachers need to keep in mind that the two main options for completing the ASQ-3 are 1) working together with parents on completing the ASQ-3 and 2) allowing parents to complete the ASQ-3 independently. Specific steps for using the ASQ-3 together with teachers and parents can be found in Appendix 9A at the end of this chapter.

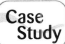

Case Study

CENTER-BASED EDUCATIONAL PROGRAM EXAMPLE

Big Little School is a local preschool program that offers developmental screening and monitoring as part of their services to children and their families enrolled in the program. The Carlson have two children enrolled at the Big Little School and have completed several questionnaires for their children in the time that their children have attended school there. When they began with Big Little School, an orientation was scheduled for the family that included an introduction to the ASQ-3. The school coordinator and teachers explained the ASQ-3 system to the family and enlisted their support and participation in completing the questionnaires. The Big Little School provides an age-appropriate questionnaire to parents while teachers at school also use the same-age questionnaire to make observations about the child's skills. At a prearranged time, such as conference time, the parents and school staff meet to compare item answers and discuss differences in parent and teacher observations.

Recently a questionnaire was completed for the Carlson's daughter Rachael using the process just described. During the meeting with Rachael's parents and teaching staff, Rachael's teacher's responses on the ASQ-3 showed that Rachael had scores in the monitoring zone in the Gross Motor and Fine Motor areas, whereas her parents' responses indicated that Rachael's scores were well above the cutoff scores in these areas. This discrepancy prompted a discussion with Rachael's parents about her comfort level in participating in gross and fine motor activities at school. Based on this discussion, Rachael's parents and teachers came up with a plan to increase Rachael's comfort in trying the various gross and fine motor activities at school. In addition, teaching staff gave Rachael's parents activities designed to be used with the ASQ-3 to work on her gross and fine motor skills at home.

PRIMARY CARE PRACTICES

Providing developmental screening in primary care practices is another effective setting for screening young children. In order to minimize office staff time, parents should be encouraged to complete the ASQ-3 at home prior to a well-child checkup. When parents contact their child's pediatrician's office to schedule a well-child visit, office staff may ask if the parent has Internet access at home. If the parent says yes, then office staff may direct him or her to complete the ASQ-3 prior to the well-child visit via the ASQ Family Access online questionnaire completion system. If the parent does not have Internet access, then he or she can be mailed the age-appropriate questionnaire and an explanation about the screening/monitoring program. When parents receive appointment reminder telephone calls prior to well-child visits, the messaging system may also include a prompt for parents to go to the web site to complete the ASQ-3 online or a reminder to complete the paper questionnaire and bring it to their appointment. Results from ASQ-3 questionnaires completed online through ASQ Family Access can be transmitted to the ASQ online management system for scoring, and the results can be placed in the child's physical file.

If parents have not completed the questionnaire prior to the well-child visit, then they should be given the ASQ-3 to complete once they arrive in the waiting room. Offices may provide paper copies of questionnaires or set up a computer station or kiosk with the ASQ-3 online completion system. In either case, the space designated for ASQ-3 completion should include any materials needed to complete the ASQ-3 (e.g., small blocks, toys). Ideally, the "ASQ-3 station" will be in a separate room that is comfortable, private, quiet, and spacious enough for the child to play with materials and demonstrate target skills.

A staff member should be appointed to assist the parents as necessary while they complete the ASQ-3. One of the advantages of the ASQ-3 system is that paraprofessionals, office staff, and assistant medical health professionals (e.g., a certified nurse assistant) can receive training and provide excellent support to parents. Support may range from directing caregivers to the ASQ-3 station to helping them complete the questionnaire by reading items and assisting them in eliciting skills from their children.

Before meeting with the primary health care provider, trained ASQ-3 support staff can meet with parents to remind them about the purpose of developmental screening, discuss the results of the completed ASQ-3, and share local community resource information related to child development. This meeting is intended to be a brief conversation (i.e., 5–10 minutes) to help parents become better informed about their child's development. Information about immediate

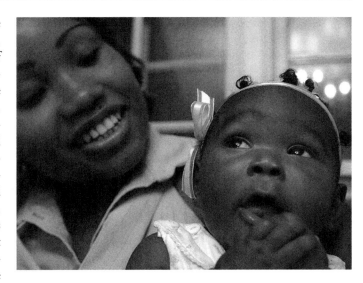

concerns as well as referrals to community agencies for more in-depth assistance may be given to parents at this time. This "touch point" is a critical one for parents, particularly for those whose children will require a referral for EI/ECSE. The designated ASQ-3 staff person should receive extensive training on how to introduce the ASQ-3, support parents in administering the ASQ-3, and score and interpret results, as well as communicating results with parents in a sensitive, supportive, and nonthreatening manner (see Chapter 6 for more information on how to talk to parents).

Screening a child with the ASQ-3 will result in one of three findings: 1) the child appears to be developing typically; 2) the child's development is questionable or in the monitoring zone in one or more areas; or 3) the child's scores fall below established cutoffs, and the child should be referred for an in-depth assessment through EI/ECSE. Office staff should be trained on interpreting and responding to each of these three results.

If the child is developing typically and the parent has no specific concerns, then the designated ASQ-3 staff will discuss and emphasize these results with the parent and provide him or her with a general developmental information packet. This packet can include age-appropriate intervention or learning activities as well as general community resources for young children.

If the child's scores are close to the cutoffs (in the monitoring zone), or if the parent has any specific concerns or questions, then the designated ASQ-3 staff should reinforce the child's developmental strengths and provide information that is tailored to the child's needs and parent's concerns. For example, if the child's development appears questionable in the Fine Motor area, then the ASQ-3 staff can provide activities that are specifically designed for fine motor practice. If a parent wants information about community child care options, then staff can refer the parent to the local child care resource and referral agency.

If a child's scores are below the cutoff in any area, then the ASQ-3 staff will discuss items marked as *not yet* to determine if the low score may be due to issues such as a child's lack of opportunity to practice skills. Staff will note any of these discussions or considerations to alert the primary health care provider to these considerations when sharing the ASQ-3 Information Summary sheet. They will discuss the areas that were below the cutoff and potential follow-up options with the parent. In some cases, such as a child's lack of opportunity to practice specific skills, the ASQ-3 staff can suggest that the parent provide practice for these skills and bring the child in for a follow-up screening in the next couple of months (or complete a follow-up questionnaire online through ASQ Family Access). When the ASQ-3 score is below the cutoff in any given area or indicates potentially significant developmental delays based on parental concerns, then parents should be encouraged to discuss these concerns with the child's primary care provider. Initial information about the local EI/ECSE agency and the services offered to children and families should also be provided.

The ASQ-3 Information Summary sheet, with any additional information noted by the ASQ-3 office staff member, should then be placed in the child's file for the primary health care provider to review. In the majority of cases, primary health care providers can simply comment on developmental progress that children have made and celebrate these accomplishments with families. When referrals are warranted, the primary care provider should discuss this with the parents and obtain consent if necessary to refer the child to the local EI/ECSE agency. It is assumed that the majority of these screenings will indicate typical development, and in most cases, there will be minimal time involved when discussing developmental issues with a child's primary health care provider.

Results from the child's developmental screening, including any referrals that were made based on screening results, should be entered into the child's medical record so that developmental progress can be monitored over time.

PRIMARY CARE PRACTICE EXAMPLE

Dr. Smith is a pediatrician who conducts ASQ-3 screenings in his office. Katie was screened with ASQ-3 during her 12-month well-child visit. Her mother filled out the ASQ-3 in the waiting room. After Dr. Smith's nurse scored the questionnaire, it was given to Dr. Smith to review before the appointment. Dr. Smith was then able to discuss the results of the ASQ-3 with Katie's parents. Based on the results of the ASQ-3, Katie was developing typically. Overall, her parents had no specific concerns. The staff at the primary care practice provided Katie's parents with age-appropriate activities to help them understand and further support Katie's development.

CONCLUSION

The purpose of this chapter has been to describe specific popular settings for using ASQ-3. Screening clinics, child care centers, center-based educational programs, and primary care practices are some examples of the variety of environments where ASQ-3 can be used.

9A

Steps for Educational Professionals Using ASQ-3 Together with Parents

ASQ-3

The following information describes how teachers and child care providers can work together with parents to administer the ASQ-3.

The first step is to obtain the date of birth for the children in the classroom. When obtaining the date of birth of children entering the classroom, it is important to determine the children's exact ages. Once this has been established, the ASQ-3 age administration chart (shown in Table 6.1 in Chapter 6 and in Table 2 in Appendix C at the end of this book) or age ranges indicated on each questionnaire can be used to determine the appropriate ASQ-3 to administer to each child.

Begin to administer ASQ-3 to the children in the classroom. Observe the children over time and create opportunities to demonstrate skills. Leave items blank that you do not have an opportunity to observe.

After administering ASQ-3, meet with or call the parents. Ideally, parents should come to a parent–teacher meeting with a completed or partially completed questionnaire. If meeting via telephone, then make sure the parent has a copy of the questionnaire in front of him or her when discussing the results.

Review items you (as the teacher) have marked *not yet*. If your observations differ from that of the parent, then determine with the parent how to ultimately mark the item, or mark the item as *sometimes*. Keep in mind that children will often do things at home before they try new skills at school and that a child may very well be performing the skill in the home environment even if you have not observed it in the classroom. Parents should have the final say as to how an item is scored.

Consider obtaining a signature on the completed questionnaire to document parent participation. One way to ensure that parents are included in the ASQ-3 process is to have parents sign a statement such as the following: *My input was gathered to complete the ASQ-3, and I believe the information is accurate.*

Discuss the Overall section questions with parents. It is important to take time to discuss the Overall questions and any parental concerns that come up during the screening process.

Score the ASQ-3 and discuss referral considerations if necessary. Discuss the scoring process and review the scores on each of the questionnaires with the parent. Together, make decisions about next steps. The ASQ-3 Parent Conference Sheet (available in English with the ASQ-3 and in Spanish with the ASQ-3 Spanish) may be a useful way to summarize the conversation and next steps discussed with parents. (The Parent Conference Sheet appears in the Supplemental Materials section of the ASQ-3 box and on the CD-ROM accompanying the ASQ-3 box.)

Provide parents with follow-up activities and resources. Parents should be able to try the activities at home with their child to encourage developmental skills and parent–child interaction. In the classroom, focus on general domain areas where children may need additional opportunities to practice skills.

10

ASQ-3 Case Examples

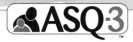

This chapter comprises a series of five case studies designed to illustrate the use of ASQ-3 across various programs and settings. They are intended to help users consider how ASQ-3 results are interpreted and to support work with families. These examples may be a useful training tool for program staff new to ASQ-3. The case studies that follow include examples of statewide screening, online developmental screening, home-based educational screening, clinic-based screening, and center-based educational screening. The following brief descriptions may be used as a guide to locate the examples that will be most relevant based on the user's needs. The case studies are as follows.

CASE STUDY 1: NICHOLAS

Case study 1 is about 3-year-old Nicholas and his parents' experiences participating in a statewide developmental monitoring program to administer ASQ-3.

CASE STUDY 2: SHANDA

Case study 2 is about Shanda, a 4-month-old girl recently adopted from India, and her family's experiences using online developmental screening.

CASE STUDY 3: GUSTAVO

Case study 3 is about Gustavo, a 2-year-old boy who is enrolled in a home visiting program.

CASE STUDY 4: ANDREA

Case study 4 is about Andrea, a 12-month-old girl whose questionnaires were administered through a clinic-based program for a well-child visit.

CASE STUDY 5: KAIDEN

Case study 5 is about Kaiden, a 15-month-old boy, and his experiences with ASQ-3 in a center-based educational program.

NICHOLAS

Statewide Screening by Mail

Nicholas is 3 years, 9 months old, and lives with his mother, father, and 6-month-old brother. Nicholas attends a local parochial preschool three times a week. He enjoys playing with trains, trucks, and cars and likes to paint and play in the sand and mud. He also likes to pretend he is a character from a favorite movie. His father works outside the home, and his mother works from home and takes care of Nicholas and his younger brother. Both sets of grandparents live in the area, see the children frequently, and provide child care and support when needed.

Nicholas's mother, Sherry, signed Nicholas and his younger brother up for Early Check, a statewide developmental monitoring program that provides developmental screening, monitoring, and follow-up to all children from age birth to 5 years. As part of the Early Check program, parents can complete an ASQ-3 for their child starting at 4 months. During this monitoring period, if a child requires a referral for further assessment, then the Early Check program staff help connect the parent to the appropriate agency. Nicholas's parents have completed the ASQ-3 by mail since he was 8 months old, although they did not return the 24 and 36 month intervals. Early Check called and left a reminder to return the questionnaires, and the staff person talked with Nicholas's mother at one point, but the office did not receive any additional questionnaires from her. Because his parents expressed an interest in continuing to receive the ASQ-3 in the mail, the family was not dropped from the monitoring program. A month before Nicholas turned 4, his mother did complete the 48 month interval and sent it back to Early Check. On the 48 month questionnaire, Nicholas scored below the cutoff point in the Communication area (see Figure 10.1). When the questionnaire was returned to Early Check, a service coordinator contacted Nicholas's parents and discussed a referral to the local ECSE agency in order to have a more comprehensive assessment conducted.

Setting/Time Factors

Nicholas's mother indicated that she was concerned about his language. She also indicated that Nicholas's preschool teacher had expressed concerns about his language because she noticed that other children were not always able to understand him. In addition, she was concerned that Nicholas's social skills may be affected by his inability to be understood by peers.

Developmental Factors

Nicholas was born 3 weeks early. During the pregnancy, his mother developed gestational diabetes, and labor was induced to avoid complications. Nicholas cooed and babbled between 5 and 6 months and said his first words at 18 months. Motor milestones included sitting independently at 6 months, crawling at 5 months, and walking at 13 months. Previous questionnaires sent to Nicholas's parents indicated no parental concerns. Nicholas's score on the Communication area of the ASQ-3 was always the lowest area (although not below the cutoff score until the 48 month interval). Nicholas's hearing was tested when he was a newborn, and his parents said that he had a number of previous ear infections. His mother also expressed concerns that Nicholas sometimes uses a "high-pitched voice," although he can use a calm voice when reminded.

Health Factors

Nicholas had to undergo oral surgery when he was 3 years old to repair severe decay in one tooth. His mother noted that Nicholas started talking more following this surgery and wondered if he had been in pain previous to having surgery. Nicholas sees a local pediatrician for well-child checkups. No general health concerns were noted by his pediatrician or parents.

Family/Cultural Factors

Nicholas' recent participation in a preschool setting has had a positive effect on his language. Nicholas has had an opportunity to practice his language skills in a setting with peers, where he is highly motivated to communicate. In addition, his mother has found support for her concerns about his language through the observations of Nicholas's preschool teacher.

Follow-Up

The Early Check service coordinator discussed referral and service options for Nicholas with his mother. Together, they decided to refer him to the local ECSE agency for an assessment. After the assessment, Nicholas's educational team—including his parents, preschool teacher, the Early Check service coordinator, and the assessment team from the local ECSE agency—met to discuss the assessment. Nicholas's communication skills were found to be significantly below age level on standardized tests. The team found he was eligible for services and recommended that he receive speech-language intervention in his preschool setting.

SHANDA

Online Developmental Screening

Shanda is a 5-month-old girl who was recently adopted from India by American parents. She has been in her new home for less than 1 month. Shanda joins two older siblings and is cared for by her maternal grandmother during the day. Shanda's birth history is unknown to her adoptive parents, although they do know that she was born near an urban orphanage and found on the doorstep of the orphanage very shortly after she was born. Her developmental milestones have not been formally assessed.

Shanda's mother was the recipient of a county-based Child Find mailing asking her to go to the ASQ Family Access online questionnaire completion system to complete a questionnaire for Shanda to see how she was developing. The purpose of this free service from the county was to provide parents with one-time developmental screening and referral as needed. Shanda's mother went to the URL indicated in the letter and followed the instructions to enter Shanda's demographic information, including her birth date and weeks premature. The system calculated that Shanda was ready for the 4 month questionnaire and presented the questionnaire on screen. The online questionnaire provided illustrations to support Shanda's mother in understanding the items, and the automated system ensured that Shanda's mother left no more than two items blank in any area. After Shanda's mother completed the questionnaire, program staff e-mailed her to thank her and provided a telephone number indicating that Shanda's mother could feel free

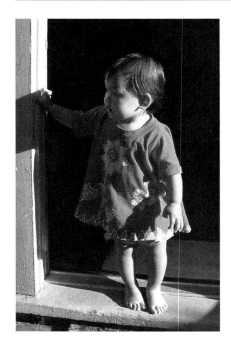

to call the Child Find program at any time; however, they would be contacting her to discuss the results within the next week. The results were returned to the Child Find program that sent Shanda's mother the letter, to finalize the questionnaire in the online management system.

Shanda's scores on the ASQ-3 (see Figure 10.2) were all in the monitoring zone (i.e., between 1 and 2 standard deviations below the mean) except for the Fine Motor area, which was below the cutoff score, suggesting a referral was warranted. Her mother also reported significant concerns on the Overall section. She reported that Shanda seems to reach only with her right arm and only rolls to her right side. When her mother was asked if anything worries her, she reported that Shanda's arms seem to be stiff and that she has jerky movements. In addition, Shanda stares at one spot often for 15 minutes or more, and she seems very quiet and does not vocalize often.

A staff person at Child Find provided a personal response to Shanda's mother, addressing her concerns and providing her with information about referrals to EI/ECSE, as well as other potential resources she was qualified to receive (e.g., WIC, Head Start). Lastly, the Child Find staff person provided Shanda's mother with a printout of intervention activities specific to Shanda's age.

Setting/Time Factors

Shanda is cared for primarily by her grandmother during the day. Her siblings are school age and return home in the afternoon. The majority of family activities occur within the home. Her parents recently joined an online chat group for new parents of adopted infants.

Developmental Factors

Although Shanda's development was not assessed previous to her adoption, her parents felt that her skills seemed typical when they first met her. Her birth weight indicated that she was born at full term, and the orphanage staff reported that she appeared in good health.

Health Factors

Shanda was given a full physical examination before leaving India and was also thoroughly assessed by her pediatrician in the United States. No remarkable conditions were noted at the time with the exception that her weight and height percentiles were lower than would be expected for an infant her age. Currently, Shanda's parents report that she is sleeping normally and takes a bottle with little difficulty.

Family/Cultural Factors

Shanda's family has numerous relatives who live in the vicinity. The extended family values kinship connections and celebrating birthdays and holidays together. Although Shanda's parents are not East Indian, they want to embrace her culture of origin and help her to connect to her roots in India as she grows. Her parents have joined an online chat and support group for parents who have adopted infants from India. In addition, they have made friends with a couple who have recently emigrated from India with their children.

Figure 10.1 (48 Month ASQ-3 Information Summary)

48 Month ASQ-3 Information Summary

45 months 0 days through 50 months 30 days

Child's name: Nicholas   Date ASQ completed: 1-15-09

Child's ID #: 0091   Date of birth: 4-13-05

Administering program/provider: Early Check

1. **SCORE AND TRANSFER TOTALS TO CHART BELOW:** See ASQ-3 User's Guide for details, including how to adjust scores if item responses are missing. Score each item (YES = 10, SOMETIMES = 5, NOT YET = 0). Add item scores, and record each area total. In the chart below, transfer the total scores, and fill in the circles corresponding with the total scores.

Area	Cutoff	Total Score	0	5	10	15	20	25	30	35	40	45	50	55	60
Communication	30.72	15				⊗									
Gross Motor	32.78	55												⊗	
Fine Motor	15.81	50											⊗		
Problem Solving	31.30	55												⊗	
Personal-Social	26.60	55												⊗	

2. **TRANSFER OVERALL RESPONSES:** Bolded uppercase responses require follow-up. See ASQ-3 User's Guide, Chapter 6.

1. Hears well? Yes NO
   Comments:

6. Family history of hearing impairment? YES No
   Comments:

2. Talks like other children his age? Yes NO
   Comments: Nicholas's teacher is worried.

7. Concerns about vision? Yes NO
   Comments:

3. Understand most of what your child says? Yes NO
   Comments:

8. Any medical problems? Yes NO
   Comments:

4. Others understand most of what your child says? YES No
   Comments: Has a high-pitched voice.

9. Concerns about behavior? Yes No
   Comments: Teacher is worried.

5. Walks, runs, and climbs like other children? Yes NO
   Comments:

10. Other concerns? Yes No
    Comments:

3. **ASQ SCORE INTERPRETATION AND RECOMMENDATION FOR FOLLOW-UP:** You must consider total area scores, overall responses, and other considerations, such as opportunities to practice skills, to determine appropriate follow-up.

If the child's total score is in the ☐ area, it is above the cutoff, and the child's development appears to be on schedule.
If the child's total score is in the ▨ area, it is close to the cutoff. Provide learning activities and monitor.
If the child's total score is in the ■ area, it is below the cutoff. Further assessment with a professional may be needed.

4. **FOLLOW-UP ACTION TAKEN:** Check all that apply.

___ Provide activities and rescreen in ___ months.

___ Share results with primary health care provider.

___ Refer for (circle all that apply) hearing, vision, and/or behavioral screening.

___ Refer to primary health care provider or other community agency (specify reason):

X Refer to early intervention/early childhood special education.

___ No further action taken at this time

___ Other (specify):

5. **OPTIONAL:** Transfer item responses (Y = YES, S = SOMETIMES, N = NOT YET, X = response missing).

	1	2	3	4	5	6
Communication	Y	S	S	Y	N	N
Gross Motor	Y	S	Y	Y	Y	Y
Fine Motor	Y	Y	Y	Y	Y	N
Problem Solving	Y	Y	Y	Y	Y	S
Personal-Social	Y	Y	Y	Y	S	Y

P101480800

Figure 10.1.   48 month ASQ-3 Information Summary Sheet for Nicholas.

Figure 10.2 (4 Month ASQ-3 Information Summary)

4 Month ASQ-3 Information Summary

3 months 0 days through 4 months 30 days

Baby's name: Shanda   Date ASQ completed: 9-1-08

Baby's ID #: 06149   Date of birth: 2-16-09

Administering program/provider: Morgan County Child Find

Was age adjusted for prematurity when selecting questionnaire? ○ Yes ⊗ No

1. **SCORE AND TRANSFER TOTALS TO CHART BELOW:** See ASQ-3 User's Guide for details, including how to adjust scores if item responses are missing. Score each item (YES = 10, SOMETIMES = 5, NOT YET = 0). Add item scores, and record each area total. In the chart below, transfer the total scores, and fill in the circles corresponding with the total scores.

Area	Cutoff	Total Score	0	5	10	15	20	25	30	35	40	45	50	55	60
Communication	34.60	40									⊗				
Gross Motor	38.41	45										⊗			
Fine Motor	29.62	15				⊗									
Problem Solving	34.98	40									⊗				
Personal-Social	33.16	40									⊗				

2. **TRANSFER OVERALL RESPONSES:** Bolded uppercase responses require follow-up. See ASQ-3 User's Guide, Chapter 6.

1. Uses both hands and both legs equally well? Yes NO
   Comments: Only uses her right arm and only rolls to her right side

5. Concerns about vision? YES No
   Comments: She stares a lot.

2. Feet are flat on the surface most of the time? Yes NO
   Comments:

6. Any medical problems? YES No
   Comments:

3. Concerns about not making sounds? YES No
   Comments: She doesn't vocalize much.

7. Concerns about behavior? YES No
   Comments:

4. Family history of hearing impairment? YES No
   Comments:

8. Other concerns? YES No
   Comments: Her arms are stiff and her movements are jerky.

3. **ASQ SCORE INTERPRETATION AND RECOMMENDATION FOR FOLLOW-UP:** You must consider total area scores, overall responses, and other considerations, such as opportunities to practice skills, to determine appropriate follow-up.

If the baby's total score is in the ☐ area, it is above the cutoff, and the baby's development appears to be on schedule.
If the baby's total score is in the ▨ area, it is close to the cutoff. Provide learning activities and monitor.
If the baby's total score is in the ■ area, it is below the cutoff. Further assessment with a professional may be needed.

4. **FOLLOW-UP ACTION TAKEN:** Check all that apply.

___ Provide activities and rescreen in ___ months.

___ Share results with primary health care provider.

___ Refer for (circle all that apply) hearing, vision, and/or behavioral screening.

X Refer to primary health care provider or other community agency (specify reason): WIC, pediatrician, Head Start.

X Refer to early intervention/early childhood special education.

___ No further action taken at this time

___ Other (specify):

5. **OPTIONAL:** Transfer item responses (Y = YES, S = SOMETIMES, N = NOT YET, X = response missing).

	1	2	3	4	5	6
Communication	Y	Y	Y	Y	S	N
Gross Motor	Y	Y	Y	Y	S	S
Fine Motor	Y	S	N	N	N	N
Problem Solving	Y	Y	Y	N	N	N
Personal-Social	Y	Y	S	Y	Y	N

P101040600

Figure 10.2.   4 month ASQ-3 Information Summary Sheet for Shanda.

Follow-Up

The Child Find staff person responded to Shanda's mother with two suggestions. First, she gave Shanda's mother the telephone number for the local early intervention program so she could make an appointment for a comprehensive assessment. Second, she suggested contacting Shanda's pediatrician to address the concerns noted in the Overall section of the questionnaire. Shanda's mother reported back that Shanda had been assessed and found eligible for services through her local center. Shanda's pediatrician ordered a battery of tests indicating that Shanda showed a "soft neurological delay" and concurred that she should be receiving early intervention services.

GUSTAVO

Home-Based Education/Home Visiting

Gustavo is a 2-year-old boy who lives with his mother and father, two sisters ages 5 and 9, and his grandmother. Gustavo likes to play with Legos and enjoys putting puzzles together. His parents report that he is very shy and often prefers to play alone in his room. Gustavo's family is enrolled in the home visiting program, Parents Ahead Now (PAN). This home visiting program provides support and information to parents and children through the Family Resource Center at Gustavo's sister's grade school. Gustavo and his family have participated in PAN for approximately 6 months. During each visit, the PAN home visitor, Gustavo's grandmother, and mother (when at home) discuss any concerns related to Gustavo's behavior. In addition, the home visitor shares toys, games, and suggested activities with the family, focused on the family's concerns and Gustavo's developmental needs.

In the PAN program the ASQ-3 is completed with the family during the home visit. The 18 and 24 month ASQ-3 were completed with Gustavo's grandmother, with the assistance of the PAN home visitor. The home visitor uses screening as a strategy to promote parent–child relationships and parent–home visitor collaboration.

Setting/Time Factors

Gustavo stays at home with his grandmother during the day while his mother and father go to work. Gustavo's grandmother does not drive and is unable to take him out during the day. Gustavo cries whenever his family goes out into the community, the doctor's office, church, or family parties. Gustavo only likes to be touched by his mother and grandmother. Gustavo often hides and clings to his mother when familiar and unfamiliar people come into his house.

Developmental Factors

Because Gustavo has been in the PAN program for 6 months, his home visitor and grandmother had previously completed the 18 month ASQ-3, and Gustavo's scores indicated that his development was on schedule; however, on the 24 month ASQ-3, he scored below the cutoff scores in the Communication, Fine Motor, and Personal-Social areas (see Figure 10.3). His grandmother reports that he doesn't want to talk and sometimes uses sign language to communicate. He also uses gestures and points. Although Gustavo's tendency to withdraw socially has been observed by his grandmother and parents, they have not wanted to pursue any interventions beyond those suggested by the PAN home visitor.

Health Factors

Gustavo's grandmother and parents have no current concerns about his health. His hearing was screened at birth and found to be normal. His parents report no concerns about his vision. Gustavo has seen a pediatrician for well-child visits, and no concerns have been indicated by his pediatrician.

Family/Cultural Factors

Gustavo's father is deaf and uses sign language to communicate. Gustavo's mother, grandmother, and sisters speak Spanish in the home. Gustavo's sisters often speak English to each other as well.

Follow-Up

The PAN home visitor, together with Gustavo's grandmother and parents, decided to pursue a referral to the local early intervention agency. Based on Gustavo's increasing wariness about other people and reluctance to speak, an assessment of his language and social skills was recommended by the PAN home visitor. The home visitor and parents also felt Gustavo might benefit from more opportunities to interact with peers. After the assessment was complete, Gustavo's early intervention team (service coordinator, evaluator, home visitor, and parents) met and determined that he did qualify for services through the early intervention program, based on communication and social delays. The team decided that home visits from an early intervention specialist together with the PAN home visitor would assist Gustavo and his family in addressing these delays. In addition, the early intervention specialist located a play group within walking distance from Gustavo's home where he will have more experience with peers.

ANDREA

Clinic-Based Well-Child Visit

Andrea is a 12-month-old girl who lives with her parents and 5-year-old brother. She currently stays at home during the day with her mother and occasionally goes along on errands. She enjoys eating and likes to sit at the dinner table with her family. During Andrea's 12 month well-child visit to the Child Health Medical Group, she was screened with the ASQ-3, which was distributed by her pediatrician, Dr. Jones. Her results on the ASQ-3 were above the cutoff scores, except in the Gross Motor area (see Figure 10.4). On the Overall section of the questionnaire, Andrea's mother indicated that Andrea will not bear weight or keep any pressure on her legs and that when she puts Andrea in a sitting position, Andrea falls over on her face without using her hands for protection. In addition, Andrea's mother notes that she is concerned because Andrea is not crawling. After Dr. Jones's nurse scored the questionnaire, the nurse gave it to Dr. Jones to review before the appointment.

Doctors at the Child Health Medical Group have a pediatric practice that emphasizes developing a relationship with parents and children over time and addressing the whole child—physical health, nutrition, development, and behavior. Developmental surveillance is conducted during all well-child visits. To formalize the process, a developmental screening tool is used at well-child visits. Parents fill out the ASQ-3 in the waiting room, and it is scored by office assistants. The pediatrician then discusses the results with parents. By starting the screening process early, parents are more knowledgeable

12 Month ASQ-3 Information Summary
11 months 0 days through 12 months 30 days

Baby's name: Andrea
Baby's ID #: 090427
Administering program/provider: Child Health Medical Group
Date ASQ completed: 3-1-09
Date of birth: 3-1-08
Was age adjusted for prematurity when selecting questionnaire?   ○ Yes   ⊗ No

1. SCORE AND TRANSFER TOTALS TO CHART BELOW: See ASQ-3 User's Guide for details, including how to adjust scores if item responses are missing. Score each item (YES = 10, SOMETIMES = 5, NOT YET = 0). Add item scores, and record each area total. In the chart below, transfer the total scores, and fill in the circles corresponding with the total scores.

Area	Cutoff	Total Score	0	5	10	15	20	25	30	35	40	45	50	55	60
Communication	15.64	55												⊗	
Gross Motor	21.49	10			⊗										○
Fine Motor	34.50	60													⊗
Problem Solving	27.32	55												⊗	
Personal-Social	21.73	60													⊗

2. TRANSFER OVERALL RESPONSES: Bolded uppercase responses require follow-up. See ASQ-3 User's Guide, Chapter 6.

1. Uses both hands and both legs equally well? Yes **NO** — Comments:
2. Plays with sounds or seems to make words? Yes **NO** — Comments:
3. Feet are flat on the surface most of the time? **YES** No — Comments: *She won't put any weight on her feet.*
4. Concerns about not making sounds? **YES** No — Comments:
5. Family history of hearing impairment? **YES** No — Comments:
6. Concerns about vision? Yes **NO** — Comments: *Her eyes cross when tired.*
7. Any medical problems? Yes **NO** — Comments: *She is small for her age.*
8. Concerns about behavior? Yes **NO** — Comments:
9. Other concerns? Yes **NO** — Comments: *When I put her in a sitting position, she falls over on her face.*

3. ASQ SCORE INTERPRETATION AND RECOMMENDATION FOR FOLLOW-UP: You must consider total area scores, overall responses, and other considerations, such as opportunities to practice skills, to determine appropriate follow-up.

If the baby's total score is in the ☐ area, it is above the cutoff, and the baby's development appears to be on schedule.
If the baby's total score is in the ▨ area, it is close to the cutoff. Provide learning activities and monitor.
If the baby's total score is in the ■ area, it is below the cutoff. Further assessment with a professional may be needed.

4. FOLLOW-UP ACTION TAKEN: Check all that apply.
___ Provide activities and rescreen in ___ months.
___ Share results with primary health care provider.
___ Refer for (circle all that apply) hearing, vision, and/or behavioral screening.
_X_ Refer to primary health care provider or other community agency (specify reason): *developmental pediatrician (for further testing)*
_X_ Refer to early intervention/early childhood special education.
___ No further action taken at this time
___ Other (specify):

5. OPTIONAL: Transfer item responses (Y = YES, S = SOMETIMES, N = NOT YET, X = response missing).

	1	2	3	4	5	6
Communication	Y	Y	Y	Y	N	S
Gross Motor	S	S	N	N	N	N
Fine Motor	Y	S	Y	Y	Y	Y
Problem Solving	Y	S	Y	Y	Y	Y
Personal-Social	Y	Y	Y	Y	Y	Y

P101120700

Figure 10.4. 12 month ASQ-3 Information Summary Sheet for Andrea.

---

24 Month ASQ-3 Information Summary
23 months 0 days through 25 months 15 days

Child's name: Gustavo
Child's ID #: 000419
Administering program/provider: Parents Ahead Now
Date ASQ completed: 2-10-09
Date of birth: 9-15-06

1. SCORE AND TRANSFER TOTALS TO CHART BELOW: See ASQ-3 User's Guide for details, including how to adjust scores if item responses are missing. Score each item (YES = 10, SOMETIMES = 5, NOT YET = 0). Add item scores, and record each area total. In the chart below, transfer the total scores, and fill in the circles corresponding with the total scores.

Area	Cutoff	Total Score	0	5	10	15	20	25	30	35	40	45	50	55	60
Communication	25.17	15				⊗									
Gross Motor	38.07	60													⊗
Fine Motor	35.16	20						⊗							
Problem Solving	29.78	45										⊗			
Personal-Social	31.54	10			⊗										

2. TRANSFER OVERALL RESPONSES: Bolded uppercase responses require follow-up. See ASQ-3 User's Guide, Chapter 6.

1. Hears well? Yes **NO** — Comments: *Screened at birth—normal range.*
2. Talks like other toddlers his age? Yes **NO** — Comments: *Doesn't talk. Sometimes uses sign language.*
3. Understand most of what your child says? Yes **NO** — Comments: *Uses gestures and points.*
4. Walks, runs, and climbs like other toddlers? **YES** No — Comments: *Cries and clings to parent.*
5. Family history of hearing impairment? **YES** No — Comments: *Father is deaf. He uses sign language.*
6. Concerns about vision? Yes **NO** — Comments:
7. Any medical problems? Yes **NO** — Comments:
8. Concerns about behavior? Yes **NO** — Comments:
9. Other concerns? Yes **NO** — Comments:

3. ASQ SCORE INTERPRETATION AND RECOMMENDATION FOR FOLLOW-UP: You must consider total area scores, overall responses, and other considerations, such as opportunities to practice skills, to determine appropriate follow-up.

If the child's total score is in the ☐ area, it is above the cutoff, and the child's development appears to be on schedule.
If the child's total score is in the ▨ area, it is close to the cutoff. Provide learning activities and monitor.
If the child's total score is in the ■ area, it is below the cutoff. Further assessment with a professional may be needed.

4. FOLLOW-UP ACTION TAKEN: Check all that apply.
___ Provide activities and rescreen in ___ months.
___ Share results with primary health care provider.
___ Refer for (circle all that apply) hearing, vision, and/or behavioral screening.
___ Refer to primary health care provider or other community agency (specify reason):
_X_ Refer to early intervention/early childhood special education.
___ No further action taken at this time
___ Other (specify):

5. OPTIONAL: Transfer item responses (Y = YES, S = SOMETIMES, N = NOT YET, X = response missing).

	1	2	3	4	5	6
Communication	Y	S	N	N	N	N
Gross Motor	Y	Y	Y	Y	Y	Y
Fine Motor	Y	Y	N	Y	Y	Y
Problem Solving	Y	Y	Y	Y	S	N
Personal-Social	Y	N	N	N	N	N

P101240800

Figure 10.3. 24 month ASQ-3 Information Summary Sheet for Gustavo.

about child development and more prepared to discuss concerns that arise as children grow older.

Setting/Time Factors

Most of Andrea's time is spent at home. Occasionally, friends bring their young children over to play. Andrea's mother feels that Andrea is bullied by these children because she cannot walk yet.

Developmental Factors

Andrea is a new patient at the Child Health Medical Group, and her mother is looking forward to completing the next questionnaire. Andrea's mother had concerns about Andrea's gross motor skills but was hoping that Andrea would eventually catch up.

Health Factors

Andrea was born at full term. Her mother has diabetes, and her pregnancy was closely monitored. Andrea's mother has indicated concern for her child's small size. She currently weighs only 14 pounds; however, she eats well, according to her mother. In addition, Andrea's eyes frequently cross when she is tired, and her mother indicates that she may need surgery later to correct this condition.

Family/Cultural Factors

Andrea's parents recently moved and have yet to develop a neighborhood support system. They are getting involved in their young son's school activities and have met a few parents with children of similar ages to their own. Andrea's father recently enrolled in college, and the family's income has been severely affected.

Follow-Up

During the well-child visit, Dr. Jones reviewed Andrea's ASQ-3 results with her mother. Together they decided that a referral to the local early intervention program was needed as well as further testing by a developmental pediatrician to rule out any metabolic disorder because of Andrea's delayed muscle development. Andrea was assessed by the local early intervention program and was found eligible for services.

KAIDEN

Center-Based Education

Kaiden is a 16-month-old toddler who lives with his mother and two sisters, ages 12 and 7. Kaiden is enrolled at Springfield Learning Center full time, where he likes to play chase and push himself on the riding toys.

Comprehensive screening is a regular component of the Springfield Learning Center, which serves children from birth to 5 years of age. At the parent orientation meeting, staff introduced the concept of screening and explained that developmental surveillance is a service provided to all families. Program coordinators work closely with teachers at the center to administer a developmental screening to all infants, toddlers, and preschoolers. Information from the assessment is used to facilitate an ongoing dialogue between the parents and teacher about the individual child. All children receive an initial general developmental screening assessment within 30 days of enrollment. If the results indicate a concern, then a conference is held with the child's parents, the teacher, the program coordinator, and a member of the center's social services staff. Dur-

16 Month ASQ-3 Information Summary 15 months 0 days through 16 months 30 days

Child's name: _Kaiden_   Date ASQ completed: _2-5-09_

Child's ID #: _03758_   Date of birth: _9-27-07_

Administering program/provider: _Springfield Learning Center_   Was age adjusted for prematurity when selecting questionnaire? ⊗ Yes ○ No

1. **SCORE AND TRANSFER TOTALS TO CHART BELOW:** See ASQ-3 User's Guide for details, including how to adjust scores if item responses are missing. Score each item (YES = 10, SOMETIMES = 5, NOT YET = 0). Add item scores, and record each area total. In the chart below, transfer the total scores, and fill in the circles corresponding with the total scores.

Area	Cutoff	Total Score	0	5	10	15	20	25	30	35	40	45	50	55	60
Communication	16.81	15													
Gross Motor	37.91	55													
Fine Motor	31.98	25													
Problem Solving	30.51	10													
Personal-Social	26.43	35													

2. **TRANSFER OVERALL RESPONSES:** Bolded uppercase responses require follow-up. See ASQ-3 User's Guide, Chapter 6.

1. Hears well?   Yes (NO)   6. Concerns about vision?   **YES** (No)
   Comments: _Lots of ear infections._   Comments:

2. Talks like other toddlers his age? Yes (NO)   7. Any medical problems?   (YES) No
   Comments: Comments: _Asthma._

3. Understand most of what your child says? Yes (NO) 8. Concerns about behavior? **YES** (No)
   Comments: Comments:

4. Walks, runs, and climbs like other toddlers? (Yes) No 9. Other concerns? **YES** (No)
   Comments: Comments:

5. Family history of hearing impairment? **YES** (No)
   Comments:

3. **ASQ SCORE INTERPRETATION AND RECOMMENDATION FOR FOLLOW-UP:** You must consider total area scores, overall responses, and other considerations, such as opportunities to practice skills, to determine appropriate follow-up.

   If the child's total score is in the ☐ area, it is above the cutoff, and the child's development appears to be on schedule.
   If the child's total score is in the ▨ area, it is close to the cutoff. Provide learning activities and monitor.
   If the child's total score is in the ■ area, it is below the cutoff. Further assessment with a professional may be needed.

4. **FOLLOW-UP ACTION TAKEN:** Check all that apply.

   ____ Provide activities and rescreen in ____ months.

   ____ Share results with primary health care provider.

   _X_ Refer for (circle all that apply) (hearing) vision, and/or behavioral screening.

   _X_ Refer to primary health care provider or other community agency (specify reason): _counseling_

   _X_ Refer to early intervention/early childhood special education.

   ____ No further action taken at this time

   ____ Other (specify): ____

5. **OPTIONAL:** Transfer item responses (Y = YES, S = SOMETIMES, N = NOT YET, X = response missing).

	1	2	3	4	5	6
Communication	Y	S	N	N	N	N
Gross Motor	Y	Y	Y	Y	Y	S
Fine Motor	Y	Y	S	N	N	S
Problem Solving	S	S	N	N	N	N
Personal-Social	Y	Y	Y	S	N	N

P1011160700

Figure 10.5. 16 month ASQ-3 Information Summary Sheet for Kaiden.

ing the conference, the staff and parents discuss the screening results and teacher and parent observations.

Kaiden was recently given the 16 month ASQ-3. His mother completed the questionnaire together with the Springfield Learning Center staff. The staff had previously observed Kaiden in the classroom and made notes before meeting with Kaiden's mother. Based on ASQ-3 results, Kaiden scored below the cutoff in the Communication, Fine Motor, and Problem Solving areas (see Figure 10.5). His score in the Personal-Social area was in the monitoring zone. When the staff and his mother discussed the ASQ-3 results, they had different scores related to his fine motor skills. Staff at the school had seen Kaiden use a marker to scribble, whereas his mother had not had the opportunity to try this with him.

Setting/Time Factors

Kaiden is in child care at Springfield Learning Center up to 40 hours a week. The family spends time together in the evenings and on the weekends. Kaiden sees his father for supervised visits once a week. His mother notices a shift in his mood after a visit with his father, who is seeking treatment for drug and alcohol addiction and anger management issues.

Health Factors

Kaiden has had numerous ear infections and has chronic fluid in his ears. His mother is worried that he cannot hear properly and that he only responds to her when she is in his line of sight. Kaiden was born 5 weeks prematurely. His mother reported that she had a very stressful pregnancy because of thyroid problems. Kaiden also has asthma and uses daily medication to control it.

Family/Cultural Factors

The family has recently separated because of ongoing domestic violence. Kaiden was bruised in an attack by his father, as were his mother and sisters, which precipitated the separation. Kaiden's mother had to seek employment to support her children. She was able to receive financial support for child care through the local Jobs to Work program.

Follow-Up

Kaiden's teacher from the Springfield Learning Center and his mother agreed that a referral to early intervention for an assessment was appropriate. His mother was also referred to a local counselor who specializes in trauma care for domestic abuse survivors. Kaiden, his mother, and his sisters will participate in these services. In addition, developmental support from the early intervention program, as well as further testing by an audiologist, will help the family address concerns about Kaiden's developmental needs.

References

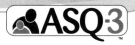

American Academy of Pediatrics. (2006). Identifying infants and young children with developmental disorders in the medical home: An algorithm for developmental surveillance and screening. *Pediatrics, 118*(1), 405–420. Available online at http://aappolicy.aappublications.org/cgi/content/full/pediatrics; 118/1/405

American Academy of Pediatrics Committee on Psychosocial Aspects of Child and Family Health. (2001). The new morbidity revisited: A renewed commitment to the psychosocial aspects of pediatric care. *Pediatrics, 108,* 1227–1230. Available online at http://aappolicy.aappublications.org/cgi/content/abstract/pediatrics;108/5/1227

Batshaw, M.L., Pellegrino, L., & Roizen, N.J. (Eds.). (2007). *Children with disabilities* (6th ed.). Baltimore: Paul H. Brookes Publishing Co.

Bayley, N. (1969). *Bayley Scales of Infant Development.* San Antonio, TX: Pearson Assessment.

Bayley, N. (1993). *Bayley Scales of Infant Development—Second Edition manual.* San Antonio, TX: Pearson Assessment.

Bayley, N. (2006). *Bayley Scales of Infant Development—Third Edition (BSID-II).* San Antonio, TX: Pearson Assessment.

Beaton, D., Bombardier, C., Guillemin, F., & Ferraz, M. (2000). Guidelines for the process of cross-cultural adaptation of self-report measure. *SPINE, 25,* 3186–3191.

Benn, R. (1993). Conceptualizing eligibility for services. In D. Bryant & M. Graham (Eds.), *Implementing early intervention* (pp. 18–45). New York: Guilford Press.

Bodnarchuk, J., & Eaton, W. (2004). Can parent reports be trusted? Validity of daily checklists of gross motor milestone attainment. *Journal of Applied Developmental Psychology, 25,* 481–490.

Bricker, D. (Ed.). (2002). *Assessment, evaluation, and programming system for infants and children (AEPS®): Vols. 1–4* (2nd ed.). Baltimore: Paul H. Brookes Publishing Co.

Bricker, D. (2004). Mental health screening in young children. *Infants and Young Children, 17*(2), 129–144.

Bricker, D., & Squires, J. (1989). Low cost system using parents to monitor the development of at risk infants. *Journal of Early Intervention, 13,* 50–60.

Bricker, D., Squires, J., Kaminski, R., & Mounts, L. (1988). The validity, reliability, and cost of a parent-completed questionnaire system to evaluate at-risk infants. *Journal of Pediatric Psychology, 13*(1), 56–68.

Casey, P., Whiteside-Mansell, L., Barrett, K., Bradley, R.H., & Gargus, R. (2006). Impact of prenatal and/or postnatal growth problems in low birth weight preterm infants on school-age outcomes: An 8-year longitudinal evaluation. *Pediatrics, 118*(3), 1078–1086.

Centers for Disease Control and Prevention. (2007, February 9). Evaluation of a methodology for collaborative multiple source surveillance network for autism spectrum disorders—Autism and Developmental Disabilities Monitoring Network, 14 sites, United States, 2002. *Morbidity and Mortality Weekly Report Surveillance Summaries, 56*(SS-1), 29–42.

Chan, B., & Taylor, N. (1998). The follow along program cost analysis in southwest Minnesota. *Infants and Young Children, 10*(4), 71–79.

Child Abuse Prevention and Treatment Act of 1974 (PL 93-247), 42 U.S.C. § 5101 *et seq.*

Dieterich, S., Landry, S., Smith, K., Swank, P., & Hebert, H. (2006). Impact of community mentors on maternal behaviors and child outcomes. *Journal of Early Intervention, 28*(2), 111–124.

Dodge, D., Colker, L., & Heroman, C. (2002). *The Creative Curriculum for preschool* (4th ed.). Washington, DC: Teaching Strategies.

Drotar, D., Stancin, T., & Dworkin, P. (2008, February 26). Pediatric developmental screening: Understanding and selecting screening instruments. Part I: Defining your practice's screening needs. Retrieved May 12, 2009, from http://www.commonwealthfund.org/General/General_show.htm?doc_id=622420

Education of the Handicapped Act Amendments of 1983, PL 98-199, 20 U.S.C. §§ 1400 *et seq.*, 97 Stat. 1357.

Education of the Handicapped Act Amendments of 1986, PL 99-457, 20 U.S.C. §§ 1400 *et seq.*

Farrell, J., & Potter, L. (Developers). (1995). *The Ages & Stages Questionnaires® on a home visit* [DVD]. Baltimore: Paul H. Brookes Publishing Co.

Fenson, L., Marchman, V.A., Thal, D.J., Dale, P.S., Reznick, J.S., & Bates, E. (2007). *The MacArthur-Bates Communicative Development Inventories (CDIs): User's guide and technical manual* (2nd ed.). Baltimore: Paul H. Brookes Publishing Co.

Frankenburg, W., K., & Bresnick, B. (1998). DENVER II Prescreening Questionnaire (PDQ II). Denver, CO: Denver Developmental Materials.

Frankenburg, W., Dodds, J., Archer, P., Bresnick, B., Maschka, P., Edelman, N., et al. (1996). *The Denver II Technical Manual.* Denver, CO: Denver Developmental Materials.

Glascoe, F. (2001). Can teachers' global ratings identify children with academic problems? *Journal of Developmental Pediatrics 22*(3), 163–168.

Glascoe, F. (2005). Screening for developmental and behavioral problems. *Mental Retardation and Developmental Disabilities Research Reviews, 11*(3), 173–179.

Glascoe, F., Foster, E., & Wolraich, M. (1997). An economic analysis of developmental detection methods. *Pediatrics 99*(6), 830–837.

Glascoe, F., & Robertshaw, N. (2007). *PEDS: Developmental Milestones professional's manual.* Nashville: Ellsworth & Vandermeer Press.

Hack, M., Taylor, H.G., Drotar, D., et al. (2005). Poor predictive validity of the Bayley scales of infant development for cognitive function of extremely low birth weight children at school age. *Pediatrics, 116,* 333–341.

Halfon, N., Regalado, M., Sareen, H., Inkelas, M., Reuland, P., Glascoe, F., et al. (2004). Assessing development in the pediatric office. *Pediatrics 113*(6), 1926–1933.

Hambleton, R., Merenda, P., & Spielberger, C. (2005). *Adapting educational and psychological tests for cross-cultural assessment.* Mahwah, NJ: Lawrence Erlbaum Associates.

Heo, K., Squires, J., & Yovanoff, P. (2008). Cross-cultural adaptation of a preschool screening instrument: Comparison of Korean and U.S. populations. *Journal of Intellectual Disability Research, 52,* 195–206.

Individuals with Disabilities Education Act Amendments (IDEA) of 1997, PL 105-17, 20 U.S.C. §§ 1400 *et seq.*

Individuals with Disabilities Education Act (IDEA) of 1990, PL 101-476, 20 U.S.C. §§ 1400 *et seq.*

Individuals with Disabilities Education Improvement Act (IDEA) of 2004, PL 108-446, 20 U.S.C. §§ 1400 *et seq.*

Jellinek, M.S., Murphy, J.M., Robinson, J., et al. (1998). Pediatric Symptom Checklist: Screening school-age children for psychosocial dysfunction. *Journal of Pediatrics, 112*(2), 201–209.

Johnson, C., Myers, S., & Council on Children with Disabilities. (2007). Management of children with autism spectrum disorder. *Pediatrics, 120,* 1162–1182.

Johnson-Martin, N.M., Attermeier, S.M., & Hacker, B. (2004). *The Carolina Curriculum for Infants and Toddlers with Special Needs* (CCITSN; 3rd ed.). Baltimore: Paul H. Brookes Publishing Co.

Keeping Children and Families Safe Act of 2003, PL 108-36, 42 U.S.C. §5101 *et seq.*

Knobloch, H., Stevens, F., & Malone, A. (1980). *Manual of developmental diagnosis: The administration and interpretation of the Revised Gesell and Amatruda Developmental and Neurological Examination.* New York: HarperCollins.

Knobloch, H., Stevens, F., Malone, A., Ellison, P., & Risemburg, H. (1979). The validity of parental reporting of infant development. *Pediatrics, 63,* 873–878.

Mardell-Czudnowski, C., & Goldenberg, D. (1998). *Developmental Indicators for the Assessment of Learning–Third Edition* (DIAL-3). Austin, TX: PRO-ED.

McCarthy, D. (1972). *McCarthy Scales of Children's Abilities.* San Antonio, TX: Pearson Assessment.

Meisels, S.J., & Atkins-Burnett, S. (2005). *Developmental screening in early childhood: A guide* (5th ed.). Washington, DC: National Association for the Education of Young Children.

Meisels, S., Marsden, D., Wiske, M., & Henderson, L. (1997). *The Early Screening Inventory–Revised* (ESI-R). Ann Arbor, MI: Rebus Inc.

Newborg, J., Stock, J., Wnek, L., Guidubaldi, J., & Svinicki, J. (1988). *Battelle Developmental Inventory.* Chicago: Riverside.

Newborg, J., Stock, J., Wnek, L., Guidubaldi, J., & Svinicki, J. (2005). *Battelle Developmental Inventory.* Chicago: Riverside.

Nickel, R.E., & Squires, J. (2000). Developmental screening and surveillance. In R.E. Nickel & L.W. Desch (Eds.), *The physician's guide to caring for children with disabilities and chronic conditions* (pp. 16–30). Baltimore: Paul H. Brookes Publishing Co.

O'Neill, L. (2007). Embodied hermeneutics: Gadamer meets Woolf in "A Room of One's Own." *Educational Theory, 57*(3), 325–337.

Sandall, S., Hemmeter, M., Smith, B., & McLean, M. (2005). *DEC recommended practices: A comprehensive guide for practical application in early intervention/early childhood special education.* Longmont, CO: Sopris West.

Shankaran, S., Johnson, Y., Langer, J., Vohr, B., Fanaroff, A., Wright, L., et al. (2004). Outcome of extremely-low-birth-weight infants at highest risk: Gestational age ≤ 24 weeks, birth weight ≤ 750 g, and 1-minute Apgar ≤ 3. *American Journal of Obstetrics and Gynecology, 191,* 1084–1091.

Squires, J., & Bricker, D. (1991). Impact of completing infant developmental questionnaires on at-risk mothers. *Journal of Early Intervention, 15*(2), 162–172.

Squires, J., & Bricker, D. (2007). *An activity-based approach to developing young children's social emotional competence.* Baltimore: Paul H. Brookes Publishing Co.

Squires, J., & Bricker, D. (with assistance from Twombly, E., Nickel, R., Clifford, J., Murphy, K., Hoselton, R., Potter, L., Mounts, L., & Farrell, J.). (2009a). *Ages & Stages Questionnaires® (ASQ-3™): A Parent-Completed Child Monitoring System* (3rd ed.). Baltimore: Paul H. Brookes Publishing Co.

Squires, J., & Bricker, D. (with assistance from Twombly, E., Nickel, R., Clifford, J., Murphy, K., Hoselton, R., Potter, L., Mounts, L., & Farrell, J.). (2009b). *Ages & Stages Questionnaires® in Spanish (ASQ-3™ Spanish): A Parent-Completed Child Monitoring System* (3rd ed.). Baltimore: Paul H. Brookes Publishing Co.

Squires, J., & Bricker, D. (2009c). *ASQ-3™ in Spanish limited upgrade.* Baltimore: Paul H. Brookes Publishing Co.

Squires, J., & Bricker, D. (2009d). *ASQ-3™ limited upgrade.* Baltimore: Paul H. Brookes Publishing Co.

Squires, J., & Bricker, D. (2009e). *ASQ-3™ quick start guide.* Baltimore: Paul H. Brookes Publishing Co.

Squires, J., & Bricker, D. (2011). *ASQ-3™ quick start guide in Spanish.* Baltimore: Paul H. Brookes Publishing Co., Inc.

Squires, J., Bricker, D., & Potter, L. (1997). Revision of a parent-completed developmental screening tool: Ages and Stages Questionnaires. *Journal of Pediatric Psychology, 22*(3), 313–328.

Squires, J., Bricker, D., & Twombly, E. (2003). *The ASQ:SE user's guide for the Ages & Stages Questionnaires®: Social-Emotional (ASQ:SE).* Baltimore: Paul H. Brookes Publishing Co.

Squires, J., Nickel, R., & Bricker, D. (1990). Use of parent-completed developmental questionnaires for Child-Find and screening. *Infants and Young Children, 3*(2), 46–57.

Squires, J., Nickel, R., & Eisert, D. (1996). Early detection of developmental problems: Strategies for monitoring young children in the practice setting. *Journal of Developmental and Behavioral Pediatrics, 17*(6), 410–427.

Squires, J., Twombly, E., & Munkres, A. (2004). *ASQ:SE in practice* [DVD]. Baltimore: Paul H. Brookes Publishing Co.

Thorndike, R., Hagen, E., & Sattler, J. (1985). *Stanford-Binet Intelligence Scale* (4th ed.). Chicago: Riverside.

Twombly, E., & Fink, G. (2013a). *ASQ-3™ Learning Activities*. Baltimore: Paul H. Brookes Publishing Co.

Twombly, E., & Fink, G. (2013b). *ASQ-3™ Learning Actividades de Aprendizaje* [ASQ-3™ Learning Activities]. Baltimore: Paul H. Brookes Publishing Co.

Twombly, E., Squires, J., & Munkres, A. (2009). *ASQ-3 scoring & referral* [DVD]. Baltimore: Paul H. Brookes Publishing Co.

Weikart, D.P., & Schweinhart, L.J. (2000). The High/Scope Curriculum for early childhood care and education. In J.L. Roopnarine & J.E. Johnson (Eds.), *Approaches to early childhood education*. Upper Saddle River, NJ: Prentice Hall.

A

Suggested Readings

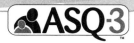

American Academy of Pediatrics. (2006). Identifying infants and young children with developmental disorders in the medical home: An algorithm for developmental surveillance and screening. *Pediatrics, 118*(1), 405–420.

Baggett, K., Warlen, L., Hamilton, J., Roberts, J., & Staker, M. (2007). Screening infant mental health indicators: An Early Head Start initiative. *Infants & Young Children, 20*(4), 300–310.

Bennett, F., Nickel, R., Squires, J., & Woodward, B. (1997). Developmental screening/surveillance. In H. Wallace, R. Biehl, R. MacQueen, & J. Blackman (Eds.), *Children with disabilities and chronic illnesses* (pp. 236–247). St. Louis: Mosby.

Bernbaum, J.C., & Batshaw, M.L. (1997). Born too soon, born too small. In M.L. Batshaw (Ed.), *Children with disabilities* (4th ed., pp. 115–139). Baltimore: Paul H. Brookes Publishing Co.

Blackman, J. (1986). *Warning signals: Basic criteria for tracking at-risk infants and toddlers.* Washington, DC: National Center for Clinical Infant Programs.

Boyce, A. (2005). Review of the Ages and Stages Questionnaires. In B.S. Plake & J.C. Impara (Eds.), *The sixteenth mental measurements yearbook* (pp. 31–36). Lincoln, NE: Buros Institute of Mental Measurements.

Bricker, D., & Littman, D. (1985). Parental monitoring of infant development. In R. McMahon & R. Peters (Eds.), *Childhood disorders: Behavioral-developmental approaches* (pp. 90–115). Levittown, PA: Brunner/Routledge.

Bricker, D., Shoen Davis, M., & Squires, J. (2004). Mental health screening in young children. *Infants & Young Children, 17*(2), 129–144.

Bricker, D., & Squires, J. (1989a). Low cost system using parents to monitor the development of at-risk infants. *Journal of Early Intervention, 13*(1), 50–60.

Bricker, D., & Squires, J. (1989b). The effectiveness of parent screening of at-risk infants: The infant monitoring questionnaires. *Topics in Early Childhood Special Education, 9*(3), 67–85.

Bricker, D., Squires, J., Kaminski, R., & Mounts, L. (1988). The validity, reliability, and cost of a parent-completed questionnaire system to evaluate at-risk infants. *Journal of Pediatric Psychology, 13*(1), 56–68.

Chan, B., & Taylor, N. (1998). The follow along program cost analysis in southwest Minnesota. *Infants & Young Children, 10*(4), 71–79.

Committee on Children with Disabilities. (2006, July). Developmental surveillance and screening of infants and young children. *Pediatrics, 108*(1), 192–196.

Diamond, K., & Squires, J. (1993). The role of parental report in the screening and assessment of young children. *Journal of Early Intervention, 17*(2), 107–115.

Dionne, C., Squires, J., & Leclerc, D. (2004, June). Psychometric properties of a developmental screening test: Using the Ages and Stages Questionnaires (ASQ) in Quebec and the US. *Journal of Intellectual Disability Research, 48*(4–5), 408.

Dobrez, D., Sasso, A.L., Holl, J., Shalowitz, M., Leon, S., & Budetti, P. (2001). Estimating the cost of developmental and behavioral screening of preschool children in general pediatric practice. *Pediatrics, 108*(4), 913–922.

Drotar, D., Stancin, T., & Dworkin, P. (2008). *Pediatric developmental screening: Understanding and selecting screening instruments.* New York: The Commonwealth Fund.

Duley, L. (2007). The Magpie Trial: A randomized trial comparing magnesium sulphate with a placebo for pre-eclampsia. Outcome for women at 2 years. *BJOG: An International Journal of Obstetrics and Gynaecology, 114,* 300–309.

Dworkin, P., & Glascoe, F. (1997). Early detection of developmental delays: How do you measure up? *Contemporary Pediatrics, 14*(4), 158–168.

Earls, M., & Hay, S. (2006). Setting the stage for success: Implementation of developmental and behavioral screening and surveillance in primary care practice—The North Carolina Assuring Better Child Health and Development (ABCD) project. *Pediatrics, 118*(1), 183–188.

Filipek, P., Accardo, P., Ashwal, S., Baranek, G.T., Cook, E.H., Jr., Dawson, G., et al. (2000). Practice parameter: Screening and diagnosis of autism. A report of the quality standards subcommittee of American Academy of Neurology and the Child Neurology Society. *Neurology, 55*(4), 468–479.

Frisk, V., Lee, E., Green, P., & Whyte, H. (2004). Deciding on a screening test for medically-at-risk children: An evidence-based approach. *IMPrint: Newsletter of the Infant Mental Health Promotion Project, 40,* 16.

Gilkerson, L., & Kopel, C. (2005). Relationship-based systems change: Illinois model for promoting social-emotional development in Part C early intervention. *Infants & Young Children, 18*(4), 349–365.

Glascoe, F.P. (2000). Evidence-based approach to developmental and behavioral surveillance using parents' concerns. *Child: Care, Health & Development, 26*(2), 137–149.

Glascoe, F., Martin, E., & Humphrey, S. (1990). Consumer reports: A comparative review of developmental screening tests. *Pediatrics, 86*(4), 547–553.

Handal, A., Lozoff, B., Breilh, J., & Harlow, S. (2007). Effects of community residence on neurobehavioral development in infants and young children in a flower-growing region of Ecuador. *Environmental Health Perspectives, 115*(1), 128–133.

Hix-Small, H., Marks, K., Squires, J., & Nickel, R. (2007). Implementing developmental screening at 12 and 24 months in a primary care pediatric office. *Pediatrics, 120*(2), 1–9.

Huberman, H. Medical and Health Research Association of New York City, Inc. (2001). *Final report. Maternal and Child Health Bureau. A randomized clinical control trial examining the feasibility of three different approaches to periodic screening of at-risk children.* Available from the author.

Janson, H. (2003). Influences on participation rate in a national Norwegian child development screening questionnaire study. *Acta Paediatrica, 92*(1), 91–96.

Janson, H., & Squires, J. (2004). Parent-completed developmental screening in a Norwegian population sample: A comparison with U.S. normative data. *Acta Paediatrica, 93*(11), 1525–1529.

Klamer, A., Lando, A., Pinborg, A., & Greisen, G. (2005, May). Ages and Stages Questionnaire used to measure cognitive deficit in children born extremely preterm. *Acta Paediatrica, 94*(9), 1327–1329.

Knobloch, H., Stevens, F., Malone, A.F., Ellison, P., & Risemburg, H. (1979). The validity of parental reporting of infant development. *Pediatrics, 63*(6), 872–878.

Kochanek, T. (1993). Enhancing screening procedures for infants and toddlers: The application of knowledge to public policy and program initiatives. In D. Bryant & M. Graham (Eds.), *Implementing early intervention: From research to effective practice* (pp. 46–66). New York: Guilford Press.

Kovanen, P., Maatta, P., Leskinen, M., & Heinonen, K. (2000, June/August). Parents as developmental screeners: The applicability of the Ages and Stages Questionnaire in Finland. *Journal of Intellectual Disability Research, 44*(3–4), 353.

Lando, A., Klamer, A., Jonsbo, J., Weiss, J., & Greisen, G. (2005, May). Developmental delay at 12 months in children born extremely preterm. *Acta Paediatrica, 94*(11), 1604–1607.

Lichtenstein, R., & Ireton, H. (1984). *Preschool screening: Identifying young children with developmental and educational problems.* San Francisco: Grune & Stratton.

Lipkin, P. (2006). Moving forward in development screening. *Pediatric News, 40*(9), 34.

Liptak, G. (1996). The pediatrician's role in caring for the developmentally disabled child. *Pediatrics in Review, 17*(6), 203–210.

Lyman, D.R., Njoroge, W., & Willis, D. (2007). Early childhood psychosocial screening in culturally diverse populations: Survey of clinical experience with Ages and Stages Questionnaires, Social-Emotional. *Zero to Three, 27*(5), 46–54.

Maternal and Child Health Bureau. (n.d.). *Developmental and behavioral pediatrics* (2nd ed.). Retrieved March, 27, 2009, from http://mchb.hrsa.gov/training/projects.asp?program=6

Meisels, S., & Shonkoff, J. (Eds.). (2000). *Handbook of early childhood intervention* (2nd ed.). New York: Cambridge University Press.

Nicol, P. (2006). Using the Ages and Stages Questionnaire to teach medical students developmental assessment: A descriptive analysis. *BMC Medical Education, 6*, 29. Retrieved March 27, 2009, from http://biomedcentral.com/1472-6920/6/29

Pinto-Martin, J., Dunkle, M., Earls, M., Fliedner, D., & Landes, C. (2004). Developmental stages of developmental screening: Steps to implementation of a successful program. *American Journal of Public Health, 95*(11), 6–10.

Printz, P.H., Borg, A. & Demarree, M.A. (2003). A look at social, emotional, and behavioral screening tools for Head Start and Early Head Start. Newton, MA: Education Development Center, Center for Children & Families. (Also available online: http://ccf.edc.org/PDF/screentools.pdf) [ASQ:SE is discussed on p. 8.]

Ringwalt, S. (2008). *Developmental screening and assessment instruments with an emphasis on social and emotional development for young children ages birth through five.* Retrieved March 27, 2009, from http://www.nectac.org/~pdfs/pubs/screening.pdf

Sameroff, A., & Fiese, B. (2000). Transactional regulation: The development ecology of early intervention. In *Handbook of early childhood intervention* (2nd ed., pp. 135–159). New York: Cambridge University Press.

Skellern, C.Y., & O'Callaghan, M. (1999, October). Parent-completed questionnaires: An effective screening instrument for developmental delay in follow-up of ex-premature infants. *Journal of Paediatrics & Child Health, 35*(5), A2.

Skellern, C.Y., Rogers, Y., & O'Callaghan, M. (2001). A parent-completed developmental questionnaire: Follow up of ex-premature infants. *Journal of Paediatrics & Child Health, 37*(2), 125–129.

Squires, J. (1996). Parent-completed developmental questionnaires: A low-cost strategy for child find and screening. *Infants & Young Children, 9*(1), 16–28.

Squires, J. (2000, June/August). Early detection of development delays: Parents as first-level screeners. *Journal of Intellectual Disability Research, 44*(3–4), 471.

Squires, J., & Bricker, D. (1991). Impact of completing infant developmental questionnaires on at-risk mothers. *Journal of Early Intervention, 15*(2), 162–172.

Squires, J., Bricker, D., Heo, K., & Twombly, E. (2001). Identification of social-emotional problems in young children using a parent-complete screening measure. *Early Childhood Research Quarterly, 16*(4), 405–419

Squires, J., Bricker, D., & Potter, L. (1997). Revision of a parent-completed developmental screening tool: Ages and Stages Questionnaires. *Journal of Pediatric Psychology, 22*(3), 313–328.

Squires, J., Bricker, D., & Twombly, E. (2004). Parent-completed screening for social emotional problems in young children: Effects of risk/disability status and gender on performance. *Infant Mental Health, 25*(1), 62–73.

Squires, J.K., Carter, A., & Kaplan, P.F. (2001, September). Developmental monitoring of children conceived by ICSI and IVF. *Fertility and Sterility, 76*(3 Suppl. 1), S145–S146.

Squires, J., Carter, A., & Kaplan, P. (2003). Developmental monitoring of children conceived by intracytoplasmic sperm injection and in vitro fertilization. *Fertility and Sterility, 79*(2), 453–454.

Squires, J.K., Kaplan, P.F., & Carter, A.M. (2000, April). Developmental monitoring of ICSI/IVF offspring. *Fertility and Sterility, 73*(4 Suppl. 1), 14S.

Squires, J., Katzev, A., & Jenkins, F. (2002, June). Early screening for developmental delays: Use of parent-completed questionnaires in Oregon's Healthy Start program. *Early Child Development and Care, 172*(3), 275–282.

Squires, J., Nickel, R., & Bricker, D. (1990). Use of parent-completed developmental questionnaires for child-find and screening. *Infants & Young Children, 3*(2), 46–57.

Squires, J., Nickel, R., & Eisert, E. (1996). Early detection of developmental problems: Strategies for monitoring young children in the practice setting. *Journal of Developmental and Behavioral Pediatrics, 17*(6), 410–427.

Squires, J., Potter, L., & Bricker, D. (1999). *The ASQ user's guide for the Ages & Stages Questionnaires®: A Parent-Completed Child-Monitoring System* (2nd ed.) [Includes technical report with research data on 2nd ed. of ASQ]. Baltimore, MD: Paul H. Brookes Publishing Co.

Squires, J., Potter, L., Bricker, D., & Lamorey, S. (1998). Parent-completed developmental questionnaires: Effectiveness with low and middle income parents. *Early Childhood Research Quarterly, 13*(2), 347–356.

Sturner, R., Layton, T., Evans, A., Funk, S., & Machon, M. (1994). Preschool speech and language screening: A review of currently available tests. *Topics in Early Childhood Special Education, 12*(2), 25–36.

Tsai, H.A., McClelland, M., Pratt, C., & Squires, J. (2006). Adaptation of the 36 month Ages and Stages Questionnaire in Taiwan. *Journal of Early Intervention, 28*(3), 213–225.

Vacca, J.J. (2005). Review of the Ages and Stages Questionnaires. In R.A. Spies & B.S. Plake (Eds.), *The sixteenth mental measurements yearbook*. Lincoln, NE: Buros Institute of Mental Measurements.

Werner, E.E., & Smith, R.S. (2004). Journeys from childhood to midlife: Risk, resilience, and recovery. *Pediatrics, 114*(2), 492.

Williams, D.L., Gelijns, A.C., Moskowitz, A.J., Weinberg, A.D., Ng, J.H., Crawford, E., et al. (2000, April). Hypoplastic left heart syndrome: Valuing the survival. *Journal of Thoracic and Cardiovascular Surgery, 119*(4 Pt. 1), 720–731.

Yovanoff, P., & Squires, J. (2006). Determining cut-off scores on a developmental screening measure: Comparison of receiver operating characteristics and item response theory approaches. *Journal of Early Intervention, 29*(1), 48–62.

B

Glossary

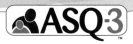

This glossary contains definitions of terminology used in this volume to discuss the screening of children.

above the cutoff An ASQ score in any developmental area that falls above the statistically derived referral cutoff point.

adjusted area score An average item score that is calculated when an item is not completed on the ASQ. An adjusted area score is computed by dividing the area's score by the number of items answered in that area.

ASQ Abbreviation for *Ages & Stages Questionnaires®*. ASQ-3™ refers specifically to *Ages & Stages Questionnaires®, Third Edition*.

ASQ:SE Abbreviation for the *Ages & Stages Questionnaires®: Social-Emotional*, a screening tool that examines social-emotional behaviors in young children.

below the cutoff An ASQ score in any developmental area that falls below the statistically derived referral cutoff point.

Child Abuse Prevention and Treatment Act (CAPTA) of 1974 (PL 93-247) A law providing federal funding to states in support of prevention, assessment, investigation, prosecution, and treatment activities and specifically directs states to provide developmental screening to all children placed in foster care.

Child Find A component of the Individuals with Disabilities Education Act (IDEA) and its amendments that requires states to identify, locate, and evaluate all children with disabilities, ages birth to 21, who are in need of early intervention or special education services.

corrected age An age correction for weeks of prematurity when the actual date of birth is 3 or more weeks earlier than the expected birth date. To calculate a corrected age, the weeks of prematurity are subtracted from the infant's chronological age.

$$\text{chronological age} - \text{number of weeks premature} = \text{corrected age}$$

For example, a child who was born 8 weeks prematurely and whose chronological age is 60 weeks will be given a corrected age of 52 weeks. The authors recommend that the corrected age be used until the infant reaches 24 months of age.

corrected date of birth (CDOB)   A chronological date correction for weeks of prematurity when the actual date of birth is more than 3 weeks earlier than the expected birthdate. To calculate CDOB, add the weeks of prematurity to the child's date of birth. (The CDOB is essentially the same as the child's original due date.)

curriculum based assessment (CBA)   Measurement that uses direct observation and recording of a student's performance as a basis for gathering information to make instructional decisions and develop intervention goals.

cutoff point   Also known as *referral cutoff point.* Empirically derived score that indicates when a child's performance is suspect and referral for further assessment is appropriate.

developmental assessment   An assessment that establishes baseline, or entry level of measurement, of a child's skills across developmental areas (e.g., communication, gross motor, fine motor, problem solving, personal-social).

developmental surveillance   An important technique used by pediatricians that includes a flexible, continual process whereby knowledgeable professionals perform skilled observations of children during the provision of health care. The components of developmental surveillance include eliciting and attending to parental concerns, obtaining a relevant developmental history, making accurate and informative observations of children, and sharing opinions and concerns with other relevant professionals. Pediatricians often use age-appropriate developmental checklists to record milestones during preventive care visits as part of developmental surveillance.

EI/ECSE   Abbreviation for *early intervention/early childhood special education.*

false positive   Those who test positive but are negative (i.e., do not have the condition).

Fine Motor   Developmental domain assessed on the ASQ focusing on hand and finger movement and coordination

Gross Motor   Developmental domain assessed on the ASQ focusing on use and coordination of arm, body, and leg movements.

identified   Also known as *screened.* Descriptive of children whose score on a screening tool, such as the ASQ, falls below the cutoff score, and who are identified as needing further assessment.

Individuals with Disabilities Education Act (IDEA)   IDEA was originally enacted by the U.S. Congress as the Education for All Handicapped Children Act of 1975 (PL 94-142) to make sure that children with disabilities have the opportunity to receive a free appropriate public education. IDEA guides how states and school districts provide special education and related services to more than 6 million eligible children with disabilities. IDEA was reauthorized in 2004 as Individuals with Disabilities Education Improvement Act of 2004 (PL 108-446).

interobserver reliability   Also known as *interrater reliability.* The degree of agreement among raters. It gives a score of how much homogeneity, or consensus, there is in the ratings given by judges.

mean (*M*)   The arithmetic average of a set of values, or distribution.

monitoring   Periodic developmental screening of young children.

monitoring zone   An empirically derived range of scores that indicate that a child's development should be monitored further over time. On the ASQ-3, scores that fall within the monitoring zone are between 1.0 and 2.0 standard deviations from the mean.

multidisciplinary team   A group of people from different disciplines and professions who work together as equal stakeholders in addressing a common challenge.

Overall   Last section of the ASQ, which asks questions about a child's overall development and about any concerns that a parent may have about his or her child's development.

overidentification   Also known as *overreferral* or *overscreening*. The proportion of children incorrectly identified as in need of further assessment by the screening tool.

paraprofessional   Job title for certain people working in the education, health care, and related fields. These individuals have obtained the required knowledge and experience to enable them to perform a task requiring significant knowledge but do not have the occupational license to perform at the professional level in the field.

Part B, Section 619, IDEA   Early childhood special education program for children ages 3–21 with disabilities.

Part C, IDEA   Early intervention program for infants and toddlers with disabilities.

percent agreement   The proportion of agreement between the screening tool and standardized assessments.

percent screened   The percentage of children who are identified as needing further assessment by a screening tool.

Personal-Social   Developmental domain assessed on the ASQ focusing on children's self-help skills and interactions with others.

positive predictive value   The probability that a child identified by the screening tool as needing further assessment will have intervention needs.

Problem Solving   Developmental domain assessed on the ASQ focusing on children's play with toys and problem-solving skills.

psychometric study   Research examining the validity, reliability, and utility of an assessment instrument.

referral   The outcome when a child's score on a screening measure such as the ASQ or when parent concerns indicate that follow up to a community agency for further assessment is warranted.

reliability   Consistency of test scores over time and between testers; the extent to which it is possible to generalize from one test result conducted by one person to test results conducted at different times or by different observers.

screening   A brief procedure to determine whether a child requires further and more comprehensive assessment.

sensitivity   The proportion of children correctly identified as needing further assessment by the screening tool and who perform below the expected level on a standardized assessment or assessment battery.

specificity   The proportion of children correctly excluded as developing typically by the screening tool and who perform at the expected level on a standardized assessment.

standard deviation (*SD*)   A measure of the dispersion of a set of values or data points.

standardized test   A test that is administered and scored in a consistent manner so that the questions and conditions for administering, scoring , and interpreting results are performed in a predetermined, standard manner.

test–retest reliability   The consistency of a measure from one time to another.

tracking   Periodic and sequential developmental screening and referral of young children for intervention services.

true positive   Those who test positive for a condition and are positive (i.e., have the condition).

underidentification   Also known as *underreferral* or *underscreening*. The proportion of children incorrectly identified as developing typically by the screening tool.

universal screening   A type of assessment that is characterized by the quick, low-cost, and repeatable testing of age-appropriate skills to all children.

validity   Extent to which a test measures what its authors claim it measures; appropriateness of the inferences that can be made from test results.

C

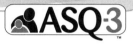

ASQ-3 Technical Report

This report offers a range of technical information about the *Ages & Stages Questionnaires®: A Parent-Completed Child Monitoring System, Third Edition (ASQ-3)*. The development of the *Ages & Stages Questionnaires (ASQ)* system, including item selection and readability, are reviewed, as are the revisions that have been made to the questionnaires. Since publishing the second edition in 1999, new data have been collected on more than 18,000 questionnaires. These data have been used to examine selected psychometric parameters of the questionnaires. In addition to describing the demographic characteristics of the samples, analyses included in this report address interobserver and test–retest reliability and measures of internal consistency. A comparison of questionnaire performance by groups of risk and nonrisk children is presented, as is the rationale for combining groups to derive the revised cutoff points for the ASQ-3. Validity analyses include descriptions of how the cutoff points were determined and of measures of concurrent validity. A final section presents a comparison between the English and Spanish versions of the questionnaires.

DEVELOPMENT OF THE ASQ

Item Selection

ASQ items were developed using a variety of sources, including standardized developmental tests, nonstandardized tests focused on early development, textbooks, and other literature containing information about early developmental milestones. Using these sources, the following criteria were used to develop items:

1. Skills were selected that easily could be observed or elicited by parents.
2. Skills were selected that were highly likely to occur in a variety of homes and child care settings.
3. Skills were selected that indexed important developmental milestones.

Once skills had been chosen, items were written using familiar, concrete words that did not exceed a sixth-grade reading level, and illustrations and examples were provided for as many items as possible.

Using this process, a large pool of potential items was created. From this pool, the six items that composed each developmental area (Communication, Gross Motor, Fine Motor, Problem Solving, and Personal-Social) for each age interval were selected. Item selection for each questionnaire interval was restricted by allowing only items that targeted a skill that occurred at the middle to low end of the developmental range for that particular chronological age interval (i.e., the developmental range of 75–100 was targeted). This range was chosen for two reasons. First, many standardized tests use 1.5–2.0 standard deviations below the mean as the lower end of the typical developmental range; therefore, it was reasoned that any child who was generally *unable* to perform items at a developmental quotient of 75–100 should be referred for further assessment. Second, it was reasoned that items above a developmental quotient of 100 would identify primarily children who were developing without problem, and, thus, the inclusion of such items would be of little help. By targeting a restricted developmental range of 75–100, it was possible to keep the questionnaires brief.

To determine the developmental quotient for each item, the following formula was used:

$$\text{(age equivalent)}/\text{(age interval of ASQ item)} \times 100 = DQ$$

The age equivalent was obtained from the source(s) of the item such as the Gesell (Knobloch, Stevens, & Malone, 1980), the Bayley Scales of Infant Development (Bayley, 1969, 2002, 2006), the Battelle Developmental Inventory (BDI; Newborg, Stock, Wnek, Guidubaldi, & Svinicki, 2004), and Developmental Resources: Behavioral Sequences for Assessment and Program Planning (Cohen & Gross, 1979). When sources varied, a developmental range was used. Table 1 contains the age equivalent and developmental quotient for each item by area for each of 20 questionnaires. As shown in Table 1, to the extent possible, each area has two items with developmental quotients of approximately 75, two items with developmental quotients of approximately 85, and two items with developmental quotients of approximately 100.

Reading Level

The ASQ was designed for use with a range of parents and other caregivers (e.g., varying income and educational levels); therefore, the reading level was kept low, and illustrations and examples were added to clarify items when possible. To ascertain the reading level of the ASQ-3 questionnaires, the Flesch Reading Ease and Flesch-Kincaid Grade Level readability measures (Microsoft Word 2007) were used. Average readability grade levels of the ASQ-3 were 4.9 for Communication, 5.6 for Gross Motor, 5.3 for Fine Motor, 5.4 for Problem Solving, 4.7 for Personal-Social, and 4.7 for the Overall section.

REVISIONS OF THE ASQ

The next section of this report reviews the revisions associated with the ASQ-3. The revisions that have occurred are discussed chronologically, beginning with the first revisions in 1991 and ending with the revisions contained in the ASQ-3 completed in 2009.

Table 1. Age equivalent and developmental quotient of items by area for each questionnaire

Questionnaire items	Communication Age	Communication DQ	Gross Motor Age	Gross Motor DQ	Fine Motor Age	Fine Motor DQ	Problem Solving Age	Problem Solving DQ	Personal-Social Age	Personal-Social DQ
2 months										
1	Newborn+	50–75	4–12 w[a]	50+	4–8 w	50–100	4–8 w	50–100	Newborn to 1 m	50–75
2	Newborn+	50–75	4 w	50+	Newborn	50+	4–8 w	50–100	Newborn	50–75
3	4–5 w[b]	50–63	4 w	50+	3–4 w	38–50	8–12 w	100–150	4 w	50
4	5–6 w	63–75	4 w	50+	4–8 w	50–100	12 w	150	5 w	63
5	8–12 w	100–125+	12 w	150	12 w	150	12 w	150	12 w	150
6	12 w	125+	12–16 w	125	12 w	125+	8–12 w	100–150	12 w	125–150
4 months										
1	12 w	75	12 w	75	12 w	75	8–12 w	75	12 w	75
2	12–16 w	75–100	12 w	75	12 w	75	12 w	75	12 w	75
3	12–16 w[b]	75–100	8–12 w	75	12 w	75	12 w	75	12 w	75
4	16 w	100	16 w	100	16 w	100	16 w	100	16 w	100
5	16 w	100	16 w	100	16 w	100	16 w	100	16 w	100
6	16 w	100	16 w	100	16 w	100	16 w	100	16 w	100
6 months										
1	16 w	62	20 w	77	20 w	77	20 w	77	20 w	77
2	20 w	77	20 w	77	20 w	77	20 w	77	20 w	77
3	24 w	92	24 w	92	24 w	92	24 w	92	24 w	92
4	24 w	92	24 w	92	24 w	92	24 w	92	24 w	92
5	28 w	107	28 w	107	28 w	107	28 w	107	28 w	107
6	28 w	107	28 w	107	28 w	107	28 w	107	28 w	107
8 months										
1	24 w	69	24 w	69	24 w	69	24 w	69	24 w	69
2	24 w	69	24 w	69	24 w	69	24 w	69	24 w	69
3	28 w	80	28 w	80	28 w	80	28 w	80	28 w	80
4	28 w	80	28 w	80	28 w	80	28 w	80	28 w	80
5	32 w	91	28–32 w	80–91	32 w	91	32 w	91	32 w	91
6	32 w	91	32 w	91	36 w	103	32 w	91	32 w	91
10 months										
1	28 w	70	28 w	70	28 w	70	28 w	70	28 w	70
2	28 w	70	28–32 w	70–80	32 w	80	32 w	80	32 w	80
3	32 w	80	32 w	80	36 w	90	32 w	80	32 w	80
4	40 w	100	40 w	100	40 w	100	40 w	100	40 w	100
5	44 w	110	40 w	100	40 w	100	40 w	100	40 w	100
6	44 w	110	44 w	110	44 w	110	44 w	110	44 w	110

(continued)

Key: DQ, developmental quotient; w, weeks; m, months.
[a]Numbers were rounded to the nearest whole numbers.
[b]Ranges are presented when the age and DQ of an item differed according to developmental sources.

Table 1. *(continued)*

Questionnaire items	Communication		Gross Motor		Fine Motor		Problem Solving		Personal-Social	
	Age	DQ	Age	DQ	Age	DQ	Age	DQ	Age	DQ
12 months										
1	32 w	67	40 w	77	40 w	77	40 w	77	40 w	77
2	40 w	77	40 w	77	40 w	77	40 w	77	40 w	77
3	44 w	85	44 w	85	44 w	85	44 w	85	44 w	85
4	44 w	85	44 w	85	48 w	92	44 w	85	44 w	85
5	48 w	92	48 w	92	48 w	92	48 w	92	48 w	92
6	52 w	100	52 w	100	52 w	100	52 w	100	52 w	100
14 months										
1	44 w	80	44 w	79	48 w	86	44 w	79	44 w	79
2	52 w	93	48 w	86	48 w	86	48 w	86	48 w	86
3	52 w	93	52 w	93	52 w	93	52 w	93	52 w	93
4	52 w	93	52–56 w	93–100	56 w	100	52 w	93	56–60 w	100–107
5	52 w	93	52 w	93	60 w	107	52 w	93	48–60 w	86–107
6	56 w	100	56 w	100	60 w	107	56 w	100	52–56 w	93–100
16 months										
1	52 w	75	52 w	75	52 w	75	52 w	75	15 m	93.75
2	52 w	75	56 w	81.25	52 w	75	52 w	75	12–15 m	75–94
3	52 w	75	52 w	75	56 w	81.25	56 w	81	52 w	75
4	56 w	81.25	56 w	81.25	15 m	93.75	56 w	81	52 w	75
5	15 m	93.75	15 m	93.75	15 m	93.75	15 m	93.75	12 m	94
6	56 w	81.25	15 m	93.75	18 m	112.5	15 m	93.75	15 m	94
18 months										
1	56 w	74	52 w	68	52 w	68	56 w	74	52 w	68
2	56 w	74	56 w	74	56 w	74	56 w	74	52 w	68
3	56 w	74	65 w	85	65 w	85	65 w	85	65 w	85
4	65 w	85	15 m	83	15 m	83	65 w	85	15 m	83
5	78 w	108	18 m	100	78 w	102	78 w	102	78 w	102
6	91 w	126	18 m	100	18 m	100	78 w	102	78 w	102
20 months										
1	15 m	75	75 w	75	15 m	75	15 m	75	15 m	75
2	15 m	75	15 m	75	15 m	75	18 m	90	15 m	75
3	18 m	90	18 m	90	18 m	90	20 m	100	18 m	90
4	18 m	90	18 m	90	18 m	90	20 m	100	18 m	90
5	21 m	105	21 m	105	21 m	105	<21 m	<105	21 m	105
6	21 m	105	21 m	105	18–24 m	90–120	24 m	120	21 m	105

22 months										
1	13 m	70	18 m	82	18 m	82	13 m	70	18 m	82
2	21 m	95	18–21 m	82–95	21 m	95	18 m	82	21 m	95
3	21 m	95	15 m	85	18–24 m	82–109	20 m	91	21 m	95
4	18–21 m	82–95	65 w	83	18 m	82	20 m	91	18–21 m	82–95
5	18–21 m	85	24 m	109	21–29 m	95–132	<21 m	<91	21 m	95
6	24 m	109	24 m	109	24 m	109	24 m	109	24 m	109
24 months										
1	18 m	75	18 m	75	18 m	75	18 m	75	18 m	75
2	18 m	75	18 m	75	18 m	75	18 m	75	18 m	75
3	21 m	87.5	21 m	87.5	18–24 m	75–100	20 m	83	21 m	87.5
4	21 m	87.5	21 m	87.5	21–29 m	87.5–121	20 m	83	21 m	87.5
5	24 m	100	24 m	100	24 m	100	24 m	100	24 m	100
6	24 m	100	24 m	100	24 m	100	24 m	100	24 m	100
27 months										
1	21 m	78	21 m	78	21 m	78	20 m	74	21 m	78
2	21 m	78	21 m	78	21–29 m	78–107	20 m	74	21 m	78
3	24 m	89	24 m	89	24 m	89	21 m	78	21 m	78
4	24 m	89	24 m	89	24 m	89	24 m	89	24 m	89
5	24 m	89	24 m	89	24 m	89	24 m	89	24 m	89
6	30 m	111	30 m	111	30 m	111	30 m	111	30 m	111
30 months										
1	21 m	70	21 m	70	21 m	70	21 m	70	21 m	70
2	21 m	70	21 m	70	24 m	80	24 m	80	24 m	80
3	24 m	80	24 m	80	24 m	80	24 m	80	24 m	80
4	24 m	80	24 m	80	30 m	100	30 m	100	30 m	100
5	30 m	100	30 m	100	30 m	100	30 m	100	30 m	100
6	30 m	100	30 m	100	30 m	100	30 m	100	30 m	100
33 months										
1	24 m	73	24 m	64	24 m	73	24 m	73	24 m	73
2	24 m	73	24 m	73	30 m	91	24 m	73	24 m	73
3	30 m	91	24 m	73	30 m	91	24 m	73	30 m	91
4	30 m	91	30 m	91	30 m	91	30 m	91	30 m	91
5	36 m	109	30 m	91	30 m	91	30 m	91	30 m	91
6	36 m	109	36 m	109	30 m	91	30 m	91	36 m	109

(continued)

Table 1. (continued)

Questionnaire items	Communication		Gross Motor		Fine Motor		Problem Solving		Personal-Social	
	Age	DQ	Age	DQ	Age	DQ	Age	DQ	Age	DQ
36 months										
1	24 m	67	24 m	67	24 m	67	24 m	67	24 m	67
2	24 m	67	24 m	67	24 m	67	24 m	67	24 m	67
3	30 m	83	30 m	83	30 m	83	30 m	83	30 m	83
4	30 m	83	30 m	83	30 m	83	30 m	83	30 m	83
5	36 m	100	36 m	100	36 m	100	36 m	100	36 m	100
6	36 m	100	36 m	100	36 m	100	36 m	100	36 m	100
42 months										
1	30 m	71	30 m	71	30 m	71	30 m	71	30 m	71
2	30 m	71	30 m	71	30 m	71	30 m	71	30 m	71
3	36 m	86	36 m	86	36 m	86	36 m	86	36 m	86
4	36 m	86	36 m	86	36 m	86	36 m	86	36 m	86
5	36–48 m	86–114	36–57 m	86–135	36–48 m	86–114	36–57 m	86–135	36–48 m	86–114
6	36–49 m	86–117	45–60 m	107–117	42 m	100	42 m	100	31–49 m	74–117
48 months										
1	40–72 m	88–150	36–57 m	75–119	36–48 m	75–100	36–48 m	75–100	36–48 m	75–100
2	54–60 m	113–125	45–60 m	94–125	36–57 m	75–108	36–57 m	75–119	48–60 m	100–125
3	30–60 m	63–125	36–48 m	75–100	48–60 m	100–125	36–53 m	75–111	36–54 m	75–113
4	48–60 m	100–125	35 m	73	48 m	100	41–53 m	85–111	48 m	100
5	36–48 m	75–100	36–48 m	75–100	48 m	100	42 m	88	42–60 m	88–125
6	36–49 m	75–102	36–72 m	75–150	48 m	100	36–44 m	75–92	31–49 m	65–102
54 months										
1	36–60 m	66–111	35 m	65	48–60 m	88–111	41–53 m	76–98	36–54 m	66–100
2	48–60 m	88–111	36–48 m	66–88	48 m	88	42 m	77	48 m	88
3	36–49 m	66–91	36–48 m	66–88	48 m	88	36–44 m	81–82	42–60 m	77–111
4	36–48 m	66–88	36–57 m	66–106	45 m	83	36–57 m	82–106	36–48 m	66–88
5	48 m	88	36–72 m	66–133	54 m	100	54 m	100	48–60 m	88–111
6	48–59 m	88–109	54–60 m	100–111	48–57 m	88–106	53–60 m	98–111	51–66 m	94–122
60 months										
1	36–48 m	60–80	36–48 m	60–80	45 m	75	36–57 m	60–75	36–48 m	60–80
2	48 m	80	36–57 m	60–95	54 m	90	41–53 m	68–88	36–54 m	60–90
3	48–59 m	80–98	36–72 m	60–120	48–57 m	80–95	54 m	90	48–60 m	80–100
4	54–60 m	90–100	54–60 m	90–100	48–60 m	80–100	60 m	100	51–66 m	85–110
5	54–60 m	90–100	60 m	100	48–60 m	80–100	53–60 m	88–100	51–66 m	85–110
6	54–60 m	90–100	60–66 m	100–110	54–66 m	90–110	60 m	100	48–62 m	80–103

First Revision

In response to validity and utility data gathered on the questionnaires (e.g., Brinker, Franzier, Lancelot, & Norman, 1989), the questionnaires were first revised in 1991. Six types of changes were made. First, a number of items were reworded to clarify meaning. These modifications were made based on feedback from project staff, interventionists, parents, nurses, and pediatricians using the questionnaires in clinic and research environments. In most cases, the modifications entailed minimal word changes. For example, "reach for a toy" was changed to "try to get a toy"; "couch or adult chair" was changed to "furniture"; and "being able to stop" was changed to "stopping." In a few cases, examples were added or modified. For example, "Does your baby play ball with you by either rolling or throwing the ball to you?" was changed to "Does your baby either roll or throw a ball back to you so that you can return it to him?" For some items, examples were changed to more available household items to facilitate completion of the questionnaires by parents. For example, "toy" and "four objects like blocks or cars" were substituted for "block" in several instances.

Second, modifications of a more extensive nature were made. In some cases, an item that was difficult to interpret was eliminated and replaced with another item. In all cases, the substituted items appeared on an ASQ at the previous or next age interval. For example, on the 20 month questionnaire, an item in the Fine Motor area was eliminated and replaced with an item from the Fine Motor area on the 24 month questionnaire.

The third change made to the questionnaires was the elimination of items with developmental quotients of 125–150. On the initial version of the questionnaires, each developmental area included one item with a developmental range of 125–150. These items were added to provide information on parents' reported tendency to overestimate their children's developmental status (cf. Gradel, Thompson, & Sheehan, 1981; Hunt & Paraskevopoulos, 1980). An analysis of parental responses to these items did not support parental overestimation of children's developmental achievements, so these items were eliminated from the questionnaires.

A fourth change was ordering the items within each developmental area according to level of difficulty. Initially, items were not arranged in developmental order on the questionnaires; however, with this revision, the items in each developmental area were arranged according to level of difficulty, beginning with the easiest items and ending with the most advanced.

A fifth modification was the addition of the 6, 18, and 48 month questionnaires. The 6 and 18 month questionnaires were constructed by taking developmentally appropriate items from the adjacent questionnaires and adding items when necessary. The 48 month questionnaire was developed by examining a variety of tests and other developmental resources and constructing test items. The same criteria for the development of the previous questionnaires were applied to items for the 48 month questionnaire.

Finally, the sixth type of revision entailed changing the name of the questionnaires from *Infant/Child Monitoring Questionnaires* to *Ages & Stages Questionnaires*. The new name was thought to be more appealing to parents and professionals.

Second Revision

A second edition of the ASQ was published in 1999. Revisions were minor, and little adjustment of the items occurred. This revision included three types of modifications: minor modification of items, format changes, and the addition of new age intervals.

The first type of revisions focused on minor wording changes and deletions to increase the clarity of items. For example, qualifying words such as *generally* or *usually* were eliminated. The second category of revisions centered on minor modification of the questionnaire format to be more user friendly.

Another type of revision involved adding eight new age intervals to the questionnaire system. From 1997 to 1998, additional intervals were completed at the 10, 14, 22, 27, 33, 42, 54, and 60 month age intervals. These intervals were added to make the ASQ series more comprehensive and to ensure that children could be screened using the ASQ at any age between 4 and 66 months.

Third Revision

The ASQ-3 was completed in 2008. For the ASQ-3, two additional questionnaire intervals were added to the ASQ series, making a total of 21 intervals across the 1- to 66-month age span. Second, the age range for administration of each questionnaire was modified so that children of any age could be continuously screened from 1 to 66 months. Administration age ranges for the ASQ-3 are listed in Table 2. Third, minor revisions were made to the existing 19 questionnaires. Fourth, additional questions were added to the Overall section to ask about behavioral concerns when applicable. Fifth, the Information Summary sheets for all intervals were revised, and a monitoring zone was added.

Addition of 2 and 9 Month Questionnaires

To assist programs in the screening of young children from birth, a 2 month ASQ-3 was developed, and data were gathered on its validity, reliability, and utility during a 2.5-year period. These data are reported in this technical report. Second, a 9 month ASQ-3 was developed primarily for use in pediatric settings, based on the American Academy of Pediatrics recommendations (2006) for screening at 9, 18, and 24 or 30 months. The 9 month ASQ-3 was derived from the items on the 10 month interval (i.e., identical items), with cutoff scores delineated for 9-month-old children (i.e., children from 9 months 0 days through 9 months 30 days). Data for the 9 month ASQ-3 are reported as appropriate in this technical report. For some analyses, the

Table 2. ASQ-3 age administration chart

Child's age	Use this ASQ-3
1 month 0 days through 2 months 30 days	2
3 months 0 days through 4 months 30 days	4
5 months 0 days through 6 months 30 days	6
7 months 0 days through 8 months 30 days	8
9 months 0 days through 9 months 30 days	9 or 10 month[a]
10 months 0 days through 10 months 30 days	10
11 months 0 days through 12 months 30 days	12
13 months 0 days through 14 months 30 days	14
15 months 0 days through 16 months 30 days	16
17 months 0 days through 18 months 30 days	18
19 months 0 days through 20 months 30 days	20
21 months 0 days through 22 months 30 days	22
23 months 0 days through 25 months 15 days	24
25 months 16 days through 28 months 15 days	27
28 months 16 days through 31 months 15 days	30
31 months 16 days through 34 months 15 days	33
34 months 16 days through 38 months 30 days	36
39 months 0 days through 44 months 30 days	42
45 months 0 days through 50 months 30 days	48
51 months 0 days through 56 months 30 days	54
57 months 0 days through 66 months 0 days	60

[a]May use the 9 or 10 month ASQ-3 with children in this age range.

9 and 10 month questionnaires are reported separately, whereas for other analyses, the 9 and 10 month questionnaire data are combined. When combined, there are 20 questionnaire intervals; when reported separately, there are 21 questionnaire intervals.

Revisions to Items

The items are the heart of the ASQ, and changes made were carefully considered and generally did not alter meanings. Item revisions such as minor rewording and inclusion of additional examples to items were made based on ASQ user feedback and statistical analyses. Statistical analyses included item response theory (IRT) modeling, in which mathematical models that scaled items according to the statistical probability of response to each item and a child's ability to complete the item were computed. Items that did not fit a developmental model were examined, and minor revisions were made to clarify items. Item changes were made across all developmental areas and age intervals (with the exception of the 2 month interval) and are of four types. The numbers of changes across questionnaire intervals are shown in Table 3.

The most frequent type of change was wording adjustments to improve the clarity of items. For example, in the Personal-Social area, the item, "Can your child put on a coat, jacket, or shirt by himself?" was changed to "Does your child put on a coat, jacket, or shirt by himself?" In the Fine Motor area, the item, "Does your baby usually pick up a small toy with only one hand?" was changed to "Does your baby pick up a small toy with only one hand?"

A second type of item revision involved deleting or adding examples that accompanied items. For example, in the Gross Motor area, the item, "While standing, does your child throw a ball *overhand* by raising his arm to shoulder height and throwing the ball forward? (Dropping the ball, letting the ball go, or throwing the ball underhand does not count)" was changed to "While standing, does your child throw a ball *overhand* by raising his arm to shoulder height and

Table 3. Number of items per questionnaire with revisions

Questionnaire interval (months)	Minor wording revisions
4	0
6	3
8	2
10	4
12	1
14	3
16	5
18	6
20	4
22	4
24	4
27	4
30	4
33	6
36	6
42	5
48	7
54	10
60	6

throwing the ball forward? (Dropping the ball or throwing the ball underhand should be scored as 'not yet')." In the Fine Motor area, the item, "Does your child thread a shoelace through either a bead or an eyelet of a shoe?" was changed to "Can your child string small items such as beads, macaroni or pasta 'wagon wheels' onto a string or shoelace?"

A third type of revision entailed changing illustrations accompanying items. For example, the illustration in the 30 month Fine Motor area for item number 4 was deleted and replaced with the correct illustration for the item: "After your child watches you draw a line from one side of the paper to the other side, ask her to make a line like yours. Do not let your child trace your line. Does your child copy you by drawing a single line in a horizontal direction?"

The final type of revision was the addition of one item to the Communication area to assist in identifying children who may have delays in expressive language. On the 12 month questionnaire interval, the following item was added: "Does your baby make two similar sounds like 'ba-ba,' 'da-da,' or 'ga-ga'? (The sounds do not need to mean anything)."

Revisions to Overall Section

The Overall section of the ASQ asks a series of general questions about children's early development. In this section, two types of changes were made. First, changes in the wording of some existing questions were made to improve the clarity of the items. For example, in the 4 month through 14 month intervals, the question, "Does your baby use both hands equally well?" was changed to "Does your baby use both hands and both legs equally well?"

Second, new questions were added to the Overall section. For example, on the 30 month through 60 month intervals, "Can other people understand most of what your child says?" was added to help ensure that infants and children who might require further assessment were identified. A question about behavioral concerns was added on all intervals that was based on our research and other studies regarding the early identification of autism spectrum disorders (ASDs). Our research suggests that parents of young children often notice anomalies in their child's behavior early on—in the first few months—far ahead of when professionals diagnose ASD in these children. Thus, asking specifically about concerns regarding a child's behavior may alert professionals to parental concerns early on and assist in the early identification of ASDs and other developmental disorders. A summary of changes to the Overall questions on the ASQ-3 can be found in Table 4.

Table 4.   Number and wording of new and revised items added to Overall section in the ASQ-3

Questionnaire intervals	Number of new items added	Item wording
4 months through 10 months	3	Does your baby use both hands and both legs equally well?
		Do you have concerns that your baby is too quiet or does not make sounds like other babies?
		Do you have concerns about your baby's behavior?
12 months and 14 months	4	Does your baby use both hands and both legs equally well?
		Does your baby play with sounds or seem to make words?
		Do you have concerns that your baby is too quiet or does not make sounds like other babies?
		Do you have concerns about your baby's behavior?
16 months through 27 months	1	Do you have concerns about your child's behavior?
30 months through 60 months	2	Can other people understand most of what your child says?
		Do you have concerns about your child's behavior?

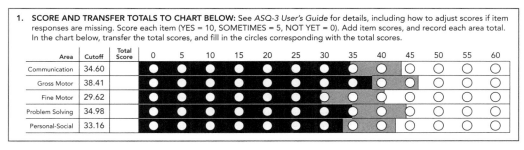

Figure 1.   Portions of the ASQ-3 Information Summary sheet, with monitoring zone shown in light gray shading.

Revisions to the Information Summary Sheet

Some sections on the Information Summary sheet were reordered to more closely follow the order of sections on the ASQ. Second, a monitoring zone (i.e., questionable area) was added to the summary profile of children's scores. A lightly shaded area located just to the right of the cutoff points (i.e., representing scores that are ≥ 1 and < 2 standard deviations from the mean) was included, as shown in Figure 1. It may be important to closely track the development of children whose ASQ-3 scores fall in this monitoring range and to provide parents/caregivers with activities to practice with these children.

Ages & Stages Questionnaires®: Social-Emotional

With the passage of the amendments to the Individuals with Disabilities Education Act (IDEA) of 1990 (PL 101-476) came a call for early detection of social or emotional problems in young children. As a complement to the ASQ, the *Ages & Stages Questionnaires: Social-Emotional (ASQ:SE)* was developed and published in 2002. This screening tool should be used in conjunction with the ASQ to identify children between 3 and 66 months of age who may need in-depth assessments of their social and emotional behavior. Eight questionnaires are available (in either English or Spanish) that address seven behavioral areas: self-regulation, compliance, communication, adaptive functioning, autonomy, affect, and interaction with people. An accompanying *User's Guide* also is available to assist professionals in the use of the ASQ:SE questionnaires, as is a DVD, *ASQ:SE in Practice* (Squires, Twombly, & Munkres, 2004).

Summary

An overall review of the modifications that have been made to the ASQ over the years suggests that most revisions have not entailed substantive changes. The majority of changes have been associated with tweaking item wording to enhance clarity. In large part, the present form and content of the questionnaires are similar to those of the original version.

PSYCHOMETRIC STUDIES OF THE ASQ

This section presents a range of empirical information collected on the questionnaires since 2004. These data were used to guide the ASQ-3 revisions. The data include 18,572 completed questionnaires for children between 1 and 66 months of age. This entire data set was used to derive new cutoff scores for the questionnaires. Subsamples of the data set were used to examine reliability and validity of the questionnaires. The respective *n*s are provided for each analysis.

Data Collection Procedures

Revisions for the ASQ-3 were based on 18,572 questionnaires completed by parents of children between 1 and 66 months of age. The numbers of questionnaires by interval are shown in Table 5 along with methods of completion (paper and web based).

Questionnaire data were collected using two methods: 1) completion of paper questionnaires and 2) completion of online, web-based questionnaires. Data were gathered between January 2004 and June 2008, across 20 ASQ intervals, as shown in Table 5. Paper questionnaires (52.4%) were completed by parents from an array of community-based programs. Web-based questionnaires (47.6%) were completed by parents who logged onto the ASQ research web site and completed demographic and research forms and questionnaires. The online questionnaires had wide geographic distribution, with the sample representing families from all 50 states and several U.S. territories.

Paper Questionnaire Completion

Paper questionnaires were completed by parents whose children attended programs for young children, including child care centers, preschools, infant programs, nonprofit organizations serving young children, medical offices conducting well-child screening, Head Start and Early Head Start programs, Healthy Start programs, home visiting programs, nonprofit organizations such as the Urban League and United Way, and IDEA Child Find programs throughout the United

Table 5. Number of questionnaires by age interval and method of completion

Questionnaire interval (months)	n for interval	Paper	Web based
2	352	4	348
4	1,824	1,428	396
6	633	134	499
8	1,362	924	438
10	899	524	375
12	2,088	1,346	742
14	811	381	430
16	1,191	748	443
18	616	158	458
20	1,278	925	353
22	404	94	310
24	1,443	1,046	397
27	559	162	397
30	953	499	454
33	546	156	390
36	1,006	414	592
42	956	342	614
48	672	209	463
54	590	131	459
60	389	108	281
		9,733	8,839
Total	18,572		

States. In addition, questionnaires were completed as part of large-scale screening projects for monitoring and identifying developmental delays in young children (e.g., at-risk monitoring projects in Idaho; Head Start and Migrant Head Start in Oregon, California, Ohio, New York, and Washington; subsidized child care programs in Florida).

For the paper questionnaires, recruitment procedures included inquiries made by the ASQ-3 research staff to 1) EI/ECSE programs in Washington, Oregon, Hawaii, and California and 2) Healthy Start, nurse home visiting, child care, and Head Start/Early Head Start programs in Ohio, Washington, California, Colorado, Minnesota, and Florida. As part of providing services, parents received a questionnaire from the provider along with a form asking for the child's demographic information and a research consent form. The questionnaire was completed either independently by the parent or with

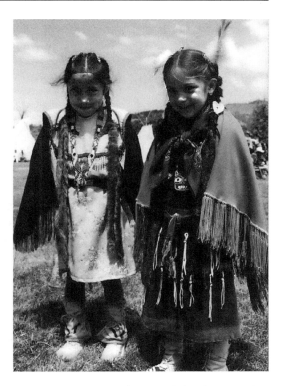

assistance from providers. The completed questionnaires were usually scored by the provider, and the results were shared with the parent or caregiver. The provider assisted the parent with referrals to community evaluation services as needed. Either hard copies of the questionnaires or deidentified computer files were sent to the research site and entered into an ASQ database. Procedures ensuring protection of human participants were approved by the University of Oregon institutional review board and were followed in all research phases.

Web-Based Questionnaire Completion

With the premise of a parent-friendly tool, the mediated ASQ research web site was designed using best practices of recruitment, data collection, and data management. The web site was produced in a hypertext markup language form that used PHP: Hypertext Preprocessor version 4.4.3 scripting to process and save data. It was tested through a variety of Windows- and Mac-compatible web browsers (i.e., Internet Explorer, Netscape, Firefox, Safari).

After consenting to participate in the online completion of the questionnaires, parents provided the required demographic information and were then given access an ASQ that matched the child's age (e.g., date of birth, corrected for prematurity up to 2 years). The electronic pages of the ASQ were an identical translation of the paper questionnaires. The parent or caregiver answered the ASQ items by clicking on the appropriate response (i.e., *yes, sometimes, not yet*). Parents received information to further facilitate and encourage caregiver–child interaction such as activity sheets or e-mail feedback from the research assistants on the ASQ research project. Follow-up services for referral were provided by the ASQ research staff when parents or caregivers requested assistance.

Several recruitment procedures were employed to encourage parents to complete the web-based questionnaires. Search engines were used so that parents or caregivers could visit the web site through descriptive words (e.g., parent help, play activities, stages of development, child research, parent education, home school, child progress). Moreover, information about web-based completion of the questionnaires was posted on sites such as http://www.daycareresource.com and http://www.craigslist.com.

Paper and Web-Based Questionnaire Completion Comparison

To test variations between the web-based and paper versions of the ASQ, statistical analyses including IRT modeling were used (for a full research report, see Yovanoff, McManus, & Squires, 2009). IRT involves mathematical models that statistically characterize the probability of response to each item in a test and the participant's ability to endorse the item. Such probabilistic response to the item is depicted by an item response function (i.e., item characteristic curve). The item characteristic curve characterizes one item from other items with three location parameters: 1) a, item discrimination; 2) b, item difficulty; and 3) c, guessing—the probability of correctly endorsing the item. IRT models include one-, two-, or three-parameter logistics models (Embretson & Reise, 2000; Ferrando & Lorenzo-Seva, 2005; Fraley, Waller, & Brennan, 2000).

The Rasch model, a one-parameter logistic model, was applied in studying differences (i.e., differential items functioning, or DIF) between web-based completed and paper completed questionnaires. The one-parameter logistic model contains only one item parameter—b, difficulty—which is free to vary between groups. It was used to examine the item response of the web-based group (focal group) in relation to that of the paper group (reference group). DIF occurs when the groups at the same ability level differ in their likelihood of endorsing an item.

The WINSTEPS Rasch Measurement version 3.64.2 computer program (Linacre, 2007) was used to analyze the questionnaire data. WINSTEPS DIF statistics imply the following: 1) web and paper groups represent the same ability—ability constant—on the same scale, and 2) item calibrations have been made at the item and ability levels. The implementation of a statistical test with a p value of .01 indicated items displaying DIF.

Out of 570 questionnaire items, the statistical findings indicated that only 60 items (10.5%) exhibited significant DIF when comparing the web-based (focal group) and paper (referent group) groups. DIF items were equally spread among all intervals (for this analysis, the 19 intervals from 4 to 60 months were used—the 2 and 9 month intevals were still under development), and, within each developmental area, they did not show all positive or negative t values, indicating no consistent pattern of differences between the same items on the web-based and paper questionnaires.

Several factors may explain the differences between web-based and paper questionnaire completion of these 60 items. First, the stationary location of computers may have interfered with parents' ability to directly observe their children demonstrating skills. Also, the location of online connections may have posed further mobility limitations. In contrast, the paper method allowed parents to go to their children either for direct observation or for hands-on activity to address specific items.

Second, it is possible that parents or caregivers navigated the web-based ASQ when their children were not present (e.g., napping or asleep during the night). In addition, completion of the web-based ASQ was limited to 1 hour, whereas the paper ASQ could be completed across a period of days at the convenience of the caregiver. These variations may explain, in part, the differential functioning of some items between the web-based and paper groups.

Third, assistance with the completion of the ASQ may have differed between the web-based and paper groups. For the most part, the web-based questionnaires seemed to be completed independently by parents or caregivers. With the paper ASQ, the probability of professional assistance was more likely. Assistance provided by home visitors and other practitioners may have influenced how items were scored.

Table 6. Gender of children

	Frequency	Percent
Male	7,819	52.6
Female	7,051	47.4
Total	14,870	100.0
Missing	268	
Total *N*	15,138	

Overall, the IRT analyses found few significant differences between web-based and paper-completed questionnaires. Only 10% of items (60 items out of 570 total) seemed to function differently when these two completion methods were compared. Differences also were both positive and negative, indicating no consistent pattern between the completion methods. Therefore, web-based and paper questionnaire data were combined for all 21 questionnaire intervals to derive the cutoff scores.

Population Sample

The data analyses that are contained in this report are based on 18,572 completed questionnaires. However, within this sample, 3,434 children had more than one completed questionnaire (e.g., 4, 8, and 12 months); therefore, the total demographic sample was 15,138 individual children.

Each parent or caregiver who completed a questionnaire was asked to complete a demographic form. Demographic data included information on gender, ethnicity, mother's education, family income, who had completed the questionnaire, and whether the child was known to have any medical or environmental risk. The demographic data for the population sample are displayed in Tables 6–11.

As shown in Table 6, the gender distribution for the sample was 53% male and 47% female. The distribution of mother's level of education is displayed in Table 7. The greatest percentage of mothers in this sample (54%) had at least 4 years of college, whereas 12% had an associate's degree, 23% had a high school education, and only 3.5% had not completed high school.

Data on family income were collected and are displayed in Table 8. The majority of the reporting caregivers indicate incomes greater than $40,000 (57%), whereas 36% reported incomes below that figure, and 7% reported not knowing.

Table 9 contains data on the person completing the questionnaires. The majority of individuals completing the questionnaires were mothers (82%). This finding is consistent with feedback from hundreds of screening professionals who report that mothers are most apt to complete the questionnaires on their children.

Table 7. Level of mother's education

	Frequency	Percent
Less than high school	387	3.5
High school	2,488	22.7
Associate's degree	1,320	12.0
4 years of college or above	5,931	54.0
Don't know	848	7.7
Total	10,974	100.0
Missing	4,164	
Total *N*	15,138	

Table 8. Family income level

	Frequency	Percent
$0–$12,000	1,417	12.8
$12,001–$24,000	1,037	9.3
$24,001–$40,000	1,524	13.7
More than $40,000	6,341	57.1
Don't know	779	7.0
Total	11,098	100.0
Missing	4,040	
Total N	15,138	

Data on the risk status of each child were collected and are displayed in Table 10. Seventy-six percent of the sample had only one or no known risk factor, whereas 19% had two risk factors, and 4% had three or more known risk factors; there are missing data for 4% of the sample. The number of children with two or more risk factors may seem high; however, it may be that children exposed to risk conditions may be referred for screening more often than children who are not.

Table 11 contains data on the ethnicity of the sample. The greatest percentage of children were white (66%); 12% were African American, and 15% were Hispanic. Asian, Native American, Hawaiian, Pacific Islander, other, and mixed ethnicity composed 5% of the sample. Table 11 also contains data from the U.S. Census estimates for 2007. These comparisons suggest that the ethnicity of this sample of children is representative of the general U.S. population.

Table 12 contains information on the number of questionnaires completed for each child in the sample. One questionnaire was completed for 86.5% of the children, 8.5% had two questionnaires completed, and the remaining 5% of the sample had three or more questionnaires completed.

Reliability Studies

Reliability studies completed on the ASQ-3 include test–retest reliability and interobserver reliability. In addition, internal consistency of ASQ-3 items was examined using correlational analyses and the Cronbach coefficient alpha (Cronbach, 1951). Each of these analyses is presented next.

Table 9. Person completing ASQ-3

	Frequency	Percent
Mother	9,092	81.7
Father	428	3.8
Guardian	54	0.5
Grandparents	165	1.5
Foster parent	40	0.4
Both parents	214	1.9
Other	496	4.5
Teacher/home visitor	456	4.1
Adoptive parent	190	1.7
Total	11,135	100.0
Missing	4,003	
Total N	15,138	

Table 10. Risk status of child

	Frequency	Percent
No known risk factor	7,809	69.0
One risk factor	838	7.4
Agency affiliation or two risk factors	2,186	19.3
Three or more risk factors	481	4.3
Total	11,314	100.0
Missing	3,824	
Total N	15,138	

Table 11. Ethnicity of children in sample compared with 2007 U.S. Census estimates

Ethnicity	n	ASQ sample percent	Census estimate for 2007[a] percent
Caucasian/white	9,122	66.4	79.9
African American	1,588	11.6	12.8
Asian/Pacific Islander	546	3.9	0.9
Native American/Alaskan	139	1.1	4.4
Latino/Hispanic	1,449	10.5	N/A
Other	146	1.1	0.0
Don't know	125	0.9	2.0
Mixed	616	4.5	
Total	13,731	100.0	100.0
Missing	1,407		
Total	15,138		
Hispanic or Latino (as per U.S. Census)	1,449	10.5	15.0
Not Hispanic or Latino	12,282	89.4	84.9
Total	13,731	100.0	

[a]*Source:* Population Division, U.S. Census Bureau, May 1, 2008.

Table 12. Number of questionnaires completed for each child

	Frequency	Percent of sample	Number of total questionnaires
1	13,094	86.5	13,094
2	1,292	8.5	2,584
3	390	2.6	1,170
4	188	1.2	752
5	105	0.7	525
6	50	0.3	300
7	13	0.1	91
8	4	0.0	32
12	2	0.0	24
Total	15,138	100.0	18,572

Test–Retest Reliability

Test–retest reliability is designed to help determine the stability of test outcomes over time. Test–retest reliability of the ASQ was examined by comparing two questionnaires completed by the same parent at a 2-week time interval. That is, parents were asked to complete the same questionnaire interval for their child twice within a 2-week time period between completions. Questionnaires completed by 145 parents were included in this analysis. Forty-two parents completed two questionnaires online, and 103 parents completed two paper questionnaires. Parents were blind to the results of the first questionnaire when they completed the second one. The two questionnaires completed by parents were then compared for agreement on classifications (i.e., screened or not screened). The percent agreement for the 145 parents was 92%. Intraclass correlations ranged from .75 to .82, indicating strong test–retest reliability across ASQ developmental areas.

Interobserver Reliability

Interobserver reliability refers to the agreement of test outcomes that have been completed by at least two independent test administrators. The interobserver reliability of the ASQ was examined by comparing questionnaires completed by parents with questionnaires completed by trained test examiners for the same children. Trained test examiners filled out a questionnaire on a child immediately after completing a standardized assessment (e.g., BDI). Interobserver reliability was derived by comparing the agreement between the classifications (i.e., screened or not screened) of 107 children based on the parents' and trainer examiners' completion of ASQ. The percent agreement between ASQ classifications between parents and trainer examiners was 93%. Intraclass correlations by area ranged from .43 to .69, suggesting robust agreement between parents and trained examiners when completing the ASQ for this group of 107 children. The Personal-Social area had the strongest agreement (.69), and the Communication area had the lowest agreement (.43). Parents and professionals may observe different samples of behavior while completing the Communication Area, thus accounting for fair intraclass correlations between parents and test administrators.

Internal Consistency

The internal consistency of the questionnaires was addressed by examining the relationship between developmental area and overall scores. Correlational analyses and Cronbach coefficient alpha (Cronbach, 1951) were calculated.

Pearson product moment correlation coefficients were calculated for developmental area scores with an overall ASQ score for 20 questionnaire age intervals. As shown in Table 13, the correlations by developmental area and overall ASQ score are consistent and generally range from .60 to .85. The one exception is the Gross Motor area, in which two correlations are below .60. All correlations are significant at $p < .01$. These findings suggest moderate to strong internal consistency between developmental areas and total test score.

Table 14 contains the correlations between developmental area scores that have been collapsed across the 20 questionnaire age intervals. Again, all correlations are significant, suggesting congruence between developmental areas as well as between developmental areas and overall ASQ scores.

Cronbach coefficient alphas were calculated for developmental area scores for 20 age intervals. Alphas are presented in Table 15 and range from .51 to .87. These alphas indicate that ASQ items have good to acceptable internal consistency.

The reliability of the questionnaires has been studied by examining the internal consistency, test–retest reliability, and interobserver reliability of the questionnaires. Internal consistency

Table 13.   Correlations between developmental area and overall ASQ-3 score

Age interval (months)	n	Communication	Gross Motor	Fine Motor	Problem Solving	Personal-Social
2	352	.81	.51	.70	.83	.81
4	1,824	.67	.71	.85	.83	.78
6	633	.64	.74	.81	.80	.80
8	1,362	.73	.69	.74	.72	.74
9[a]	160	.72	.68	.65	.64	.70
10[a]	739	.79	.72	.67	.74	.79
12	2,088	.78	.66	.68	.74	.80
14	811	.78	.66	.81	.78	.79
16	1,191	.73	.57	.74	.76	.78
18	616	.75	.60	.71	.74	.74
20	1,278	.75	.64	.73	.80	.76
22	404	.79	.67	.78	.79	.79
24	1,443	.77	.67	.69	.77	.81
27	559	.84	.66	.75	.83	.78
30	953	.79	.64	.78	.82	.76
33	546	.84	.66	.80	.83	.84
36	1,006	.80	.66	.81	.81	.78
42	956	.82	.68	.82	.84	.80
48	672	.79	.71	.82	.80	.81
54	590	.81	.68	.81	.75	.77
60	389	.77	.75	.84	.72	.71
Total	18,572					

Note: All correlations are significant at $p < .01$. Total number of questionnaires completed = 18,572.
[a]9 month interval data are a subset of 10 month data.

analyses have indicated strong relationships across items and within areas on the questionnaires. The questionnaires also achieved substantial test–retest and interobserver reliability. Parents' evaluations of their children using the questionnaires were consistent over time. In addition, professional examiners' agreement with parental evaluations of children on the questionnaires was consistently high.

Validity

Studies of the validity of the ASQ-3 are described here, beginning with a comparison of performance on the questionnaires by nonrisk and risk groups. The next section describes the procedures used to determine the screening cutoff points for each interval. This section is followed by de-

Table 14. Correlations between developmental area scores collapsing (combining all intervals) across questionnaires and with overall ASQ-3 scores

Area	Area				
	Communication	Gross Motor	Fine Motor	Problem Solving	Personal-Social
Communication					
Gross Motor	.33				
Fine Motor	.36	.36			
Problem Solving	.50	.37	.52		
Personal-Social	.54	.41	.46	.53	
Overall	.76	.65	.73	.78	.79

Note: All correlations are significant at $p < .01$.

Table 15. Standardized alphas by area and age interval

Age interval (months)	n	Communication	Gross Motor	Fine Motor	Problem Solving	Personal-Social
2	352	.76	.57	.56	.78	.51
4	1,194	.60	.64	.73	.73	.60
6	602	.57	.61	.70	.70	.61
8	1,328	.69	.68	.70	.69	.54
10	446	.69	.81	.71	.69	.67
12	2,035	.68	.82	.55	.61	.63
14	481	.73	.87	.60	.70	.63
16	1,176	.70	.81	.64	.66	.59
18	592	.74	.77	.58	.54	.56
20	1,002	.77	.71	.57	.53	.58
22	399	.80	.72	.57	.56	.61
24	1,371	.80	.64	.51	.53	.58
27	546	.78	.68	.65	.61	.58
30	935	.75	.62	.75	.65	.65
33	537	.76	.62	.77	.69	.65
36	982	.71	.69	.77	.69	.61
42	950	.72	.68	.76	.72	.66
48	667	.80	.69	.76	.70	.68
54	586	.83	.73	.79	.75	.71
60	387	.66	.72	.83	.78	.67

Note: Analyses include only questionnaires with no missing items.

tailing the investigation of concurrent validity. The final section addresses a preliminary comparison between the English- and Spanish-language versions of the ASQ-3.

Nonrisk and Risk Groups

A sample of 18,572 questionnaires for children between the ages of 1 and 66 months (shown in Table 5) was used to determine the cutoff scores for the ASQ-3. The demographic information on this sample is presented in Tables 6–11. This sample contains both nonrisk and risk children. Subjects in the risk sample included infants and young children from families who met one or more of the following criteria: 1) extreme poverty (according to family income level, as defined

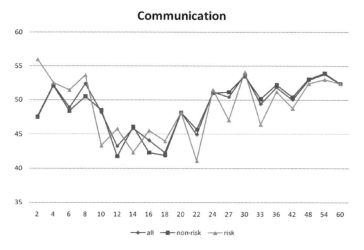

Figure 2. Risk and nonrisk samples for the Communication area.

Gross Motor

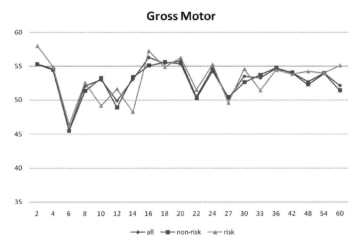

Figure 3. Risk and nonrisk samples for the Gross Motor area.

by federal guidelines, 100% poverty level); 2) maternal age of 19 years or younger at the time of the infant's birth; 3) maternal education less than 12th grade; 4) parents who had experienced involvement with child protective services for abuse and/or neglect of their children; 5) medical risk, including prematurity ($<$ 39 weeks' gestation); and 6) infant's birth weight less than 3 pounds, 5 ounces.

As noted in Table 10, 19% of this sample had two or more risk factors, and 4% had three or more known risk factors. Figures 2–6 contain graphic comparisons of the mean scores by developmental area for the nonrisk, risk, and combined samples. As expected, an examination of these graphs shows that the means for the risk group were generally, but not always, lower than the means for the nonrisk group. Some anomalies did occur. For example, at the 2 month age interval, the risk group had consistently higher means than the nonrisk group did; however, this is likely attributable to the small number of risk infants at this age interval (n = 5). Also, at the 14 month interval, large mean differences in favor of the nonrisk group occurred, which, again, may be a function of a small number of risk children in this interval (n = 52).

From studies on the second edition of the ASQ (Squires, Potter, & Bricker, 1999), it was determined that including both the risk and nonrisk samples was more representative of a gen-

Fine Motor

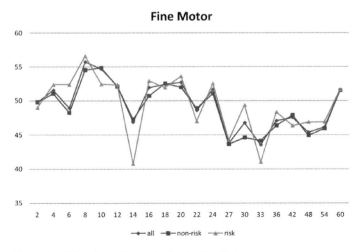

Figure 4. Risk and nonrisk samples for the Fine Motor area.

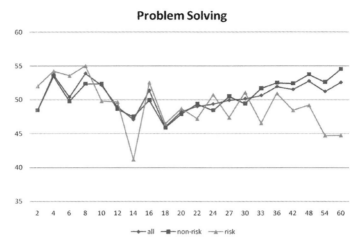

Figure 5. Risk and nonrisk samples for the Problem Solving area.

eral population and provided the most accurate cutoff scores (Squires et al., 1999). The method used to test this question was an analytic technique called relative (or receiver) operating characteristic (ROC). The ROC, based on statistical decision theory, has been used in a variety of disciplines, including human perception and decision making (Green & Swets, 1966). The ROC provides estimates of the probabilities of decision outcomes by revealing the reciprocal relationship between the true positive, true negative, false positive, and false negative probabilities that can be attained by shifting the decision criteria (i.e., cutoff points).

Based on the reported range of ROCs by group, it was determined that points derived by using means and standard deviations from the combined risk and nonrisk groups provided the most accurate cutoff scores (Squires et al., 1999). This decision had practical implications because agencies responsible for screening often do not know the risk status of the population to be screened. Adopting the combined risk and nonrisk referral cutoffs seemed the most appropriate for screening programs.

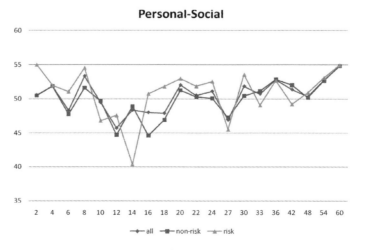

Figure 6. Risk and nonrisk samples for the Personal-Social area.

Determining Cutoff Scores

For the ASQ-3, risk and nonrisk groups were combined for all analyses and determination of age interval cutoff scores. The challenge, as with all screening measures, was to select scores that maximized accuracy and minimized error. This challenge was addressed in two ways. The first strategy was to develop a matrix showing the conditional probabilities that existed at each cutoff score for 2, 1.5, and 1 standard deviations and to generate a ROC curve that displayed the probabilities at each cutoff score.

A matrix for each questionnaire interval was created using the cutoff scores at 2, 1.5, and 1 standard deviations from the mean. This matrix included several computations that were generated using a contingency table. Cutoff scores for developmental areas were included, along with conditional probabilities that were computed. A sample matrix for the 48 month questionnaire can be found in Table 16 with the following conditional probabilities: 1) sensitivity, 2) specificity, 3) false positive proportion, 4) false negative proportion, 5) underidentification, and 6) overidentification. (For definitions and computational formulas, see Chapter 6.)

Table 17 shows combined conditional probabilities across the intervals. As expected, when the cutoff became less conservative (i.e., 1.5 or 1 standard deviations from the mean), the over-referral rate increased as the underidentification rate decreased. The cutoff score of 2 standard deviations, although not perfect, seemed the most balanced cutoff point in terms of the true positive and false positive proportions.

The second strategy entailed determining the percentage of children identified at each of the cutoff scores that were 2, 1.5, and 1 standard deviations below the mean. Targets of 12%–16% of children identified in one developmental area (i.e., one area below the cutoff score) and 2%–7% identified in two or more areas were adopted as the desired percentages to be identified for further assessment at each age interval. These figures were based on U.S. Census Bureau and Centers for Disease Control and Prevention prevalence data related to developmental disabilities in young children (Cornell University, 2003–2009; U.S. Census Bureau, 2004).

Table 16. Conditional probabilities for 48 month ASQ-3

Standard deviation(s) below the mean	Developmental matrix area	Cutoff	Sensitivity	Specificity	False positive	False negative	Underidentified	Overidentified
2.0	Communication	30.72	0.83	0.91	0.09	0.17	0.09	0.04
	Gross Motor	32.78						
	Fine Motor	15.81						
	Problem Solving	31.30						
	Personal-Social	26.60						
1.5	Communication	36.27	0.96	0.82	0.18	0.04	0.02	0.09
	Gross Motor	37.76						
	Fine Motor	23.19						
	Problem Solving	36.67						
	Personal-Social	32.54						
1.0	Communication	41.82	1.00	0.73	0.27	0.00	0.00	0.13
	Gross Motor	42.74						
	Fine Motor	30.58						
	Problem Solving	42.04						
	Personal-Social	38.47						

Note: Values are cutoff points by standard deviation units and accompanying conditional probabilities for the 48 month questionnaire (*n* = 45 for validity analyses).

Table 17. Conditional probabilities across questionnaire intervals by cutoff point for all questionnaires (*n* = 579 for validity analyses)

Standard deviation(s) below the mean	Sensitivity	Specificity	False positive	False negative	Underidentified	Overidentified
2.0	0.86	0.86	0.14	0.14	0.06	0.08
1.5	0.94	0.72	0.28	0.06	0.02	0.16
1.0	0.98	0.59	0.41	0.02	0.01	0.23

For every questionnaire interval, ROC analyses and percentages of children identified in one and two domains were studied. Based on these comparisons, a referral cutoff point of 2 standard deviations below the mean across all 21 questionnaire intervals was chosen.

Monitoring Zone

For the ASQ-3, a monitoring zone of 1–2 standard deviations below the mean score in each domain was highlighted on the ASQ-3 Information Summary sheet forms, as shown previously in Figure 1. This monitoring zone was added to alert ASQ-3 users that children who are not identified as needing follow-up assessment (i.e., with scores that were 2 standard deviations below the mean) might, nevertheless, benefit from targeted interventions. Children whose scores are 1–2 standard deviation units below the mean score in any developmental area should be monitored and given follow-up activities for practicing skills in these areas. In addition, these children should be rescreened at regular intervals. The monitoring zones and cutoff scores are presented in Table 18. (Scores that fall within the monitoring zone are ≥ 1 but < 2 standard deviations from the mean.)

Concurrent Validity

Concurrent validity was measured by comparing the classification of children based on their performance on a standardized test with their classification based on their performance on the ASQ-3. Agreement meant that the ASQ-3 had assigned a child to the same classification as the standardized test had; disagreement meant that the ASQ-3 classification did not match the standardized test's classification.

Two groups of children were included in this analysis: those tested for eligibility for IDEA services and those not receiving services and presumed to be developing without problems—hereafter called the *typical group*. The identified group (*n* = 257) participated in EI/ECSE programs in Oregon, New York, and California, and the typical group (*n* = 322) was recruited from child care centers, preschool programs, and Internet advertising for research participants. In most cases, the standardized measure used was the BDI, first and second editions (Newborg, Stock, Wnek, Guidubaldi, & Svinicki, 1984, 2004). The BDI was administered and scored by trained examiners.

For the identified group, test data were gathered from children's files and included scores and classifications that were based on both the ASQ-3 and BDI. For the typical group, the ASQ-3 was completed by parents/caregivers, and a trained examiner administered the BDI.

A child's performance on the standardized test was designated as *identified* if the child's scaled BDI score was equal to or less than 75 on any scale or subscale. This score was chosen because a child scoring at or below this point is likely to be functioning below developmental expectations for his or her chronological age and should be seen for further diagnostic assessment. In addition, a delay of 1.5–2 standard deviations on a standardized test meets eligibility criteria

Table 18. ASQ-3 means, standard deviations, and cutoff scores

Question-naire interval	Communication					Gross Motor					Fine Motor					Problem Solving					Personal-Social				
	Mean	SD	1.0 SD[a]	1.5 SD	2.0 SD[b]	Mean	SD	1.0 SD[a]	1.5 SD	2.0 SD[b]	Mean	SD	1.0 SD[a]	1.5 SD	2.0 SD[b]	Mean	SD	1.0 SD	1.5 SD	2.0 SD[b]	Mean	SD	1.0 SD	1.5 SD	2.0 SD[b]
2	47.62	12.42	35.19	28.98	22.77	55.32	6.74	48.58	45.21	41.84	49.80	9.82	39.98	35.07	30.16	48.48	11.93	36.55	30.59	24.62	50.57	8.43	42.14	37.92	33.71
4	52.28	8.84	43.44	39.02	34.60	54.63	8.11	46.52	42.46	38.41	51.58	10.98	40.60	35.11	29.62	53.79	9.41	44.38	39.68	34.98	51.92	9.38	42.54	37.85	33.16
6	48.90	9.63	39.27	34.46	29.65	45.64	11.69	33.95	28.10	22.25	48.93	11.90	37.04	31.04	25.14	50.41	11.35	39.06	33.39	27.72	48.31	11.48	36.83	31.08	25.34
8	52.40	9.67	42.73	37.90	33.06	52.09	10.74	41.35	35.98	30.61	55.75	7.80	47.95	44.05	40.15	53.92	8.87	45.05	40.61	36.17	53.35	8.75	44.60	40.22	35.84
9	38.55	12.29	26.26[c]	20.12	13.97	46.72	14.45	32.27	25.05	17.82	52.31	10.49	41.82	36.58	31.32	49.51	10.39	39.11	33.92	28.72	42.47	11.78	30.69	24.80	18.91
10	48.17	12.65	35.52	29.19	22.87	53.02	11.47	41.54	35.81	30.07	54.72	8.38	46.36	42.16	37.97	52.19	9.84	42.35	37.43	32.51	49.49	11.12	38.37	32.81	27.25
12	43.22	13.79	29.43[c]	22.53	15.64	49.92	14.22	35.71	28.60	21.49	52.22	8.86	43.36	38.93	34.50	48.99	10.84	38.16	32.74	27.32	45.73	12.00	33.73	27.73	21.73
14	45.85	14.23	31.63	24.51	17.40	53.09	13.64	39.44	32.62	25.80	46.87	11.91	34.97	29.01	23.06	47.08	12.26	34.82	28.69	22.56	48.34	12.58	35.76	29.47	23.18
16	44.08	13.64	30.45	23.63	16.81	56.31	9.20	47.11	42.52	37.91	51.96	9.99	41.97	36.98	31.98	51.39	10.44	40.95	35.73	30.51	48.01	10.79	37.22	31.83	26.43
18	42.30	14.62	27.68[c]	20.37	13.06	55.46	9.04	46.42	41.90	37.38	52.44	9.06	43.38	38.85	34.32	45.99	10.13	35.86	30.80	25.74	47.90	10.35	37.55	32.37	27.19
20	48.14	13.82	34.32	27.41	20.50	55.82	7.96	47.85	43.87	39.89	52.73	8.34	44.39	40.22	36.05	48.24	9.70	38.54	33.69	28.84	52.04	9.34	42.70	38.03	33.36
22	44.94	15.95	28.99[c]	21.01	13.04	50.48	11.37	39.11	33.43	27.75	48.58	9.49	39.09	34.35	29.61	49.02	9.86	39.16	34.23	29.30	50.54	10.24	40.31	35.19	30.07
24	51.23	13.03	38.20	31.69	25.17	54.73	8.33	46.40	42.23	38.07	51.70	8.27	43.43	39.30	35.16	49.40	9.81	39.59	34.69	29.78	51.14	9.80	41.34	36.44	31.54
27	50.43	13.21	37.22	30.62	24.02	50.27	11.13	39.14	33.58	28.01	43.74	12.66	31.08	24.75	18.42	49.95	11.16	38.79	33.20	27.62	46.92	10.82	36.11	30.71	25.31
30	53.81	10.25	43.56	38.43	33.30	53.54	8.70	44.84	40.49	36.14	46.78	13.76	33.02	26.14	19.25	50.18	11.55	38.63	32.85	27.08	51.87	9.93	41.94	36.98	32.01
33	49.38	12.01	37.37	31.37	25.36	53.28	9.24	44.04	39.42	34.80	43.52	15.62	27.90	20.09	12.28	50.65	11.86	38.78	32.86	26.92	50.74	10.89	39.85	34.40	28.96
36	51.88	10.44	41.43	36.21	30.99	54.68	8.84	45.84	41.42	36.99	47.07	14.50	32.57	25.32	18.07	51.97	10.84	41.13	35.71	30.29	52.82	8.74	44.07	39.70	35.33
42	50.02	11.48	38.54	32.80	27.06	54.03	8.88	45.15	40.71	36.27	47.55	13.87	33.68	26.75	19.82	51.54	11.72	39.82	33.96	28.11	51.39	10.13	41.25	36.29	31.12
48	52.92	11.10	41.82	36.27	30.72	52.71	9.97	42.74	37.76	32.78	45.35	14.77	30.58	23.19	15.81	52.78	10.74	42.04	36.67	31.30	50.34	11.87	38.47	32.54	26.60
54	53.79	10.97	42.82	37.34	31.85	53.98	9.40	44.58	39.88	35.18	46.12	14.40	31.72	24.52	17.32	51.25	11.56	39.68	33.90	28.12	52.77	10.22	42.55	37.44	32.33
60	52.42	9.62	42.80	37.00	33.19	52.17	10.44	41.72	36.50	31.28	51.57	12.52	39.05	32.79	26.54	52.59	11.30	41.29	35.64	29.99	54.84	7.89	46.96	43.01	39.07

Key: SD, standard deviation.
[a]Scores in the monitoring zone are ≥ 1.0 but < 2.0 SD below the mean. Scores higher than the monitoring zone indicate typical development. Scores in the monitoring zone may need further investigation.
[b]Scores ≤ referral cutoff (2.0 SD below mean) indicate a possible delay in development (further assessment with a professional is recommended).
[c]The monitoring zones for these four ASQ-3 intervals were adjusted slightly to 30.00.

established by many states for entrance into EI/ECSE programs (http://www.NECTAC.org). (Although 75 is 2.5 points less than the BDI 1.5-SD cutoff score of 77.5, 75 was the mean cutoff score used for BDI eligibility decisions.)

A child's performance on the ASQ was considered identified if his or her score was at or below the cutoff score of 2 standard deviations below the mean in one or more developmental areas. One of the following four outcomes was possible:

1. Both tests classified the child as typical.
2. Both tests classified the child as identified.
3. The standardized measure classified the child as typical, and the questionnaire classified him or her as identified.
4. The questionnaire classified the child as typical, and the standardized measure classified him or her as identified.

Agreement between the BDI and ASQ-3 classifications for the total group of 579 children across all questionnaires is shown in Figure 7. An examination of these data suggests that the ASQ-3 has moderate to high agreement with BDI classifications. These findings are important because they provide objective evidence that, in most cases, ASQ-3 results will accurately identify children who require further assessment but will *not* identify those who are developing typically as needing further assessment. Users of the ASQ-3 can be relatively confident that ASQ-3 results will identify those children whose development is suspect and those whose development is falling within typical developmental norms.

Contingency tables containing agreement between the BDI and the ASQs by combined age intervals (2–12, 14–24, 27–36, and 42–60 months) can be found in Figure 8. Age intervals are combined for this report to simplify the reporting of results because of the numerous intervals in the ASQ-3. Contingency tables showing validity agreement for the 20 separate intervals (9 and 10 month intervals were combined) can be found at http://www.agesandstages.com.

Spanish Translation of the ASQ-3

Extensive review and revision have been undertaken in the development of the Spanish translation of the ASQ-3. The Spanish version of the second edition of the ASQs was reviewed by several experts in pediatrics and also by developmental pediatricians and practitioners working with

		Eligibility status		
		Eligible	Typical	Total
Status determined by ASQ-3	Eligible	217	47	264
	Typical	35	280	315
	Total	252	327	579

Sensitivity	Specificity	False positive	False negative	Percent agreement	Under-identified	Over-identified
86.1%	85.6%	14.4%	13.9%	85.8%	6.0%	8.1%

Figure 7.   Overall concurrent validity for aggregated 20 questionnaire intervals (9- and 10-month intervals were combined for this analysis).

2–12 months

		Eligibility status		
		Eligible	Typical	Total
Status determined by ASQ-3	Eligible	33	6	39
	Typical	6	63	69
	Total	39	69	108

Sensitivity	Specificity	False positive	False negative	Percent agreement	Under-identified	Over-identified
84.6%	91.3%	8.7%	15.4%	88.9%	5.6%	5.6%

14–24 months

		Eligibility status		
		Eligible	Typical	Total
Status determined by ASQ-3	Eligible	66	23	98
	Typical	8	81	92
	Total	74	104	178

Sensitivity	Specificity	False positive	False negative	Percent agreement	Under-identified	Over-identified
89.2%	77.9%	22.1%	10.8%	82.6%	4.5%	12.9%

27–36 months

		Eligibility status		
		Eligible	Typical	Total
Status determined by ASQ-3	Eligible	85	13	98
	Typical	14	78	92
	Total	99	91	190

Sensitivity	Specificity	False positive	False negative	Percent agreement	Under-identified	Over-identified
85.9%	85.7%	14.3%	14.1%	85.8%	7.4%	6.8%

42–60 months

		Eligibility status		
		Eligible	Typical	Total
Status determined by ASQ-3	Eligible	33	5	38
	Typical	7	58	65
	Total	40	63	103

Sensitivity	Specificity	False positive	False negative	Percent agreement	Under-identified	Over-identified
82.5%	92.1%	7.9%	17.5%	88.3%	6.8%	4.9%

Figure 8. Agreement between ASQ-3 and eligibility status, collapsed by age grouping.

young children and families who speak numerous Spanish dialects (e.g., Nicaraguan, Mexican, Argentinean). Translation errors that were found in the Spanish second edition of the ASQ were corrected, and minor wording changes and substitutions were made. The experts suggested these changes and revisions to develop a translation that could be used across a variety of Spanish dialects. Items also were reworded to match the changes in items and format made in the ASQ-3 English version. To date, analyses suggest similar cutoff scores when comparing the Spanish risk and English risk samples, with a few exceptions; differences appeared in both positive and negative directions. Data will continue to be gathered on the ASQ-3 and will be posted at www.agesandstages.com.

CONCLUSION

This report describes the latest revisions that have been made to the ASQ and also presents the most recent empirical information gathered on the questionnaires. The second edition of the ASQ appeared in 1999, and during the ensuing years, the authors and research staff have accumulated information that suggested minor changes to the questionnaires would improve their accuracy and functionality. These changes have necessitated the collection of additional data on the psychometric characteristics of the modified questionnaires.

Examining the validity and reliability of a screening measure is essential to understanding and appreciating its strengths and weaknesses. All screening measures make errors; however, users should have confidence in the measure's accuracy (i.e., underidentification and overidentification of children is low). The data present in this report should provide the user with the assurance that in most cases, children will be accurately screened and that the screening can be conducted at a modest cost.

The ASQ system is built on the premise that early identification is essential to maximally effective intervention with young children and their families. A critical feature of early identification is universal and ongoing developmental screening of young children. The ASQ provides practitioners and researchers a measure that is low cost to use and reliable in its identification of children who require further in-depth assessment.

REFERENCES

American Academy of Pediatrics. (2006). Identifying infants and young children with developmental disorders in the medical home: An algorithm for developmental surveillance and screening. *Pediatrics, 118*(1), 405–420. Available online at http://aappolicy.aappublications.org/cgi/content/full/pediatrics;118/1/405

Bayley, N. (1969). *Bayley Scales of Infant Development.* San Antonio, TX: The Psychological Corporation.

Bayley, N. (2002). *Bayley III Scales of Infant Development.* San Antonio, TX: The Psychological Corporation.

Bayley, N. (2006). *Bayley Scales of Infant Development* (3rd ed.). San Antonio, TX: The Psychological Corporation.

Brinker, R., Franzier, W., Lancelot, B., & Norman, J. (1989). Identifying infants from the inner city for early intervention. *Infants and Young Children, 2*(1), 49–58.

Cohen, M., & Gross, P. (1979). *Developmental resources: Behavioral sequences for assessment and program planning* (Vols. I–II). New York: Grune & Stratton.

Cornell University. (2003–2009). *Disability statistics.* Retrieved from http://www.ilr.cornell.edu/edi/disabilitystatistics/links.cfm

Cronbach, L. (1951). Coefficient alpha and the internal structure of tests. *Psychometrika, 16*(3), 297–334.

Embretson, S., & Reise, S. (2000). *Item response theory for psychologists.* Mahwah, NJ: Lawrence Erlbaum Associates.

Ferrando, P., & Lorenzo-Seva, U. (2005). IRT-related factor analytic procedures for testing the equivalence of paper-and-pencil and internet-administered questionnaires. *Psychological Methods, 10*(2), 193–205.

Fraley, R., Waller, N., & Brennan, K. (2000). An item-response theory analysis of self-report measures of adult attachment. *Journal of Personality and Social Psychology, 78*(2), 350–365.

Gradel, K., Thompson, M., & Sheehan, R. (1981). Parental and professional agreement in early childhood assessment. *Topics in Early Childhood Special Education, 1*(2), 31–39.

Green, D., & Swets, J. (1966). *Signal detection theory and psychophysics.* New York: Wiley.

Hunt, J., & Paraskevopoulos, J. (1980). Children's psychological development as a function of the accuracy of their mothers' knowledge of their abilities. *Journal of Genetic Psychology, 136*(2), 285–298.

Individuals with Disabilities Education Act (IDEA) of 1990, PL 101-476, 20 U.S.C. §§ 1400 *et seq.*

Knobloch, H., Stevens, F., & Malone, A.F. (1980). *Manual of developmental diagnosis: The administration and interpretation of the revised Gesell and Amatruda developmental and neurological examination.* New York: Harper & Row.

Linacre, J.M. (2007). WINSTEPS (Version 3.64.2) [Computer software]. Chicago: Winsteps.com.

Newborg, J., Stock, J.R., Wnek, L., Guidubaldi, J., & Svinicki, J. (1984). *Battelle Developmental Inventory.* Itasca, IL: Riverside.

Newborg, J., Stock, J., Wnek, L., Guidubaldi, J., & Svinicki, J. (2004). *Battelle Developmental Inventory.* Chicago, IL: Riverside Publishing.

Squires, J., Potter, L., & Bricker, D. (1999). *Ages and Stages Questionnaires user's guide* (2nd ed.). Baltimore: Paul H. Brookes Publishing Co.

Squires, J., Twombly, E., & Munkres, A. (2004). *ASQ:SE in practice* [DVD]. Baltimore: Paul H. Brookes Publishing Co.

U.S. Census Bureau. (2004). *American Community Survey.* Available online at http://www.census.gov/acs/www/index.html

Yovanoff, P., McManus, S., & Squires, J. (2009). *Web-based and paper-pencil administration of a developmental questionnaire for young children: Score interpretation using item response theory.* Available from University of Oregon, Early Intervention Program, Eugene.

D

Letters and Forms

ASQ·3

PARENT LETTERS/FORMS (IN ENGLISH)

Parent Welcome Letter
Parent Consent Form
Demographic Information Sheet
Parent ASQ-3 Questionnaire Cover Letter
Parent Feedback Letter: Typical
Parent Feedback Letter: Monitoring
Parent Feedback Survey

PARENT LETTERS/FORMS (IN SPANISH)

Parent Welcome Letter
Parent Consent Form
Demographic Information Sheet
Parent ASQ-3 Questionnaire Cover Letter
Parent Feedback Letter: Typical
Parent Feedback Letter: Monitoring
Parent Feedback Survey

PHYSICIAN/PROFESSIONAL LETTERS (IN ENGLISH)

Physician Information Letter
Physician Results Letter

SCREENING/MONITORING PROGRAM FORMS (IN ENGLISH)

ASQ-3 Master List
Implementation Progress Worksheet

Throughout this volume, a number of sample forms and letters to the parents and physicians of children participating in an ASQ monitoring program, are provided. This appendix contains photocopiable versions of these items. To assist program staff who serve Spanish-speaking families, the forms and letters intended for use by parents have been translated into Spanish and are provided in this appendix. The forms and letters intended for use by physicians and programs have not been translated into Spanish. Purchasers of the ASQ-3 are granted permission to photocopy the blank letters and forms in this appendix (please see the Photocopying Release on p. xxi).

Dear Parent/Caregiver:

Welcome to our screening and monitoring program. Because your child's first 5 years of life are so important, we want to help you provide the best start for your child. As part of this service, we provide the Ages & Stages Questionnaires, Third Edition (ASQ-3), to help you keep track of your child's development. A questionnaire will be provided every 2-, 4-, or 6-month period. You will be asked to answer questions about some things your child can and cannot do. The questionnaire includes questions about your child's communication, gross motor, fine motor, problem solving, and personal-social skills.

If the questionnaire shows that your child is developing without concerns, we will provide some activities designed for use with ASQ-3 to encourage your child's development and will provide the next questionnaire at the appropriate time.

If the questionnaire shows some possible concerns, we will contact you about getting a more involved assessment for your child. Information will only be shared with other agencies with your written consent.

We look forward to your participation in our program!

Sincerely,

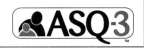

Consent Form

The first 5 years of life are very important for your child because this time sets the stage for success in school and later life. During infancy and early childhood, your child will gain many experiences and learn many skills. It is important to ensure that each child's development proceeds well during this period.

Please read the text below and mark the desired space to indicate whether you will participate in the screening/monitoring program.

◯ I have read the information provided about the Ages & Stages Questionnaires®, Third Edition (ASQ-3™), and I wish to have my child participate in the screening/monitoring program. I will fill out questionnaires about my child's development and will promptly return the completed questionnaires.

◯ I do not wish to participate in the screening/monitoring program. I have read the provided information about the Ages & Stages Questionnaires®, Third Edition (ASQ-3™), and understand the purpose of this program.

_____

Parent's or guardian's signature

_____

Date

Child's name: _____

Child's date of birth: _____

If child was born 3 or more weeks prematurely, # of weeks premature: _____

Child's primary physician: _____

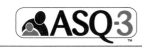

Demographic Information Sheet

Today's date: _____

Child's name (first /middle/last): _____

Child's date of birth (MM/DD/YYYY): _____ / _____ / _____

If child was born prematurely, # of weeks premature: _____

Child's gender: ◯ Male ◯ Female

Child's ethnicity: _____

Child's birth weight (pounds/ounces): _____

Parent/primary caregiver's name (first/middle/last): _____

Relationship to child: _____

Street address: _____

City: _____

State/Province: _____ ZIP/Postal code: _____

Home telephone: _____ Work telephone: _____

Cell/other telephone: _____

E-mail address: _____

Child's primary language: _____

Language(s) spoken in the home: _____

Child's primary care physician: _____

Clinic/location/practice name: _____

Clinic/practice mailing address: _____

City: _____

State/Province: _____ ZIP/Postal code: _____

Telephone: _____ Fax: _____

E-mail address: _____

Please list any medical conditions that your child has: _____

Please list any other agencies that are involved with your child/family: _____

_____

_____

Program Information

Child ID #: _____

Date of admission to program: _____

Child's adjusted age in months and days (if applicable): _____

Program ID #: _____

Program name: _____

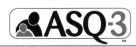

Dear Parent/Caregiver:

Thank you for participating in our child screening/monitoring program. The enclosed questionnaire from the Ages & Stages Questionnaires®, Third Edition (ASQ-3™), is a screening tool that will provide a quick check of your child's development. The information you supply will help reveal your child's strengths, uncover any areas of concern, and determine if there are community resources or services that may be useful for your child or your family.

We'd like to ask you first to fill out the enclosed family information sheet, which helps us be sure we have the most up-to-date information possible. Then, please try the activities on the questionnaire with your child and record what you see and any concerns you'd like to share.

Section 1: The first section of ASQ-3 includes five developmental areas. Each area has six questions that go from easier to more difficult skills. Your child may be able to do some but not all of the items. Read each question and mark

    Yes if your child is performing the skill

    Sometimes if your child is performing the skill but doesn't yet do it consistently

    Not yet if your child does not perform the skill yet

Here is a brief description of the five developmental areas screened with ASQ-3:

    Communication: Your child's language skills, both what your child understands and what he or she can say

    Gross motor: How your child uses his or her arms and legs and other large muscles for sitting, crawling, walking, running, and other activities

    Fine motor: Your child's hand and finger movement and coordination

    Problem solving: How your child plays with toys and solves problems

    Personal-social: Your child's self-help skills and interactions with others

Section 2: The Overall section asks important questions about your child's development and any concerns you may have about your child's development. Answer questions by marking **yes** or **no,** and if indicated, please explain your response.

Have fun completing this questionnaire with your child, and make sure he or she is rested, fed, and ready to play before you try the activities! Please be sure to send back the questionnaire within 2 weeks. If you have any questions or concerns, please contact me.

Sincerely,

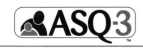

Dear Parent/Caregiver:

Thank you for completing the recent questionnaire from the Ages & Stages Questionnaires®, Third Edition (ASQ-3™), for your child. Your responses on the questionnaire show that your child's development appears to be progressing well.

Enclosed are activities designed for use with the ASQ that you may use to encourage your child's development.

You'll receive another questionnaire in _____ months. Please remember that it is very important to complete all items and return each questionnaire as soon as you finish it. Feel free to call us if you have any questions.

Sincerely,

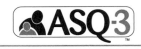

Dear Parent/Caregiver:

Thank you for completing the recent questionnaire from the Ages & Stages Questionnaires®, Third Edition (ASQ-3™), for your child. Your responses on the questionnaire show that your child's development should be monitored for a period of time. However, your child may benefit from playing some games and practicing skills in certain areas. We have included some suggestions for activities and games you can play with your child.

Enclosed are activities designed to be used with the ASQ that you may use to encourage your child's development.

We also suggest that you complete another ASQ-3 questionnaire _____ months. We will contact you with a reminder and send you an ASQ-3 questionnaires at that time.

Please get in touch if you have any questions.

Sincerely,

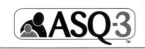

Dear Parent,

Would you please take a few minutes to evaluate our questionnaires? We appreciate your participation in our program and hope that our services have been helpful to you.

Please circle the number that best expresses your opinion.

1. Approximately how many minutes did it take you to fill out each questionnaire? _____ minutes. Did you consider this amount of time:

very little time			too much time
1	2	3	4

    Comments:

2. Did the questionnaires alert you to skills your child has or activities your child could do that you were not sure about?

very few			very many
1	2	3	4

    Comments:

3. After filling out the questionnaires, did you have any new ideas about how to interact or play with your child?

very few			very many
1	2	3	4

    Comments:

4. Were any items unclear or difficult to understand?

very few			very many
1	2	3	4

    Comments:

5. Did you enjoy participating in this program?

very little			very much
1	2	3	4

    Comments:

If you have any further comments about the questionnaires, please write them on the back of this form.

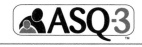

Estimados padres de familia o guardián,

Bienvenido/a a nuestro programa. Los primeros 5 años de vida son muy importantes para su(s) niño(s) porque éste es el periodo en el que se forma el marco que determinará su éxito en la escuela y, más adelante, en la vida. Durante la infancia, su(s) niño(s) tendrá(n) muchas experiencias y adquirirá(n) muchas habilidades. Es importante asegurarse de que todos los niños vayan desarrollándose de una forma sana durante este periodo.

Como parte de nuestro programa, le ofrecemos los Ages & Stages Questionnaires®, 3ª Edición (ASQ-3™), para ayudarle a monitorear el desarrollo de su niño/a. Nuestro deseo es ayudarle a proveer el mejor comienzo para su niño/a, y con gusto les invitamos a participar.

Usted recibirá un cuestionario de ASQ-3 en intervalos regulares que corresponden a la edad que tenga su niño/a. Cada cuestionario contiene una serie de preguntas sobre las habilidades de su niño/a en 5 áreas: comunicación, motora gruesa, motora fina, resolución de problemas, y socio-individual. A usted se le pedirá que intente hacer varias actividades con su niño/a, y que conteste las preguntas en base a las observaciones que hace de las habilidades actuales que tiene su niño/a.

Si los resultados del cuestionario muestran que el desarrollo de su niño/a está bien, le proporcionaremos actividades diseñadas para usarse con el ASQ-3 con el fin de seguir motivando un desarrollo sano, y le daremos el siguiente cuestionario en el momento apropiado.

Si los resultados muestran una área que nos da motivo de preocupación, le contactaremos para programar una evaluación más completa de su niño/a. No se compartirá la información con otras agencias a menos que usted nos lo autorice por escrito.

¡Esperamos con entusiasmo su participación en nuestro programa!

Cordialmente,

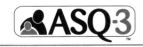

Hoja de autorizacion

Los primeros 5 años de vida son muy importantes para su niño porque éste es el periodo en el que se forma el marco que determinará su éxito en la escuela y, más adelante, en la vida. Durante la infancia, su niño tendrá muchas experiencias y adquirirá muchas habilidades. Es importante asegurarse de que todos los niños vayan desarrollándose de una forma sana durante este periodo.

Favor de leer el texto abajo y marcar con una palomita (✓) la casilla apropiada para indicar si usted acepta participar en el programa de evaluación/monitoreo.

○ He leído la información provista sobre los Ages & Stages Questionnaires®, 3ª Edición (ASQ-3™), y acepto que mi niño participe en el programa de evaluación/monitoreo. Completaré los cuestionarios sobre el desarrollo de mi niño y los devolveré al programa lo más pronto que pueda.

○ No acepto participar en el programa de evaluación/monitoreo. He leído la información provista sobre los Ages & Stages Questionnaires®, 3ª Edición (ASQ-3™), y me ha quedado claro el propósito de este programa.

_____

Firma del padre/madre o tutor

_____

Fecha

Nombre del niño/a: _____

Fecha de nacimiento del niño/a: _____

Si nació 3 semanas o más antes de la fecha proyectada, # de semanas que se adelantó:

_____

Médico familiar del niño/a: _____

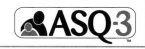

Información demográfica

Fecha de hoy: _____

Nombre del niño/a (primero/segundo/apellidos): _____

Fecha de nacimiento del niño/a (DD/MM/AAAA): _____ / _____ / _____

Si nació 3 semanas o más antes de la fecha proyectada, # de semanas que se adelantó: _____

Sexo del niño/a: ◯ Masculino   ◯ Femenino

Origen étnico del niño/a:_____

Peso al nacer del niño/a (libras/onzas): _____

Nombre del padre/madre o adulto a cargo (primero/segundo/apellidos):_____

_____

Parentesco con el niño/a: _____

Dirección: _____

Ciudad: _____

Estado/Provincia: _____   ZIP/ Código postal: _____

Teléfono de casa: _____   Teléfono de trabajo: _____

Teléfono celular/otro #: _____

Dirección de correo electrónico: _____

Idioma principal del niño/a: _____

Idioma(s) que se habla(n) en casa: _____

Nombre del médico familiar del niño/a: _____

Nombre de la clínica o consultorio/ubicación: _____

Dirección de la clinica o consultorio: _____

Ciudad: _____

Estado/Provincia: _____   ZIP/ Código postal: _____

Teléfono: _____   Fax: _____

Dirección de correo electrónico: _____

Favor de enumerar cualquier enfer medad que tenga su niño/a: _____

Favor de escribir el nombre de cualquier otra agencia al servicio del niño/la familia:

_____

_____

Información del programa

de identificación del niño: _____

Fecha de ingreso al programa: _____

Edad ajustada del niño en meses y días (si corresponde): _____

de identificación del programa: _____

Nombre del programa: _____

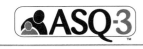

Estimados padres de familia o guardián:

Gracias por su participación en nuestro programa de evaluación/monitoreo de desarrollo infantil. El cuestionario que le proporcionamos es parte de la serie Ages & Stages Questionnaires®, 3ª Edición (ASQ-3™), y es una herramienta de evaluación que le permitirá vigilar el desarrollo de su niño/a de manera fácil y rápida. La información que usted provea nos permitirá detectar cuáles son las áreas de más fortaleza en el desarrollo de su niño/a, nos revelará si existen áreas de preocupación, y nos ayudará a determinar qué recursos de la comunidad le pueden ser útiles a usted o a su familia.

Quisiéramos pedirle primero que complete la hoja adjunta de información familiar, para asegurarnos de que los datos de nuestros archivos estén actualizados. Después, le invitamos a tratar de hacer las actividades del cuestionario con su niño/a, y a anotar sus observaciones, así como cualquier preocupación que desee mencionar.

Sección 1: La primera sección de ASQ-3 incluye cinco áreas de desarrollo. Para cada una de estas áreas, se pide que conteste seis preguntas que van de las habilidades más fáciles hasta las más complicadas. Es posible que su niño/a pueda hacer algunas de las actividades, pero no todas. Lea cada pregunta y marque

Sí si su niño/a hace la actividad

A veces si su niño/a hace la actividad pero todavía no la hace con regularidad

Todavía no si su niño/a aún no ha hecho la actividad

A continuación le proporcionamos una breve descripción de las cinco áreas de desarrollo que se evalúan con ASQ-3:

Comunicación: Las habilidades verbales de su niño/a, que incluyen la comprensión (lo que entiende) y la expresión (lo que puede decir)

Motora gruesa: La manera en que su niño/a utiliza los brazos, las piernas y los otros músculos grandes para sentarse, gatear, caminar, correr, y para hacer otras actividades

Motora fina: Los movimientos y la coordinación de las manos y los dedos

Resolución de problemas: La manera en que su niño/a juega con los juguetes y cómo soluciona problemas

Socio-individual: Las habilidades que tiene su niño/a de ayudarse a sí mismo/a y cómo interactúa con las demás personas

Sección 2: La sección titulada Observaciones Generales contiene preguntas importantes sobre el desarrollo de su niño/a y sobre cualquier preocupación que usted pueda tener al respecto. Para contestar las preguntas, marque *sí* o *no*, y si se le indica, por favor explique su respuesta.

¡Diviértase al completar este cuestionario con su niño/a, y asegúrese de que su niño/a haya descansado y comido y que esté listo/a para jugar antes de intentar hacer las actividades juntos! Le pedimos que devuelva el cuestionario dentro de 2 semanas. Si tiene cualquier preocupación o pregunta, no dude en comunicarse con conmigo.

Cordialmente,

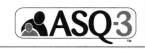

Estimados padres de familia o guardián:

Gracias por completar el cuestionario reciente de los Ages & Stages Questionnaires®, 3ª Edición (ASQ-3™), sobre su niño/a. Sus respuestas al cuestionario muestran que el desarrollo de su niño/a parece estar bien hasta ahora.

Hemos incluido algunas actividades diseñadas para usarse con el ASQ que usted puede hacer con su niño/a para ayudar a fomentar un desarrollo saludable.

Usted recibirá otro cuestionario en _____ meses. Por favor, tenga presente que es muy importante contestar todas las preguntas del cuestionario y devolvérnoslo tan pronto como lo haya completado. No dude en llamarnos si tiene cualquier pregunta.

Cordialmente,

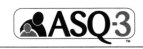

Estimados padres de familia o guardián:

Gracias por haber completado el cuestionario más reciente de los Ages & Stages Question-naires®, 3a Edición (ASQ-3™), sobre su niño. Sus respuestas al cuestionario indican que se debe monitorear el desarrollo de su niño/a por un periodo de tiempo.

Hemos incluido en esta carta algunas actividades diseñadas para usarse con el ASQ. Usted puede hacerlas con su niño/a para ayudar a fomentar un desarrollo saludable.

También, le recomendamos que complete otro cuestionario ASQ-3 en _____ meses. Le mandaremos un recordatorio, así como un nuevo cuestionario ASQ-3 cuando llegue el momento.

Por favor, no dude en comunicarse con nosotros si tiene cualquier pregunta.

Cordialmente,

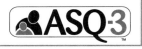

Estimado/a padre o madre de familia,

Le agradecemos su participación en el programa y esperamos que nuestros servicios le hayan sido de ayuda. ¿Podría tomar unos momentitos para evaluar nuestros cuestionarios?

Favor de trazar un círculo alrededor del número que mejor expresa su opinión.

1. Aproximadamente, ¿cuántos minutos tardó en completar cada cuestionario? _____ minutos. Le pareció que esto fue:

Muy poco tiempo			Demasiado tiempo
1	2	3	4

   Comentarios:

2. Al completar los cuestionarios, ¿reconoció habilidades que su niño/a tiene o notó algunas actividades que él/ella puede hacer que usted no había notado hasta ahora?

Muy pocas			Muchas
1	2	3	4

   Comentarios:

3. Después de completar los cuestionarios, ¿se le ocurrieron nuevas ideas de cómo interactuar o jugar con su niño/a?

Muy pocas			Muchas
1	2	3	4

   Comentarios:

4. ¿Había preguntas que le parecieron difíciles de entender?

Muy pocas			Muchas
1	2	3	4

   Comentarios:

5. ¿Disfrutó la experiencia de participar en el programa?

Poco			Mucho
1	2	3	4

   Comentarios:

Si usted tiene comentarios adicionales sobre los cuestionarios, favor de escribirlos al dorso de este formulario.

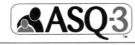

Dear Physician:

The parents or caregivers of your patient, _____,
have agreed to complete the Ages & Stages Questionnaires®, Third Edition (ASQ-3™),
as part of our developmental screening/monitoring program.

The ASQ-3 is a developmental screening and monitoring system designed for children
from birth through age 5. More information on use of ASQ-3 in a medical setting can be
found at www.agesandstages.com.

Parents or guardians are asked to respond to questions on the ASQ-3 about their child's
development at 2-, 4-, or 6-month intervals from birth to 5 years. They answer items
about activities their child can or cannot do. If the child obtains a score below the established cutoff on a questionnaire, the parent or guardian and the child's physician are notified so that further developmental support or assessment can be scheduled.

If you would like more information about our program, please feel free to contact me.

Sincerely,

_____

Child's name: _____

Parent/caregiver name(s): _____

Program name: _____

Program contact name: _____

Program telephone/e-mail: _____

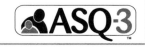

Dear Physician:

The ASQ-3 is a developmental screening and monitoring system designed for children from birth through age 5. More information on use of ASQ-3 in a medical setting can be found at www.agesandstages.com.

A questionnaire from the Ages & Stages Questionnaires®, Third Edition (ASQ-3™), was recently completed for your patient as follows:

Child's name: _____

Child's date of birth: _____

Date completed: _____

Questionnaire completed by: _____

○ The child's ASQ-3 scores are above the established cutoffs, and the child's development appears to be on schedule at this time. Our agency will continue to monitor this child's development.

○ This child's ASQ-3 scores were close to the established cutoffs (within the "monitoring zone"). We have informed the parents or caregivers that their child's progress will be monitored in the coming months.

○ The child's scores are below the established cutoffs in the following area(s):

   ○   Communication

   ○   Gross Motor

   ○   Fine Motor

   ○   Problem Solving

   ○   Personal-Social

   Further assessment with a professional may be needed. We have informed the parents or caregivers that their child would likely benefit from further assessment or developmental support, and we have referred them to the appropriate agency

Please contact us if you have any questions.

Sincerely,

ASQ-3 Master List

Program name/site: _____

Child name	Child ID #	Parent consent on file	Demographic information sheet	Physician participation letter	2 month ASQ-3	4 month ASQ-3	6 month ASQ-3	8 month ASQ-3	9 month ASQ-3	10 month ASQ-3	12 month ASQ-3	14 month ASQ-3	16 month ASQ-3	18 month ASQ-3	20 month ASQ-3	22 month ASQ-3	24 month ASQ-3	27 month ASQ-3	30 month ASQ-3	33 month ASQ-3	36 month ASQ-3	42 month ASQ-3	48 month ASQ-3	54 month ASQ-3	60 month ASQ-3

Instructions: After filling in the program name and site, program staff should be diligent in keeping the ASQ-3 Master List up to date. Every child who is participating in the program should be listed by name and ID number on this form or on one like it. In the spaces provided next to the child's name, record the date(s) any item in the top row was completed. For the questionnaires, program staff may also want to note S after the date for a Spanish questionnaire or "IC" for a questionnaire that was returned incomplete and therefore could not be scored. Programs that use the ASQ online management system (ASQ Pro, ASQ Enterprise) do not need to maintain an ASQ-3 Master List on paper (the information is stored in the online system instead).

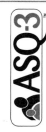

Implementation Progress Worksheet

Use the following scale for progress rating(s): 0, not applicable; 1, not begun; 2, partially begun or implemented; 3, fully completed or implemented.

Tasks	Actions					Projected completion date	Progress rating
	Personnel needs	Information needs	Supplies and equipment needs	Person/ agency responsible			
Phase I: Planning the screening/monitoring program							
1. Communicate with community partners.							
2. Include parental perspectives.							
3. Involve health care providers.							
4. Determine target population.							
5. Finalize goals and objectives.							
6. Determine program resources.							
7. Determine administration methods and settings.							
8. Determine depth and breadth of system.							
9. Select referral criteria.							
Phase II: Preparing, organizing, and managing the screening program							
10. Create a management system.							
11. Prepare questionnaires.							
12. Develop forms, letters, and a referral guide.							
13. Articulate screening policies and procedures.							
14. Provide staff training and support.							

(continued)

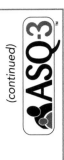

Implementation Progress Worksheet (continued)

Tasks	Actions					Progress rating
	Personnel needs	Information needs	Supplies and equipment needs	Person/ agency responsible	Projected completion date	
Phase III: Administering and scoring ASQ-3 and following up						
15. Select the appropriate ASQ-3 age interval.						
16. Assemble ASQ-3 materials.						
17. Support parents' completion of ASQ-3.						
18. Score the ASQ-3 and review the Overall section.						
19. Interpret ASQ-3 scores.						
20. Determine type of follow-up.						
21. Communicate results with families.						
Phase IV: Evaluating the screening/monitoring program						
22. Assess progress in establishing and maintaining the screening/monitoring program.						
23. Evaluate the program's effectiveness.						

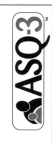

E

Materials List

The Materials List specifies toys and other materials needed to complete the ASQ-3. Each questionnaire interval is listed across the top; necessary materials are listed in the far left column. Under each questionnaire interval, a dot indicates that a particular item is needed to complete the questionnaire. Most items listed are portable and can be brought to the home or waiting room. There are a few items (e.g., steps, chair, stroller, shopping cart, wagon) that are difficult to transport. For these particular items, other objects may be substituted.

Many programs using the ASQ-3 in a home visit format have assembled toy kits with the assistance of this Materials List. Some of the items listed are likely to be found in a family home (i.e., cup, clothing), but the home visitor may find it useful to bring novel items from a toy kit to encourage child and parent participation. It also may be helpful to parents to have items on this list available in waiting rooms where parents are completing the ASQ-3.

ASQ-3 Materials List

ASQ INTERVAL	2	4	6	8	9	10	12	14	16	18	20	22	24	27	30	33	36	42	48	54	60
Puzzle—five- to seven-piece interlocking																			•		
Clothing with button/zipper																		•	•	•	•
Clothing—socks, hats, shoes								•	•						•	•	•	•	•	•	•
Clothing—coat, jacket, or shirt					•	•	•	•	•	•	•	•	•	•	•	•	•	•	•	•	•
Clothing—loose-fitting pants							•	•							•	•			•	•	•
Baby bottle		•			•	•	•	•	•	•	•	•	•								
Book with pictures					•	•	•	•	•	•	•	•	•	•	•	•	•	•	•		
Chair					•	•	•	•	•	•	•			•	•	•	•				
Cheerios or other small food			•		•	•	•	•	•	•		•					•			•	•
Scissors—child safe																				•	
Coloring book																				•	
Container (box or bowl)					•			•	•	•											•
Cookies or crackers				•	•	•															
Crib rail or supportive furniture				•	•	•	•														
Cup				•	•	•	•		•	•	•	•	•	•							
Doll or stuffed animal					•			•	•	•	•	•	•		•	•	•	•		•	•
Fork													•	•							
Ladder with rungs																					
Ball—large									•	•	•	•		•	•	•	•	•	•	•	•
Ball—small							•	•	•	•		•	•	•	•	•	•	•	•	•	•
Mirror	•		•	•											•	•	•	•			
Paper					•	•									•	•	•	•	•	•	•
Pencil, marker, pen, or crayon										•	•	•			•	•	•	•	•	•	•
String or shoelace					•	•	•								•	•	•				
Beads—1"–2"															•	•	•	•			
Blocks—1"–2"											•	•		•	•	•	•	•			
Wagon, stroller, or other toy on wheels															•	•	•				
Spoon									•	•	•	•		•	•	•	•	•	•		
Toy—small, easy to grasp	•		•	•	•	•	•	•	•	•	•			•	•						•
Windup toy or jar with lid												•		•	•	•					
Steps															•	•	•	•			
Light switch															•	•	•	•			
Toothbrush and toothpaste																			•	•	
Soap, water, and/or towel											•				•	•			•	•	•

ASQ-3™ User's Guide by Squires, Twombly, Bricker, & Potter. © 2009 Paul H. Brookes Publishing Co. All rights reserved.

F

Intervention Activities

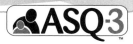

The intervention activities include games and other fun events for parents and caregivers and their young children. The activities are provided in English and Spanish. Each sheet contains activities that correspond to ages in the ASQ-3 intervals: 1–4 months old, 4–8 months old, 8–12 months old, 12–16 months old, 16–20 months old, 20–24 months old, 24–30 months old, 30–36 months old, 36–48 months old, 48–60 months old, and 60–66 months old. These sheets can be photocopied and used in monitoring programs in a variety of ways. The intervention activities are also available on the CD-ROM that accompanies the ASQ-3 (the activities are provided in English with the English version of the ASQ-3 and Spanish with the ASQ-3 Spanish).

The intervention activities suggestions can be mailed or given to parents with the ASQ-3, or they can be attached to a feedback letter along with the ASQ-3 results. They can be printed or enlarged onto colored paper. Parents can be encouraged to post the sheets on their refrigerator door or bulletin board and to try activities with their young children as time allows. If a child has difficulties in a particular developmental area, a service provider can star or underline certain games that might be particularly useful for parents to present. Similarly, service providers and family members can modify the activities to make them match the family's cultural setting and available materials. ***As with all activities for young children, these intervention activities should be supervised by an adult at all times.***

The intervention activities for 4- to 36-month-olds were compiled by Davidson, J., & Cripe, J. (1987). *Intervention activities*. Eugene: University of Oregon Infant Monitoring Project.

Activities for Infants 1–4 Months Old

Talk softly to your baby when feeding him, changing his diapers, and holding him. He may not understand every word, but he will know your voice and be comforted by it.	When you see your baby responding to your voice, praise and cuddle her. Talk back to her and see if she responds again.	Take turns with your baby when he makes cooing and gurgling sounds. Have a "conversation" back and forth with simple sounds that he can make.	Sing to your baby (even if you don't do it well). Repetition of songs and lullabies helps your baby to learn and listen.	With your baby securely in your arms or in a front pack, gently swing and sway to music that you are singing or playing on the radio.
Place a shatterproof mirror close to your baby where she can see it. Start talking, and tap the mirror to get her to look. The mirror will provide visual stimulation. Eventually your baby will understand her reflection.	Rock your baby gently in your arms and sing "Rock-a-bye Baby" or another lullaby. Sing your lullaby and swing your baby to the gentle rhythm.	Put a puppet or small sock on your finger. Say your baby's name while moving the puppet or sock up and down. See whether he follows the movement. Now move your finger in a circle. Each time your baby is able to follow the puppet, try a new movement.	With your baby on her back, hold a brightly colored stuffed animal above her head, in her line of vision. See if she watches the stuffed animal as you move it slowly back and forth.	Make sure your baby is positioned so that you can touch his feet. Gently play with his toes and feet, tickling lightly. Add the "This Little Piggy Went to Market" rhyme, touching a different toe with each verse.
Rest your baby, tummy down, on your arm, with your hand on her chest. Use your other hand to secure your baby—support her head and neck. Gently swing her back and forth. As she gets older, walk around to give her different views.	Hold your baby in your lap and softly shake a rattle on one side of his head, then the other side. Shake slowly at first, then faster. Your baby will search for the noise with his eyes.	Place your baby on her tummy with head to one side, on a blanket/towel on carpeted floor. Lie next to her to provide encouragement. Until she has the strength, have her spend equal time facing left and right. Make "tummy time" a little longer each day. Closely watch your baby in case she rests her face on the floor, which could restrict breathing. As her strength grows, she will be able to lift her head and push up on her arms, leading to rolling and crawling.	Lay your baby on his back and touch his arms and legs in different places. Make a "whooping" sound with each touch. Your baby may smile and anticipate the next touch by watching your hand. When you make each sound, you can also name the part of the body you touch.	In nice weather, take your baby on a nature walk through a park or neighborhood. Talk about everything you see. Even though she might not understand everything, she will like being outside and hearing your voice.
Read simple books to your baby. Even if he does not understand the story, he will enjoy being close and listening to you read.	With white paper and a black marker, create several easy-to-recognize images on each piece of paper. Start with simple patterns (diagonal stripes, bull's eyes, checkerboards, triangles). Place the pictures so that your baby can see them (8"–12" inches from her face). Tape these pictures next to her car seat or crib.	Lay your baby on his back on a soft, flat surface such as a bed or a blanket. Gently tap or rub your baby's hands and fingers while singing "Pat-a-Cake" or another nursery rhyme.	Gently shake a rattle or another baby toy that makes a noise. Put it in your baby's hand. See if she takes it, even for a brief moment.	Hold your baby closely, or lay him down on a soft, flat surface. Be close enough (8"–12") so that he can see you. Face to face, start with small movements (stick out your tongue, open your mouth with a wide grin). If you are patient, your baby may try to imitate you. As he gets older, you can try larger body movements with your head, hands, and arms. You can also try to imitate your baby.

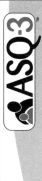

Activities for Infants 4–8 Months Old

Put a windup toy beside or behind your baby. Watch to see if your baby searches for the sound.	While sitting on the floor, place your baby in a sitting position inside your legs. Use your legs and chest to provide only as much support as your baby needs. This allows you to play with your baby while encouraging independent sitting.	Gently rub your baby with a soft cloth, a paper towel, or nylon. Talk about how things feel (soft, rough, slippery). Lotion feels good, too.	Let your baby see herself in a mirror. Place an unbreakable mirror on the side of your baby's crib or changing table so that she can watch. Look in the mirror with your baby, too. Smile and wave at your baby.
Common household items such as measuring spoons and measuring cups make toys with interesting sounds and shapes. Gently dangle and shake a set of measuring spoons or measuring cups where your baby can reach or kick at them. Let your baby hold them to explore and shake, too.	Fill a small plastic bottle (empty medicine bottle with child-proof cap) with beans or rice. Let your baby shake it to make noise.	Make another shaker using bells. Encourage your baby to hold one in each hand and shake them both. Watch to see if your baby likes one sound better than another.	Place your baby on her tummy with favorite toys or objects around but just slightly out of reach. Encourage her to reach out for toys and move toward them.
Play voice games. Talk with a high or low voice. Click your tongue. Whisper. Take turns with your baby. Repeat any sounds made by him. Place your baby so that you are face to face—your baby will watch as you make sounds.			
Fill an empty tissue box with strips of paper. Your baby will love pulling them out. (Do not use colored newsprint or magazines; they are toxic. Never use plastic bags or wrap.)	Safely attach a favorite toy to a side of your baby's crib, swing, or cradle chair for him to reach and grasp. Change toys frequently to give him new things to see and do.	Place your baby in a chair or car seat, or prop her up with pillows. Bounce and play with a flowing scarf or a large bouncing ball. Move it slowly up, then down or to the side, so that your baby can follow movement with her eyes.	With your baby lying on his back, place a toy within sight but out of reach, or move a toy across your baby's visual range. Encourage him to roll to get the toy.
Give your baby a spoon to grasp and chew on. It's easy to hold and feels good in the mouth. It's also great for banging, swiping, and dropping.			Play Peekaboo with hands, cloth, or a diaper. Put the cloth over your face first. Then let your baby hide. Pull the cloth off if your baby can't. Encourage her to play. Take turns.
Place your baby in a chair or car seat to watch everyday activities. Tell your baby what you are doing. Let your baby see, hear, and touch common objects. You can give your baby attention while getting things done.	Your baby will like to throw toys to the floor. Take a little time to play this "go and fetch" game. It helps your baby to learn to release objects. Give baby a box or pan to practice dropping toys into.	Once your baby starts rolling or crawling on her tummy, play "come and get me." Let your baby move, then chase after her and hug her when you catch her.	Place your baby facing you. Your baby can watch you change facial expressions (big smile, poking out tongue, widening eyes, raising eyebrows, puffing or blowing). Give your baby a turn. Do what your baby does.
Place your baby on your knee facing you. Bounce him to the rhythm of a nursery rhyme. Sing and rock with the rhythm. Help your baby bring his hands together to clap to the rhythm.			

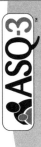

Activities for Infants 8–12 Months Old

ASQ-3

Let your baby feed himself. This gives your baby practice picking up small objects (cereal, cooked peas) and also gives him experience with textures in his hands and mouth. Soon your baby will be able to finger feed an entire meal.

A good pastime is putting objects in and out of containers. Give your baby plastic containers with large beads or blocks. Your baby may enjoy putting socks in and out of the sock drawer or small cartons (Jell-O, tuna or soup cans) on and off shelves.

Mirrors are exciting at this age. Let your baby pat and poke at herself in the mirror. Smile and make faces together in the mirror.

Your baby will begin using his index fingers to poke. Let your baby poke at a play telephone or busy box. Your baby will want to poke at faces. Name the body parts as your baby touches your face.

Your baby will be interested in banging objects to make noise. Give your baby blocks to bang, rattles to shake, or wooden spoons to bang on containers. Show your baby how to bang objects together.

Read baby books or colorful magazines by pointing and telling your baby what is in the picture. Let your baby pat pictures in the book.

Play hide-and-seek games with objects. Let your baby see you hide an object under a blanket, diaper, or pillow. If your baby doesn't uncover the object, just cover part of it. Help your baby find the object.

Play ball games. Roll a ball to your baby. Help your baby, or have a partner help him roll the ball back to you. Your baby may even throw the ball, so beach balls or Nerf balls are great for this game.

Put toys on a sofa or sturdy table so that your baby can practice standing while playing with the toys.

Find a big box that your baby can crawl in and out of. Stay close by and talk to your baby about what she is doing. "You went in! Now you are out!"

Let your baby play with plastic measuring cups, cups with handles, sieves and strainers, sponges, and balls that float in the bathtub. Bath time is a great learning time.

Play Pat-a-Cake with your baby. Clap his hands together or take turns. Wait and see if your baby signals you to start the game again. Try the game using blocks or spoons to clap and bang with.

Your baby will play more with different sounds like "la-la" and "da-da." Copy the sounds your baby makes. Add a new one and see if your baby tries it, too. Enjoy your baby's early attempts at talking.

Turn on a radio or stereo. Hold your baby in a standing position and let your baby bounce and dance. If your baby can stand with a little support, hold her hands and dance like partners.

Play imitation games like Peekaboo and So Big. Show pleasure at your baby's imitations of movements and sounds. Babies enjoy playing the same games over and over.

Let your baby make choices. Offer two toys or foods and see which one your baby picks. Encourage your baby to reach or point to the chosen object. Babies have definite likes and dislikes!

New places and people are good experiences for your baby, but these can be frightening. Let your baby watch and listen and move at her own speed. Go slowly. Your baby will tell you when she is ready for more.

Make a simple puzzle for your baby by putting blocks or Ping-Pong balls inside a muffin pan or egg carton.

You can make a simple toy by cutting a round hole in the plastic lid of a coffee can. Give your baby wooden clothes pins or Ping-Pong balls to drop inside.

Say "hi" and wave when entering a room with your baby. Encourage your baby to imitate. Help your baby wave to greet others. Waving "hi" and "bye" are early gestures.

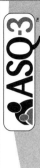

Activities for Infants 12–16 Months Old

ASQ:3

Babies love games at this age (Pat-a-Cake, This Little Piggy). Try different ways of playing the games and see if your baby will try it with you. Hide behind furniture or doors for Peekaboo; clap blocks or pan lids for Pat-a-cake.	Make puppets out of a sock or paper bag—one for you and one for your baby. Have your puppet talk to your baby or your baby's puppet. Encourage your baby to "talk" back.	To encourage your baby's first steps, hold your baby in standing position, facing another person. Have your baby step toward the other person to get a favorite toy or treat.	Give your baby containers with lids or different compartments filled with blocks or other small toys. Let your baby open and dump. Play "putting things back." This will help your baby learn how to release objects where he wants them.	Loosely wrap a small toy in a paper towel or facial tissue without tape. Your baby can unwrap it and find a surprise. Use tissue paper or wrapping paper, too. It's brightly colored and noisy.
Babies enjoy push and pull toys. Make your own pull toy by threading yogurt cartons, spools, or small boxes on a piece of yarn or soft string (about 2 feet long). Tie a bead or plastic stacking ring on one end for a handle.	Tape a large piece of drawing paper to a table. Show your baby how to scribble with large nontoxic crayons. Take turns making marks on the paper. It's also fun to paint with water.	Arrange furniture so that your baby can work her way around a room by stepping across gaps between furniture. This encourages balance in walking.	Babies continue to love making noise. Make sound shakers by stringing canning rims together or filling medicine bottles (with child-proof caps) with different-sounding objects like marbles, rice, salt, bolts, and so forth. Be careful to secure lids tightly.	This is the time your baby learns that adults can be useful! When your baby "asks" for something by vocalizing or pointing, respond to his signal. Name the object your baby wants and encourage him to communicate again—taking turns with each other in a "conversation."
Play the naming game. Name body parts, common objects, and people. This lets your baby know that everything has a name and helps her begin to learn these names.	Make an obstacle course with boxes or furniture so that your baby can climb in, on, over, under, and through. A big box can be a great place to sit and play.	Let your baby help you clean up. Play "feed the wastebasket" or "give it to Mommy or Daddy."	Make a surprise bag for your baby to find in the morning. Fill a paper or cloth bag with a soft toy, something to make a sound, a little plastic jar with a screw-top lid, or a book with cardboard pages.	Play "pretend" with a stuffed animal or doll. Show and tell your baby what the doll is doing (walking, going to bed, eating, dancing across a table). See if your baby will make the doll move and do things as you request. Take turns.
Cut up safe finger foods (do not use foods that pose a danger of your baby's choking) in small pieces and allow your baby to feed himself. It is good practice to pick up small things and feel different textures (bananas, soft crackers, berries).	Let your baby "help" during daily routines. Encourage your baby to "get" the cup and spoon for mealtime, to "find" shoes and coat for dressing, and to "bring" the pants or diaper for changing. Following directions is an important skill for your baby to learn.	Your baby is learning that different toys do different things. Give your baby a lot of things to roll, push, pull, hug, shake, poke, turn, stack, spin, and stir.	Most babies enjoy music. Clap and dance to the music. Encourage your baby to practice balance by moving forward, around, and back. Hold her hands for support, if needed.	Prepare your baby for a future activity or trip by talking about it beforehand. Your baby will feel like a part of what is going on rather than being just an observer. It may also help reduce some fear of being "left behind."

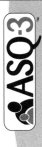

Activities for Toddlers 16–20 Months Old

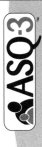ASQ·3

Toddlers love to play in water. Put squeezable objects in the bathtub, such as sponges or squeeze bottles, along with dump-and-pour toys (cups, bowls).	Toddlers are excited about bubbles. Let your toddler try to blow bubbles or watch you blow bubbles through a straw. Bubbles are fun to pop and chase, too.	Pretend play becomes even more fun at this age. Encourage your toddler to have a doll or stuffed toy do what he does—walk, go to bed, dance, eat, and jump. Include the doll in daily activities or games.	Make instant pudding together. Let your toddler "help" by dumping pudding, pouring milk, and stirring. The results are good to eat or can be used for finger painting.	Use boxes or buckets for your toddler to throw bean bags or balls into. Practice overhand release of the ball or bean bag.
Play Hide and Seek. Your toddler can hide with another person or by herself for you to find. Then take your turn to hide and let your toddler find you.	Toddlers love movement. Take him to the park to ride on rocking toys, swings, and small slides. You may want to hold your toddler in your lap on the swing and on the slide at first.	Sing action songs together such as "Ring Around the Rosy," "Itsy-Bitsy Spider," and "This Is the Way We Wash Our Hands." Do actions together. Move with the rhythm. Wait for your toddler to anticipate the action.	Put favorite toys in a laundry basket slightly out of reach of your toddler or in a clear container with a tight lid. Wait for your toddler to request the objects, giving her a reason to communicate. Respond to her requests.	Your toddler may become interested in "art activities." Use large nontoxic crayons and a large pad of paper. Felt-tip markers are more exciting with their bright colors. Let your toddler scribble his own picture as you make one.
A favorite pull toy often is a small wagon or an old purse for collecting things. Your toddler can practice putting objects in and out of it. It can also be used to store favorite items.	Make a picture book by putting common, simple pictures cut from magazines into a photo album. Your toddler will enjoy photos of herself and family members. Pictures of pets are favorites, too.	Toddlers are interested in playing with balls. Use a beach ball to roll, throw, and kick.	Play the "What's that?" game by pointing to clothing, toys, body parts, objects, or pictures and asking your toddler to name them. If your toddler doesn't respond, name it for him and encourage imitation of the words.	Fill a plastic tub with cornmeal or oatmeal. Put in kitchen spoons, strainers, measuring cups, funnels, or plastic containers. Toddlers can fill, dump, pour, and learn about textures and use of objects as tools. Tasting won't be harmful.
Toddlers will begin putting objects together. Simple puzzles (separate pieces) with knobs are great. Putting keys into locks and letters into mailbox slots is fun, too.	Get two containers (coffee cups or cereal bowls) that look the same and a small toy. Hide the toy under one container while your toddler watches. Ask her, "Where did it go?" Eventually you can play the old shell game (moving the containers after you hide the toy).	Help your toddler sort objects into piles. He can help you sort laundry (put socks in one pile and shirts in another). Play "clean up" games. Have your toddler put toys on specified shelves or boxes.	Save milk cartons or gelatin or pudding boxes. Your toddler can stack them to make towers. You can also stuff grocery bags with newspapers and tape them shut to make big blocks.	Lay out your toddler's clothes on the bed before dressing. Ask her to give you a shirt, pants, shoes, and socks. This is an easy way to learn the names of common items.

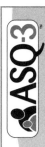

Activities for Toddlers 20–24 Months Old

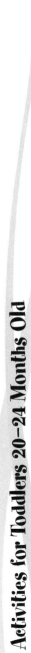

Toddlers enjoy looking at old pictures of themselves. Tell simple stories about him as you look at the pictures. Talk about what was happening when the picture was taken.

A good body parts song is "Head, Shoulders, Knees, and Toes." Get more detailed with body parts by naming teeth, eyebrows, fingernails, and so forth.

Make grocery sack blocks by filling large paper grocery sacks about half full with shredded or crumpled newspaper. Fold the top of the sack over and tape it shut. Your toddler will enjoy tearing and crumpling the paper and stuffing the sacks. The blocks are great for stacking and building. Avoid newsprint contact with mouth. Wash hands after this activity.

Playing beside or around other children the same age is fun but usually requires adult supervision. Trips to the park are good ways to begin practicing interacting with other children.

Cut a rectangular hole in the top of a shoebox. Let your toddler insert an old deck of playing cards or used envelopes. The box is easy storage for your toddler's "mail."

Make your toddler an outdoor "paint" set by using a large wide paint brush and a bowl or bucket of water. Your toddler will have fun "painting" the side of the house, a fence, or the front porch.

"Dress up" clothes offer extra practice for putting on and taking off shirts, pants, shoes, and socks. Toddlers can fasten big zippers and buttons.

Play the "show me" game when looking at books. Ask your toddler to find an object in a picture. Take turns. Let your toddler ask you to find an object in a picture. Let him turn the pages.

Set up your own bowling game using plastic tumblers, tennis ball cans, or empty plastic bottles for bowling pins. Show your toddler how to roll the ball to knock down the pins. Then let your toddler try.

Turn objects upside down (books, cups, shoes) and see if your toddler notices they're wrong and turns them back the right way. Your toddler will begin to enjoy playing "silly" games.

Put small containers, spoons, measuring cups, funnels, a bucket, shovels, and a colander into a sandbox. Don't forget to include cars and trucks to drive on sand roads.

Add a few Ping-Pong balls to your toddler's bath toys. Play a "pop up" game by showing your toddler how balls pop back up after holding them under the water and letting go.

Many everyday items (socks, spoons, shoes, mittens) can help your toddler learn about matching. Hold up an object, and ask if she can find one like yours. Name the objects while playing the game.

Give your toddler some of your old clothes (hats, shirts, scarves, purses, necklaces, sunglasses) to use for dress up. Make sure your toddler sees herself in the mirror. Ask her to tell you who is all dressed up.

Rhymes and songs with actions are popular at this age. "Itsy-Bitsy Spider," "I'm a Little Teapot," and "Where Is Thumbkin?" are usual favorites. Make up your own using your toddler's name in the song.

Clean plastic containers with push or screw-on lids are great places to "hide" a favorite object or treat. Toddlers will practice pulling and twisting them to solve the "problem" of getting the object. Watch to see if your toddler asks you to help.

Hide a loudly ticking clock or a softly playing transistor radio in a room and have your child find it. Take turns by letting him hide and you find.

Use plastic farm animals or stuffed animals to tell the Old McDonald story. Use sound effects!

Make your own playdough by mixing 2 cups flour and 3/4 cup salt. Add 1/2 cup water and 2 tablespoons salad oil. Knead well until it's smooth; add food coloring, and knead until color is fully blended. Toddlers will love squishing, squeezing, and pounding the dough.

Make a book by pasting different textures on each page. Materials such as sandpaper, feathers, cotton balls, nylon, silk, and buttons lend themselves to words such as rough, smooth, hard, and soft.

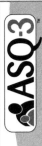

Add actions to your child's favorite nursery rhymes. Easy action rhymes include "Here We Go 'Round the Mulberry Bush," "Jack Be Nimble," "This Is the Way We Wash Our Clothes," "Ring Around the Rosy," and "London Bridge."	During sandbox play, try wetting some of the sand. Show your child how to pack the container with the wet sand and turn it over to make sand structures or cakes.	Wrap tape around one end of a piece of yarn to make it stiff like a needle and put a large knot at the other end. Have your child string large elbow macaroni, buttons, spoons, or beads. Make an edible necklace out of Cheerios.	Children at this age love outings. One special outing can be going to the library. The librarian can help you find appropriate books. Make a special time for reading (like bedtime stories).	Play a jumping game when you take a walk by jumping over the cracks in the sidewalk. You may have to hold your child and help him jump over at first.
Take time to draw with your child when she wants to get out paper and crayons. Draw large shapes and let your child color them in. Take turns.	Children at this age love to pretend and really enjoy it when you can pretend with them. Pretend you are different animals, like a dog or cat. Make animal sounds and actions. Let your child be the pet owner who pets and feeds you.	Add an old catalog or two to your child's library. It's a good "picture" book for naming common objects.	Give your child soap, a washcloth, and a dishpan of water. Let your child wash a "dirty" doll, toy dishes, or doll clothes. It's good practice for hand washing and drying.	Make "sound" containers using plastic Easter eggs or pantyhose eggs. Fill eggs with noisy objects like sand, beans, or rice and tape the eggs shut. Have two eggs for each sound. Help your child match sounds and put them back in an egg carton together.
Show your child how to make snakes or balls or how to roll out pancakes with a small rolling pin using playdough. Use large cookie cutters to make new playdough shapes.	Try a new twist to fingerpainting. Use whipping cream on a washable surface (cookie sheet, Formica table). Help your child spread it around and draw pictures with your fingers. Add food coloring to give it some color.	Your child will begin to be able to make choices. Help him choose what to wear each day by giving a choice between two pairs of socks, two shirts, and so forth. Give choices at other times like snack or mealtime (two kinds of drink, cracker, etc.).	Enhance listening skills by playing compact discs or cassettes with both slow and fast music. Songs with speed changes are great. Show your child how to move fast or slow with the music. (You might find children's cassettes at your local library.)	Children can find endless uses for boxes. A box big enough for your child to fit in can become a car. An appliance box with holes cut for windows and a door can become your child's playhouse. Decorating the boxes with crayons, markers, or paints can be a fun activity to do together.
Play "Follow the Leader." Walk on tiptoes, walk backward, and walk slow or fast with big steps and little steps.		Action is an important part of a child's life. Play a game with a ball where you give directions and your child does the actions, such as "Roll the ball." Kick, throw, push, bounce, and catch are other good actions. Take turns giving the directions.	Make an obstacle course using chairs, pillows, or large cartons. Tell your child to crawl over, under, through, behind, in front of, or between the objects. Be careful arranging so that the pieces won't tip and hurt your child.	Collect little and big things (balls, blocks, plates). Show and describe (big/little) the objects. Ask your child to give you a big ball, then all of the big balls. Do the same for little. Another big/little game is making yourself big by stretching your arms up high and making yourself little by squatting down.

ASQ-3™ User's Guide by Squires, Twombly, Bricker, & Potter. © 2009 Paul H. Brookes Publishing Co. All rights reserved.

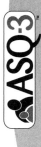

Activities for Children 30–36 Months Old

Tell or read a familiar story and pause frequently to leave out a word, asking your child to "fill it in." For example, Little Red Riding Hood said, "Grandmother, what big _____ you have."

Teach somersaults by doing one yourself first. Then help your child do one. Let her try it alone. Make sure furniture is out of the way. You may want to put some pillows on the floor for safety.

Give a cup to your child. Use bits of cereal or fruit and place one in your child's cup ("one for you") and one in your cup ("one for me"). Take turns. Dump out your child's cup and help count the pieces. This is good practice for early math skills.

Put an old blanket over a table to make a tent or house. Pack a "picnic" sack for your camper. Have your child take along a pillow on the "camp out" for a nap. Flashlights are especially fun.

Get a piece of butcher paper large enough for your child to lie on. Draw around your child's body to make an outline. Don't forget fingers and toes. Talk about body parts and print the words on the paper. Let your child color the poster. Hang the poster on a wall in your child's room.

Children at this age may be interested in creating art in different ways. Try cutting a potato in half and carving a simple shape or design for your child to dip in paint and then stamp onto paper.

Add water to tempera paint to make it runny. Drop some paint on a paper and blow through a straw to move the paint around the paper, or fill an old roll-on deodorant bottle with watered-down paint. Your child can roll color onto the paper.

Trace around simple objects with your child. Use cups of different sizes, blocks, or your child's and your hands. Using felt-tip markers or crayons of different colors makes it even more fun.

Have your child help you set the table. First, have your child place the plates, then cups, and then napkins. By placing one at each place, he will learn one-to-one correspondence. Show your child where the utensils should be placed.

Collect empty boxes (cereal, TV dinners, egg cartons) and help your child set up her own grocery store.

Help your child learn new words to describe objects in everyday conversations. Describe by color, size, and shape (the blue cup, the big ball). Also, describe how things move (a car goes fast, a turtle moves slowly) and how they feel (ice cream is cold, soup is hot).

Make your own puzzles by cutting out magazine pictures of whole people. Have your child help glue pictures onto cardboard. Cut pictures into three pieces by cutting curvy lines. Head, trunk, and legs make good pieces for your child to put together.

Dribble different colors of paint in the middle or on one side of a paper. Fold the paper in half. Let your child open the paper to see the design it makes.

A good game for trips in the car is to play a matching game with a set of Old Maid cards. Place a few different cards in front of your child. Give him a card that matches one displayed and ask him to find the card like the one you gave him.

Cut pictures out of magazines to make two groups such as dogs, food, toys, or clothes. Have two boxes ready and put a picture of a dog in one and of food in the other. Have your child put additional pictures in the right box, helping her learn about categories.

Cut a stiff paper plate to make a hand paddle and show your child how to use it to hit a balloon. See how long your child can keep the balloon in the air or how many times he can hit it back to you. This activity helps develop large body and eye–hand coordination. Always carefully supervise when playing with balloons.

To improve coordination and balance, show your child the "bear walk" by walking on hands and feet, keeping the legs and arms straight. Try the "rabbit hop" by crouching down and then jumping forward.

Encourage your child to try the "elephant walk," bending forward at the waist and letting your arms (hands clasped together) swing freely while taking slow and heavy steps. This is great to do with music.

Make a poster of your child's favorite things using pictures from old magazines. Use safety scissors and paste or a glue stick to allow your child to do it independently, yet safely.

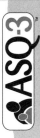

Activities for Children 36–48 Months Old

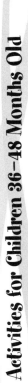

Make a book "about me" for your child. Save family pictures, leaves, magazine pictures of a favorite food, and drawings your child makes. Put them in a photo album, or glue onto sheets of paper and staple together to make a book.	Make a bird feeder using peanut butter and bird seed. Help your child find a pine cone or a piece of wood to spread peanut butter on. Roll in or sprinkle with seeds and hang in a tree or outside a window. While your child watches the birds, ask her about the number, size, and color of the different birds that visit.	Grow a plant. Choose seeds that sprout quickly (beans or peas), and together with your child place the seeds in a paper cup, filling almost to the top with dirt. Place the seeds 1/2 inch under the soil. Put the cup on a sunny windowsill and encourage your child to water and watch the plant grow.
While cooking or eating dinner, play the "more or less" game with your child. Ask who has more potatoes and who has less. Try this using same-size glasses or cups, filled with juice or milk.	Cut out some large paper circles and show them to your child. Talk with your child about things in her world that are "round" (a ball, the moon). Cut the circle in half, and ask her if she can make it round again. Next, cut the circle into three pieces, and so forth.	During bath time, play Simon Says to teach your child names of body parts. First, you can be "Simon" and help your child wash the part of his body that "Simon says." Let your child have a turn to be "Simon," too. Be sure to name each body part as it is washed and give your child a chance to wash himself.
When your child is getting dressed, encourage her to practice with buttons and zippers. Play a game of Peekaboo to show her how buttons go through the holes. Pretend the zipper is a choo-choo train going "up and down" the track.	Practice following directions. Play a silly game where you ask your child to do two or three fun or unusual things in a row. For example, ask him to "Touch your elbow and then run in a circle" or "Find a book and put it on your head."	Encourage your child's "sharing skills" by making a play corner in your home. Include only two children to start (a brother, sister, or friend) and have a few of the same type of toys available so that the children don't have to share all of the time. Puppets or blocks are good because they encourage playing together. If needed, use an egg or oven timer with a bell to allow the children equal time with the toys.
Find large pieces of paper or cardboard for your child to draw on. Using crayons, pencils, or markers, play a drawing game where you follow his lead by copying exactly what he draws. Next, encourage your child to copy your drawings, such as circles or straight lines.	When reading or telling a familiar story for bedtime, stop and leave out a word. Wait for your child to "fill in the blank."	Make a necklace you can eat by stringing Cheerios or Froot Loops on a piece of yarn or string. Wrap a short piece of tape around the end of the string to make a firm tip for stringing.

Before bedtime, look at a magazine or children's book together. Ask your child to point to pictures as you name them, such as "Where is the truck?" Be silly and ask him to point with an elbow or foot. Ask him to show you something that is round or something that goes fast.	Play a matching game. Make two sets of 10 or more pictures. You can use pictures from two copies of the same magazine or a deck of playing cards. Lay the pictures face up and ask your child to find two that are the same. Start with two picture sets and gradually add more.
Talk about the number 3. Read stories that have 3 in them (The Three Billy Goats Gruff, Three Little Pigs, The Three Bears). Encourage your child to count to 3 using similar objects (rocks, cards, blocks). Talk about being 3 years old. After your child gets the idea, move up to the numbers 4, 5, and so forth as long as your child is interested.	Put out several objects that are familiar to your child (brush, coat, banana, spoon, book). Ask your child to show you which one you can eat or which one you wear outside. Help your child put the objects in groups that go together, such as "things that we eat" and "things that we wear."
Listen for sounds. Find a cozy spot, and sit with your child. Listen and identify all of the sounds that you hear. Ask your child if it is a loud or soft sound. Try this activity inside and outside your home.	Make an adventure path outside. Use a garden hose, rope, or piece of chalk and make a "path" that goes under the bench, around the tree, and along the wall. Walk your child through the path first, using these words. After she can do it, make a new path or have your child make a path.
Listen and dance to music with your child. You can stop the music for a moment and play the "freeze" game, where everyone "freezes," or stands perfectly still, until you start the music again. Try to "freeze" in unusual positions for fun.	Make long scarves out of fabric scraps, old dresses, or old shirts by tearing or cutting long pieces. Use material that is lightweight. Hold on to the edge of the scarf, twirl around, run, and jump.

ASQ-3™ User's Guide by Squires, Twombly, Bricker, & Potter. © 2009 Paul H. Brookes Publishing Co. All rights reserved.

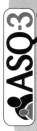 **ASQ-3**™

Activities for Children 48–60 Months Old

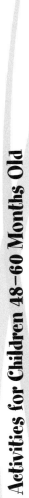

Play the "who, what, and where" game. Ask your child who works in a school, what is in a school, and where is the school. Expand on your child's answers by asking more questions. Ask about other topics, like the library, bus stop, or post office.

When you are setting the table for a meal, play the "what doesn't belong" game. Add a small toy or other object next to the plate and eating utensils. Ask your child if she can tell you what doesn't belong here. You can try this game any time of the day. For example, while brushing your child's hair, set out a brush, barrette, comb, and a ball.

Let your child help prepare a picnic. Show him what he can use for the picnic (bread, peanut butter, and apples). Lay out sandwich bags and a lunch box, basket, or large paper bag. Then go have fun on the picnic.

On a rainy day, pretend to open a shoe store. Use old shoes, paper, pencils, and a chair to sit down and try on the shoes. You can be the customer. Encourage your child to "write" your order down. Then she can take a turn being the customer and practice trying on and buying shoes.

Play the "guess what will happen" game to encourage your child's problem-solving and thinking skills. For example, during bath time, ask your child, "What do you think will happen if I turn on the hot and cold water at the same time?" or "What would happen if I stacked the blocks to the top of the ceiling?"

Play "bucket hoops." Have your child stand about 6 feet away and throw a medium-size ball at a large bucket or trash can. For fun outdoors on a summer day, fill the bucket with water.

Write your child's name often. When your child finishes drawing a picture, be sure to put his name on it and say the letters as you write them. If your child is interested, encourage him to name and/or to copy the letters. Point out the letters in your child's name throughout the day on cereal boxes, sign boards, and books.

Invite your child to play a counting game. Using a large piece of paper, make a simple game board with a straight path. Use dice to determine the count. Count with your child, and encourage her to hop the game piece to each square, counting each time the piece touches down.

Make a person with playdough or clay using sticks, buttons, toothpicks, beads, and any other small items. Start with a playdough (or clay) head and body and use the objects for arms, legs, and eyes. Ask your child questions about his person.

Encourage your child to learn her full name, address, and telephone number. Make it into a singing or rhyming game for fun. Ask your child to repeat it back to you when you are riding in the car or on the bus.

Cut out three small, three medium, and three large circles. Color each set of circles a different color (or use colored paper for each). Your child can sort the circles by color or by size. You can also ask your child about the different sizes. For example, ask your child, "Which one is smallest?" Try this game using buttons removed from an old shirt.

Go on a walk and pick up things you find. Bring the items home and help your child sort them into groups. For example, groups can include rocks, paper, or leaves. Encourage your child to start a collection of special things. Find a box or special place where he can display the collection.

Play a picture guessing game. Cover a picture in a familiar book with a sheet of paper and uncover a little at a time until your child has guessed the picture.

Let your child help you prepare a meal. She can spread peanut butter and jelly, peel a banana, cut with a butter knife, pour cereal, and add milk (using a small container). Never give her a task involving the stove or oven without careful supervision.

"Write" and mail a letter to a friend or relative. Provide your child with paper, crayons or pencil, and an envelope. Let your child draw, scribble, or write; or he can tell you what to write down. When your child is finished, let him fold the letter to fit in the envelope, lick, and seal. You can write the address on the front. Be sure to let him decorate the envelope as well. After he has put the stamp on, help mail the letter.

Play "circus." Find old, colorful clothes and help your child put on a circus show. Provide a rope on the ground for the high wire act, a sturdy box to stand on to announce the acts, fun objects for a magic act, and stuffed animals for the show. Encourage your child's imagination and creativity in planning the show. Don't forget to clap.

Take a pack of playing cards and choose four or five matching sets. Lay the cards out face up, and help your child to find the pairs. Talk about what makes the pairs of cards the "same" and "different."

Make bubbles. Use 1/4 cup dishwashing liquid (Dawn or Joy works best) and 2 2/3 cups water. Use straws to blow bubbles on a cookie sheet. Or make a wand by stringing two pieces of a drinking straw onto a string or piece of yarn. Tie the ends of the string together to make a circle. Holding onto the straw pieces, dip the string in the bubble mixture. Pull it out and gently move forward or backward. You should see lovely, big bubbles.

Make a bean bag to catch and throw. Fill the toe of an old sock or pantyhose with 3/4 cup dry beans. Sew the remaining side or tie it off with a rubber band. Play "hot potato" or simply play catch. Encourage your child to throw the ball overhand and underhand.

Pretend to be an animal. Encourage your child to use her imagination and become a kitty. You can ask, "What do kitties like to eat?" or "Where do kitties live?" Play along, and see how far the game can go.

Activities for Children 60–66 Months Old

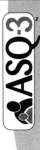 ASQ-3

Make a nature collage. Collect leaves, pebbles, and small sticks from outside and glue them on a piece of cardboard or stiff paper. (Cereal and cracker boxes can be cut up and used as cardboard.)	Practice writing first names of friends, toys, and relatives. Your child may need to trace the letters of these names at first. Be sure to write in large print letters.	Encourage dramatic play. Help your child act out his favorite nursery rhyme, cartoon, or story. Use large, old clothes for costumes.	Play simple ball games such as kickball. Use a large (8"–12") ball, and slowly roll it toward your child. See if your child can kick the ball and run to "first base."	When reading stories to your child, let her make up the ending, or retell favorite stories with "silly" new endings that she makes up.
Let your child help you with simple cooking tasks such as mashing potatoes, making cheese sandwiches, and fixing a bowl of cereal. Afterward, see if he can tell you the order that you followed to cook and mash the potatoes or to get the bread out of the cupboard and put the cheese on it. Supervise carefully when your child is near a hot stove.	Play "20 Questions." Think of an animal. Let your child ask 20 yes/no questions about the animal until she guesses what animal it is. (You may need to help your child to ask yes/no questions at first.) Now let your child choose an animal and you ask the 20 questions. You can also use other categories such as food, toys, and people.	You can play "license plate count-up" in the car or on the bus. Look for a license plate that contains the number 1. Then try to find other plates with 2, 3, 4, and so forth, up to 10. When your child can play "count-up," play "count-down," starting with the number 9, then 8, 7, 6, and so forth, down to 1.	Practice pretend play or pantomime. Here are some things to act out: 1) eating hot pizza with stringy cheese; 2) winning a race; 3) finding a giant spider; 4) walking in thick, sticky mud; and 5) making footprints in wet sand.	Make a simple concentration game with two or three pairs of duplicate playing cards (two king of hearts), or make your own cards out of duplicate pictures or magazine ads. Start with two or three pairs of cards. Turn them face down and mix them up. Let your child turn two cards over to see if they match. If they don't, turn the cards face down again. You can gradually increase to playing with more pairs of cards.
Make an obstacle course either inside or outside your home. You can use cardboard boxes for jumping over or climbing through, broomsticks for laying between chairs for "limbo" (going under), and pillows for walking around. Let your child help lay out the course. After a couple of practice tries, have him complete the obstacle course as quickly as possible. Then try hopping or jumping the course.	After washing hands, practice writing letters and numbers in pudding or thinned mashed potatoes spread on a cookie sheet or cutting board. Licking fingers is allowed!	Play mystery sock. Put a common household item in a sock. Tie off the top of the sock. Have your child feel the sock and guess what is inside. Take turns guessing what's inside.	Make color rhymes. Take turns rhyming a color and a word: blue, shoe; red, bed; yellow, fellow. You can also rhyme with names (Dad, sad; Jack, sack). Take turns with the rhyming.	Make an "I can read" poster. Cut out names your child can read—fast-food restaurant names, names from cereal cartons, and other foods. You can write your child's name, names of relatives, and names of friends on pieces of paper and put them on the poster. Add to the poster as your child learns to read more names.
Play "what doesn't belong?" Let your child find the word that doesn't belong in a list of six or seven spoken words. The one that doesn't belong can be the word that doesn't rhyme or the word that is from a different category. Some examples are 1) fly, try, by, coat, sigh, my; 2) Sam, is, ram, am, spam, ham; 3) red, orange, purple, green, yellow, beetle; 4) spoon, fork, shirt, pan, spatula, knife. Have your child give three to four words with one that doesn't belong.	Make puppets out of ice cream sticks, paper bags, socks, or egg carton cups. Decorate the puppets with yarn, pens, buttons, and colored paper. Make a puppet stage by turning a coffee table or card table on its side. Be the audience while your child crouches behind the table and puts on a puppet show.	Play the "memory" game. Put five or six familiar objects on a table. Have your child close her eyes. Remove one object, and rearrange the rest. Ask your child which object is missing. Take turns finding the missing object.	Play the old shell game. Get four cups or glasses that you cannot see through. Find a small ball, object, or edible item such as a raisin or cracker that fits under the cups. Have your child watch as you place the object under one of the cups and move all of the cups around. Have your child try to remember which cup the object is under. Have your child take a turn moving the objects while you guess.	Play "mystery sound." Select household items that make distinct sounds such as a clock, cereal box, metal lid (placed on a pan), and potato chip bag. Put a blindfold on your child and have him try to guess which object made the sound. Take turns with your child.

ASQ-3™ User's Guide by Squires, Twombly, Bricker, & Potter. © 2009 Paul H. Brookes Publishing Co. All rights reserved.

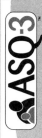

ACTIVIDADES PARA BEBÉS DE ENTRE 1 Y 4 MESES DE EDAD

Hable con su bebé en un tono bajo y suave al darle de comer, cambiarla, o cuando la cargue en brazos. Puede que no entienda todo lo que le dice, pero sí reconocerá su voz y se sentirá reconfortada al escucharla.	Cuando vea que su bebé reaccione al sonido de su voz, festéjelo y hágale nuevo para ver si le vuelve a responder.	Cuando su bebé balbucee o gorjee, tome turnos con ella para "comunicarse". "Converse" con ella hablando y respondiendo con sonidos sencillos que ella pueda hacer.	Cántele a su bebé (aunque crea que no sabe cantar). Repetir las canciones de cuna y las rimas infantiles le ayuda a escuchar y a aprender.	Tome a su bebé en brazos o póngalo en el canguro o mochila porta-bebé, asegurándose de que esté bien sujetado. Baile con su bebé, haciendo movimientos suaves al ritmo de la música de la radio o de las melodías que usted le canta.
Acueste a su bebé en su cuna. Ate o sostenga un espejo irrompible a un lado de la cuna donde ella alcance a verlo. Empiece a hablarle, y dé unos golpecitos al espejo para que lo mire. El espejo será un estimulo visual. Después de un tiempo su bebé entenderá lo que es su reflejo.	Meza a su bebé suavemente en sus brazos y cántele "A la rurru niño" o cualquier otra canción de cuna. Entone la melodía y balancéelo ligeramente de lado a lado al compás de la canción.	Póngase un títere de mano (botita o calcetín de bebé) en el dedo. Diga el nombre de su bebé mientras que mueve el dedo hacia arriba y hacia abajo. Vea si ella sigue el movimiento con la vista. Ahora, mueva su dedo como formando un círculo. Cada vez que su bebé logre seguir el movimiento del títere, intente hacer un movimiento diferente.	Cuando está acostado boca arriba su bebé, sostenga un animalito de peluche de colores llamativos encima de su cabeza, donde él lo alcance a ver. Vea si lo mira mientras que usted lo mueve lentamente de lado a lado.	Ponga a su bebé en una posición que le permita tocarle los pies. Juegue delicadamente con sus pies y los dedos del pie, haciéndole cosquillitas. Dígale la rima infantil "Este cerdito fue al mercado" tocándole los dedos del pie uno por uno con cada frase.
Recueste a su bebé boca abajo sobre su brazo, poniéndole la mano en el pecho y sosteniéndole la cabeza y cuello con la otra mano para que se sienta segura. En esta posición, balancéela delicadamente de lado a lado. Cuando sea más grande, camine por la casa con ella en esta posición para que vea diferentes espacios.	Siéntese con su bebé en su regazo y suene ligeramente una sonaja, primero de un lado de su cabeza y después del otro. Suene la sonaja lentamente al principio, luego más rápido. Su bebé seguirá el ruido con su mirada.	Acueste a su bebé boca abajo sobre una cobija en la alfombra, con la cabeza hacia un lado. Póngase en el piso a un lado de ella. Haga que pase el mismo lapso de tiempo con la cabeza hacia la derecha y después hacia la izquierda. Cada día aumente el tiempo que está boca abajo con su bebé hasta que ella pueda alzar la cabeza y extender sus brazos para levantar el tronco, facilitando que empiece a rodar y a gatear. No le deje recostar la cara sobre el piso, lo cual podría sofocarla.	Acueste a su bebé boca arriba y tóquele los brazos y las piernas en sitios distintos. Haga pequeños sonidos como "cuchi-cuchi" cada vez que lo toque. Puede que su bebé sonría y que le mire la mano, anticipando que lo vuelva a tocar. Cada vez que haga un sonido, también puede nombrar la parte del cuerpo que está tocando.	Cuando haga buen tiempo, saque a su bebé a caminar por el parque o por la vecindad. Platíquele sobre todo lo que vea. Aunque no pueda entenderlo todo, a su bebé le encantará estar afuera y escuchar el sonido de su voz.
Léale un libro sencillo a su bebé. Aunque no entienda la historia, disfrutará el rato estando junto a usted y escuchando su voz mientras lee.	Con unas hojas de papel blanco y un marcador de color negro, dibuje varias imágenes que sean fáciles de reconocer en cada hoja. Al principio, use formas sencillas (una raya diagonal, el centro de un blanco, un patrón en forma de tablero de damas, un triángulo). Coloque los dibujos de manera que su bebé los pueda ver (a unas 8–12 pulgadas o 20–30 centímetros de distancia de su cara). Con cinta adhesiva, pegue los dibujos cerca de su cuna o de su sillita de bebé para el coche.	Acueste a su bebé boca arriba sobre una superficie plana y blanda como una cama o una cobija. Frote sus manos y dedos ligeramente mientras que le canta "Palmas, palmitas" o cualquier otra canción infantil.	Suene ligeramente una sonaja u otro juguete de bebé que produzca ruido. Colóquelo en la mano de su bebé. Vea si lo agarra, aunque sea por un momentito breve.	Cargue en brazos a su bebé, o acuéstela en una superficie plana y blanda. Póngase cerca de ella (8–12 pulgadas o 20–30 cms.) para que lo/la alcance a ver. Estando así, cara a cara, haga movimientos pequeños (saque la lengua, déle una gran sonrisa). Puede ser que su bebé intente imitarle. Al principio, use movimientos pequeños, pero después, puede intentar este juego usando movimientos más exagerados con la cabeza, las manos, y los brazos. También podría intentar imitarla usted a ella.

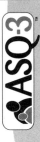

ACTIVIDADES PARA BEBÉS DE ENTRE 4 Y 8 MESES DE EDAD

Ponga un juguete de cuerda al lado o detrás de su bebé. Preste atención para ver si su bebé intenta identificar de dónde proviene el sonido.	Déle a su bebé una cuchara para que la agarre y la muerda. Una cuchara es fácil de sujetar y provoca una sensación agradable en la boca. También es excelente para hacer ruido, intentar golpear cosas, y para dejarla caer.	Siéntese en el suelo y ponga a su bebé sentada entre sus piernas. Si su bebé necesita apoyo, utilice sus piernas o su pecho para acomodarla bien. Esta es una buena posición para jugar con ella e incentivarla a que se siente de forma independiente.	Frote con cuidado el cuerpo de su bebé con un paño suave o con una toalla de papel. Dígale en voz alta qué textura tienen estos objetos (suave, áspero, resbaladizo). También puede untar un poco de crema en la piel de su bebé e indicarle la textura de ésta.	Deje que su bebé se mire en un espejo. Ponga un espejo irrompible al costado de la cuna de su bebé o en la mesa de cambiar pañales para que se pueda ver. Véase usted en el espejo al mismo tiempo que su bebé, sonría y hágale señales con la mano.
Los objetos caseros comunes como las cucharas y las tazas de plástico para medir pueden ser buenos juguetes para su bebé, ya que su forma y el ruido que hacen son interesantes. Agite u oscile ligeramente unas cucharas para medir en un lugar dónde su bebé pueda intentar alcanzarlas o darles paditas. Deje también que su bebé las toque y que las agite.	Juegue con la voz. Háblele a su bebé en tonos altos y bajos, haga un chasquido con la lengua o susurre. Después escuche los sonidos que su bebé hace y repítalos. Coloque a su bebé de manera que esté enfrente de usted—su bebé lo/la mirará cuando usted haga sonidos.	Llene una botella pequeña de plástico (frasco de medicina con tapa a prueba de niños) con frijoles o arroz. Deje que su bebé la agite para hacer ruido.	Haga otra sonaja usando cascabeles dentro de una botella pequeña con tapa a prueba de niños. Incentive a su bebé a sujetar una sonaja en cada mano y a agitar ambas. Preste atención para ver si a su bebé le gusta más un sonido que otro.	Coloque a su bebé sobre su barriguita con sus juguetes u objetos favoritos a su alrededor, pero ligeramente fuera de su alcance. Motívela a que trate de moverse para llegar a los juguetes.
Llene una caja de pañuelos de papel con tiras de papel. Su bebé disfrutará mucho sacándolas de la caja. (No utilice papel de periódico ni revistas a colores ya que la tinta puede ser tóxica. No use nunca bolsas ni envoltorios de plástico.)	Ate firmemente uno de los juguetes favoritos de su bebé al lado de su cuna (o de su mecedora o de su silla para balancearse) para que intente moverse hacia él y agarrarlo. Cambie frecuentemente los juguetes para que su bebé vea y haga cosas nuevas.	Ponga a su bebé en una silla, en una sillita para el coche o siéntela entre almohadas para que pueda verlo/la a usted. Use una bufanda o una pelota grande para moverla lentamente enfrente de ella. Muévala hacia arriba, luego hacia abajo y después, a los lados para que su bebé pueda seguir el movimiento con los ojos.	Con su bebé acostado sobre la espalda, coloque un juguete de manera que pueda verlo pero no tocarlo, o mueva un juguete dentro del campo visual de su bebé. Motívelo a rodar para llegar al juguete.	Juegue a las escondidas (picabú) con las manos, un paño, o un pañal. Tápese la cara con el paño, y después deje que su bebé se esconda detrás de éste. Incentive a su bebé a jugar, pero si no puede llevarse el paño a la cara, retíreselo. Tomen turnos para esconderse.
Siente a su bebé en una silla o en su sillita para el coche para que observe las actividades diarias que usted hace. Háblele sobre lo que usted está haciendo. Deje que su bebé vea, oiga, y toque objetos comunes. Usted puede prestar atención a su bebé mientras hace otras cosas.	Ponga a su bebé sobre su rodilla de manera que quede mirando hacia usted. Mézcala o hágala brincar mientras le canta o recita rimas infantiles. Ayude a su bebé a juntar las manos para aplaudir con el ritmo de la canción.	A su bebé le gustará tirar juguetes al suelo. Tómese un poco de tiempo para jugar a este juego de "ir y buscar". Esto ayudará a su bebé a aprender a soltar objetos. Ponga una caja o una cacerola enfrente de su bebé para que suelte los juguetes dentro de ésta.	Una vez que la bebé empiece a rodar o a gatear sobre su barriguita, juegue a "ven por mí". Deje que su bebé se mueva, luego vaya detrás de ella, y abrácela cuando la alcance.	Coloque a su bebé mirando hacia usted. Su bebé puede mirarlo/la mientras usted cambia sus expresiones faciales (sonrisa grande, sacar la lengua, ojos que se ensanchan, arquear las cejas, dar resoplidos o soplar). Déle un turno a su bebé. Imite usted lo que haga su bebé.

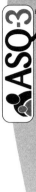
ACTIVIDADES PARA BEBÉS DE ENTRE 8 Y 12 MESES DE EDAD

Deje que su bebé coma, sin ayuda. Esto le permitirá aprender a tomar objetos pequeños entre los dedos (como cereal o arvejas cocidas) y también le permitirá sentir texturas nuevas en las manos y en la boca. En poco tiempo, su bebé podrá hacer solito toda una comida usando los dedos.	A su bebé le gustará hacer ruido al golpear un objeto con otro. Déle a su bebé cubos (bloques) para golpear, una sonaja para agitar, o cucharas de madera para golpear con recipientes de la cocina. Muéstrele a su bebé cómo golpear un objeto con el otro.	Un juego divertido es meter y sacar objetos de un recipiente. Déle a su bebé recipientes de plástico con pelotitas o cubos grandes para que practique esta actividad. También le podría gustar meter y sacar calcetines del cajón o meter y sacar envases o cajas pequeñas (como de gelatina, de atún o de sopa) de la despensa.	Su bebé empezará a usar su dedo índice para tocar objetos con el dedo. Deje que su bebé toque sus juguetes, tales como un teléfono de plástico, con el dedo índice. También deje que le toque la cara y nómbrele la parte que le toca.
Ponga juguetes en un sofá o mesa sólida para que su bebé pueda practicar cómo ponerse de pie mientras juega con los juguetes.	Ponga una caja grande con la apertura hacia un lado para que su bebé pueda entrar y salir gateando. Quédese cerca e indíquele a su bebé la acción que está haciendo. "Entraste y ahora has salido".	Léale libros para bebés o revistas con imágenes coloridas a su bebé. Indíquele las imágenes con el dedo y cuéntele lo que representan. Deje que su bebé toque las imágenes del libro.	Juegue a la pelota con su bebé. Ruede una pelota hacia su bebé y ayúdele o pida a otra persona que le ayude al bebé a rodar la pelota de vuelta. Es posible que su bebé le lance la pelota; por esta razón, las pelotas de playa, o pelotas de espuma ("Nerf") son excelentes para este juego.
Encienda la radio o el equipo de música. Sujete a su bebé con las manos alrededor de su cintura y deje que dé saltitos y baile. Si su bebé puede permanecer de pie con poco apoyo, tome sus manos y baile como pareja.	Inicie juegos como "las palmaditas" y otros juegos de imitación. Cuando su bebé imite los movimientos o sonidos que hace usted, felicítelo y hágale mimos. A los bebés les encanta repetir los mismos juegos una y otra vez.	Mientras la baña, deje que su bebé juegue con tazas para medir, tazas con asas, coladeras, esponjas, y pelotas que flotan en la tina. La hora de bañarse es un momento excelente para aprender.	Su bebé empezará a jugar haciendo diferentes sonidos como "ma-ma" o "pa-pa". Imite los sonidos que haga su bebé. Agregue un sonido nuevo para ver si su bebé intenta copiarlo. Disfrute de estos primeros intentos de hablar del bebé.
Haga un rompecabezas sencillo para su bebé poniendo cubos o pelotas de ping-pong adentro de moldes para hacer panecillos o colocándolos en los compartimentos de un cartón de huevo.	Usted puede hacer un juguete sencillo cortando un agujero redondo en la tapa de plástico de una lata de café. Déle a su bebé ganchos para tender ropa o pelotas de ping-pong para que las meta por el agujero de la tapa.	Diga "Hola" y salude con la mano cuando entre en un cuarto con su bebé. Incentive a su bebé a imitarlo/la y ayúdela a saludar con la mano a otras personas. Saludar con la mano para decir "hola" y "adiós" es uno de los primeros gestos que hacen los bebés.	Déle opciones a su bebé para que aprenda a escoger. Ofrézcale dos juegos o alimentos y vea cuál elige. Enséñele cómo señalar el objeto que elige o cómo moverse hacia él. ¡Los bebés definitivamente tienen sus preferencias!
			La gente y los lugares nuevos son buenas experiencias para su bebé, pero pueden asustarla. Deje que vea, escuche, y se mueva a su propio ritmo en un espacio nuevo o con gente nueva. Vaya despacio, su bebé le dirá cuándo esté lista para más estímulos.

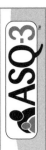

ACTIVIDADES PARA BEBÉS DE ENTRE 12 Y 16 MESES DE EDAD

A los bebés les fascinan los juegos a esta edad ("Las escondidas", "Las palmaditas", "Este cerdito"). Haga diferentes variantes de estos juegos y vea si su bebé los intente con usted. Escóndase detrás de los muebles o puertas para jugar a las escondidas. Golpee un par de cubos o tapaderas de cacerola entre sí para jugar a las palmaditas.

Haga títeres con un calcetín o con una bolsa de papel—uno para usted y otro para su bebé. Haga que su títere le hable a su bebé o al títere de su bebé. Incentive a su bebé a "contestar".

Incentive a su bebé a que dé sus primeros pasos. Sujete al bebé de pie, frente a otra persona que tenga su juguete o comida favorita en las manos. Haga que su bebé camine hacia la otra persona para obtener el juguete o la comida.

Déle a su bebé recipientes con tapas y con diferentes compartimentos que tengan cubos u otros juguetes pequeños. Deje que su bebé quite las tapas y que vuelque o saque los juguetes. Después, enséñele como volver a poner las cosas en su sitio. Este juego le enseñará a la bebé a poner o a acomodar objetos en el lugar donde ella desea.

Envuelva holgadamente un juguete pequeño en una toalla de papel o en un pañuelo sin usar cinta. Déselo al bebé para que trate de desenvolverlo y así encontrar una sorpresa. También puede utilizar papel de china o papel para envolver, ya que ambos tienen colores llamativos y hacen ruido.

A los bebés les gusta jugar con juguetes que se empujan o que se jalan. Haga su propio juguete para jalar uniendo cartones de yogur, carretes de hilo, o cajas pequeñas con una cuerda suave o trozo de estambre (de 2 pies o 60 centímetros de longitud) aproximadamente). Ate un anillo de plástico o cuenta en uno de los extremos para que se pueda usar como asa.

Pegue un pedazo grande de papel para dibujar a una mesa con cinta adhesiva. Enseñe a su bebé cómo hacer garabatos con crayones grandes que no sean tóxicos. Dibujen sobre el papel tomando turnos. También es divertido pintar con agua.

Coloque los muebles de manera que su bebé pueda desplazarse por el cuarto pasando por los espacios abiertos que queden entre los muebles. Esto permite el desarrollo del equilibrio al caminar.

En esta etapa, a los bebés les sigue gustando hacer ruido. Haga sonajas atando con una cuerda los anillos que se usan en las tapas de los frascos para hacer conservas. O llene pequeñas botellas como frascos de medicamento (con tapas a prueba de niños) con objetos que hagan diferentes sonidos como bolitas (canicas), arroz, sal, etc. Asegúrese de apretar firmemente las tapas.

¡Esta es la etapa en que su bebé aprende que los adultos pueden ser útiles! Cuando su bebé "pida" algo vocalizando o señalando con el dedo, responda a lo que le pide. Nombre el objeto que su bebé quiere e incentívela a que intente comunicarse nuevamente. Hable con ella tomando turnos en una "conversación".

Juegue al "juego de los nombres". Nombre partes del cuerpo, objetos comunes y gente. Esto le permite a su bebé saber que todas las cosas tienen un nombre y le ayuda a empezar a aprender estos nombres.

Haga una especie de carrera de obstáculos usando cajas o muebles de manera que su bebé pueda meterse, subirse, pasar por encima, por debajo o por en medio de ellos. Una caja grande puede ser un sitio magnífico para sentarse y jugar.

Deje que su bebé le ayude a limpiar. Juegue a "poner cosas en el cesto de basura" o "dárselas a mamá o papá".

Deje una bolsa llena de sorpresas en un lugar accesible a su bebé para que ella la encuentre por la mañana. La bolsa puede contener una toalla o una servilleta de papel, un juguete blando, algo que haga ruido, un tarro pequeño de plástico con tapa de rosca o un libro con páginas de cartón.

Juegue al juego de "imaginemos" con un animal o muñeco de peluche. Haga que el muñeco realice diferentes acciones y dígale al bebé lo que el muñeco está haciendo (caminando, yendo a la cama, comiendo, bailando en la mesa). Vea si su bebé hace que el muñeco se mueva y si hace con el muñeco lo que usted le indica. Tomen turnos con el muñeco.

Corte alimentos que sean seguros para comer con los dedos (no use comidas que lo puedan sofocar o atragantar) en pedazos pequeños y deje que su bebé coma solo. Es bueno que el bebé practique tomar cosas pequeñas y entre los dedos y sentir las diferentes texturas (plátanos, galletas blandas, frutas pequeñas).

Deje que su bebé le "ayude" durante sus tareas cotidianas. Incentive a su bebé a "traer" su vaso y su cuchara a la mesa a la hora de la comida, así como a "buscar" los zapatos y el abrigo para vestirse o "traer" sus pantalones o pañales para que la cambie. Es importante que su bebé aprenda a seguir instrucciones.

Su bebé está aprendiendo que distintos juguetes hacen cosas diferentes. Déle a su bebé una variedad de objetos que pueda rodar, empujar, jalar, abrazar, sacudir, golpear, amontonar, girar, y revolver.

A la mayoría de los bebés les gusta la música. Aplauda y baile con él al son de la música. Ayude al bebé a que ejercite su equilibrio moviéndose hacia adelante, hacia atrás y dando vueltas. Tómelo de las manos para darle apoyo en caso de que sea necesario.

Prepare a su bebé para una actividad o viaje futuro hablando con ella de la actividad o viaje de antemano. Su bebé se sentirá parte de lo que está ocurriendo en vez de ser una simple observadora. Esto también puede ayudarla a reducir su miedo o ansiedad de que la vayan a "dejar".

ASQ-3™ User's Guide by Squires, Twombly, Bricker, & Potter. © 2009 Paul H. Brookes Publishing Co. All rights reserved.

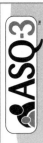

ACTIVIDADES PARA NIÑOS DE ENTRE 16 Y 20 MESES DE EDAD

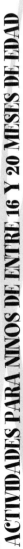

A los niños pequeños les fascina jugar con agua. Ponga objetos que se puedan "apretar o exprimir" en la bañera, tales como esponjas o botellas de plástico flexibles. Otros juguetes interesantes son las tazas o tazones de plástico, ya que los niños pueden llenarlos y vaciarlos con el agua de la tina.	A los niños pequeños les fascinan las burbujas. Deje que su niña forme burbujas soplando a través de una pajita (popote) o que observe cómo usted sopla las burbujas. También es divertido reventar las burbujas o perseguirlas.	El juego de "imaginemos" se hace aún más divertido en esta etapa. Motive a su niño a que use un animal o muñeco de peluche para actuar las actividades que el niño hace diariamente, por ejemplo: caminar, ir a la cama, bailar, comer, y saltar. Incluya al muñeco en las actividades o juegos diarios.	Preparen un budín de cajita juntos. Deje que su niña pequeña le "ayude" a prepararlo ya sea vertiendo el budín, echando la leche o mezclando. El budín preparado se puede comer o se puede usar para pintar con los dedos.	Utilice cajas o cubetas para que su niño pequeño meta almohadillas (saquitos de tela rellenos de arroz o frijoles) o pelotas. Practique con el niño cómo lanzar la pelota o la almohadilla por encima de del hombro.
Juegue al "Escondite". Su niña pequeña puede esconderse sola o con otra persona para que usted la busque. Después usted puede esconderse y dejar que su niña lo/la encuentre.	A los niños pequeños les fascina moverse. Llévelo al parque para que se suba a los columpios, a las resbaladillas pequeñas o al bimbalete. Mientras el niño aprende cómo equilibrarse en estos juegos, usted puede sostenerlo entre sus piernas.	Canten canciones en las que se usan algunas partes del cuerpo para actuar la canción tales como "Witzi, bitzi araña (La araña pequeñita)" o "El patito chiquito". Canten la canción juntas, muévanse al ritmo y hagan las acciones de la canción. Espere a que su niña anticipe la acción.	Ponga los juguetes favoritos de su niño en un cesto de ropa para lavar que esté ligeramente fuera de su alcance o en un recipiente transparente con una tapa ajustada. Espere a que su niño le pida los objetos con el fin de estimularlo a que se comunique. Responda a lo que le pida.	Su niña pequeña podría estar interesada en "actividades artísticas". Dibuje con ella utilizando crayones grandes que no sean tóxicos y un cuaderno grande. Deje que su niña haga su propio dibujo, mientras que usted hace otro También puede utilizar marcadores con punta de fieltro ya que tienen colores brillantes que pueden ser más interesantes.
A los niños pequeños les gusta mucho jugar con carretillas o con algún bolso viejo en él que pueden meter cosas. Su niño puede practicar la acción de meter y sacar objetos, poniendo y sacando juguetes u otras cosas en la carretilla o en el bolso. También puede usarlos para guardar sus artículos favoritos.	Haga un libro de fotografías con su niña. Puede usar fotografías comunes y sencillas de revistas o pegar fotos de la familia. Su niña disfrutará de las fotos en las que ella salga, así como de las fotos del resto de la familia. También puede poner fotos de las mascotas.	A los niños pequeños les interesa jugar con pelotas. Utilice una pelota inflable de playa para hacerla rodar, lanzarla, o patearla.	Juegue al juego de "¿Qué es eso?" señalando con la mano ropa, juguetes, partes del cuerpo, objetos, o fotografías y pidiendo a su niña que nombre lo que usted señala. Si su niña no responde, nombre usted los objetos y motívela a imitar las palabras.	Llene una tina de plástico con harina de maíz o con avena. También ponga, dentro de ésta, cucharas, coladeras, embudos, o tazas de plástico. Los niños podrán llenar los utensilios con la harina o la avena y después vaciarlos. De esta manera aprenderán cómo darles función de herramientas a diferentes objetos y también aprenderán sobre texturas. Además podrán probar la harina o la avena sin ningún riesgo a la salud.
Los niños pequeños empezarán a tratar de ensamblar un objeto con otro. Los rompecabezas sencillos para niños (que tienen pequeñas perillas al centro de la pieza para sacarla con facilidad de su lugar) son excelentes. Otros juegos de este tipo son meter llaves en cerraduras y poner cartas en el buzón de correo.	Consiga dos recipientes iguales (tazas de café o tazones de cereal) y un juguete pequeño. Esconda el juguete debajo de uno de los recipientes mientras su niño observa. Pregúntele, "¿dónde está?" Cuando el niño esté listo, podrá jugar al "juego de las tazas" que consiste en esconder el juguete y mover las tazas después de esconderlo.	Ayude a su niña a clasificar objetos, agrupándolos según la categoría. Por ejemplo, ella le puede ayudar a ordenar la ropa lavada haciendo un montoncito de calcetines y otro de camisas. También pueden hacer juegos de "limpieza". Pídale a su niña que ponga sus juguetes en estantes o cajas específicas.	Guarde los envases de cartón de la leche, o las cajas vacías de gelatina o de budín. Su niño pequeño podrá usarlos para hacer torres poniendo los envases uno encima del otro. Usted también puede llenar las bolsas de papel del supermercado con periódico y sellarlas con cinta adhesiva para hacer bloques grandes.	Extienda la ropa de su niña sobre la cama antes de vestirla. Pídale que le dé una camisa, pantalones, zapatos, y calcetines. Este es un método sencillo para aprender los nombres de artículos comunes.

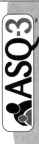 **ASQ-3**

ACTIVIDADES PARA NIÑOS DE ENTRE 20 Y 24 MESES DE EDAD

Los niños pequeños disfrutan de ver fotografías de cuando eran más pequeños. Cuando esté mirando fotos con su niño, cuéntele historias sencillas sobre él. Háblele de las cosas que estaban pasando cuando se tomó la foto.	Corte una ranura rectangular en la tapa de una caja de zapatos. Deje que su niña inserte las cartas de un juego de baraja viejo por la ranura. También puede usar sobres de carta usados. La caja es un lugar fácil para guardar el "correo" de su niña.	Haga su propio juego de bolos usando vasos de plástico, envases de pelotas de tenis, o botellas de plástico vacías. Enséñele a su niño cómo hacer rodar la bola para derribar los bolos. Después, deje que su niño lo intente.	Muchos artículos que se usan todos los días (calcetines, cucharas, zapatos, guantes) pueden ser útiles para enseñarle a su niña a hacer pares. Enséñele un objeto y pídale a la niña que encuentre otro objeto similar al suyo. Nombre los objetos mientras realiza el juego.	Esconda un reloj con un "tictac" ruidoso o un radio de transistores a un volumen bajo en un cuarto, y haga que su niño lo busque. Después, deje que él esconda el objeto y usted debe buscarlo. Tomen turnos escondiendo y encontrando los objetos.
Cántele a su niña una canción que hable de las diferentes partes del cuerpo, por ejemplo: "Hombros, pies, rodillas y la cabeza". Después nombre otras partes del cuerpo como los dientes, las cejas, las uñas de los dedos, etc.	Junte materiales para que su niño juegue a ser "pintor". Déle una brocha grande y una cubeta u otro recipiente hondo para que "pinte" el exterior de la casa. Su niño disfrutará de "pintar" las paredes de la casa, una cerca, o la terraza.	Ponga algunos objetos boca abajo (libros, tazas, zapatos) y observe si su niña se da cuenta de que están mal colocados y les da la vuelta para ponerlos en la posición correcta. Su niña empezará a disfrutar este tipo de juegos que son algo absurdos o bobos.	Dé a su niño pequeño algunas de sus prendas de vestir viejas (sombreros, camisas, bufandas, bolsos, collares, gafas de sol) para que se las pruebe. Llévelo a un espejo para que se vea y pregúntele quién es la persona que está tan bien vestida.	Use animales de granja de plástico o animales de peluche para contar la historia del "Viejo McDonald". ¡Haga los ruidos de los animales para cantar la canción!
Su niño disfrutará de hacer bloques de bolsas de papel de supermercado. Primero, llénenlas hasta la mitad con periódicos cortados en tiras o arrugado. Luego, doble la parte superior de la bolsa y ciérrela con cinta adhesiva. Cuando los bloques estén listos, su niño podrá ponerlos uno encima del otro para construir cosas. *Evite que la boca entre en contacto con el papel periódico ya que la tinta puede ser tóxica. Lávense las manos después de esta actividad.*	Una buena actividad es ponerse diferentes tipos de ropa o disfrazarse. Esta actividad permite que los niños practiquen todas las acciones asociadas a vestirse, tales como ponerse y quitarse la camisa, los pantalones, los zapatos, y los calcetines, así como abrochar y desabrochar botones y subir y bajar cierres (cremalleras).	Ponga recipientes pequeños, cucharas, tazas de plástico, embudos, una cubeta, palas y un colador en un arenero (cajón de arena). También ponga algunos autos y camiones de juguete para manejar en las carreteras de arena que su niño puede construir.	Las rimas y canciones, en las que los niños siguen la letra con movimientos de las manos, cara o cuerpo, son populares a esta edad. Un ejemplo es "Witzi, bitzi araña (La araña pequeñita)". Usted podría crear sus propias canciones usando el nombre de su niña en la canción.	Haga su propia plastilina para jugar mezclando dos tazas de harina y 3/4 de taza de sal. Añada 1/2 taza de agua y 2 cucharadas de aceite de cocina. Amase bien hasta que desaparezcan los grumos, añada colorante comestible, y amase hasta que el color haya quedado completamente mezclado. A los niños les fascinará aplastar, estrujar, y golpear la masa.
Jugar con o al lado de otros niños de la misma edad es divertido, pero normalmente requiere la supervisión de un adulto. Las idas al parque son una buena manera de empezar a practicar cómo relacionarse con otros niños.	Juegue al juego de "muéstrame" con su niña cuando estén viendo libros juntas. Pida a su niña que encuentre un objeto en una ilustración. Después deje que su niña le pida que busque un objeto en una ilustración. Sigan tomando turnos y deje que la niña le de vuelta a las páginas.	Añada varias pelotas de ping-pong a los juguetes del baño de su niño. Muéstrele cómo las pelotas salen rápidamente por sí solas a la superficie después de sujetarlas debajo del agua. A su niño le encantará este juego.	Los botes de plástico transparente con tapas de presión o de rosca son excelentes para "esconder" un objeto o algo de comer que le guste a su niña. Déle un bote con un objeto o golosina adentro a su niña para que practique cómo desenroscar las tapas y así conseguir el objeto. Esté atento/a para ver si su niña le pide ayuda.	Haga un libro pegando materiales de diferentes texturas en cada página. Los materiales como el papel de lija, las plumas, las bolas de algodón, la tela nylon, la seda, y los botones están asociados a palabras tales como *áspero, suave, duro,* y *blando.*

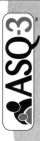

ACTIVIDADES PARA NIÑOS DE ENTRE 24 Y 30 MESES DE EDAD

Actúe o añada acciones a las canciones infantiles favoritas de su niña. Cualquier canción típica para esta edad resulta apropiada, como "Pin Pón", "Un elefante se balanceaba" o "Era un gato grande." Puede encontrar más canciones infantiles en el sitio Internet www.guiainfantil.com	Juegue al "tiro al blanco" usando una cubeta o caja grande y bolsitas de frijoles o pelotas. Cuente con su niño cuántas veces atinan en el blanco. Una pelota de estambre o unos calcetines enrollados también son apropiados para este juego.	Envuelva uno de los extremos de un trozo de estambre con cinta adhesiva para que quede rígido como si fuera una aguja y haga un nudo grande en el otro extremo (que quede sin cinta). Haga que su niña ensarte macarrones anchos y grandes, botones, cucharas, o cuentas en el trozo de estambre. También puede hacer un collar comestible con un cereal en forma de aritos como "Cheerios".	A los niños les fascina hacer excursiones a esta edad. Una excursión especial puede ser ir a la biblioteca; el bibliotecario puede ayudarle a encontrar libros apropiados. Reserve un tiempo especial para la lectura (por ejemplo, antes de ir a dormir).	Cuando vaya de paseo con su niña, salte con ella por encima de las grietas de la acera. Quizá tendrá que sujetar a su niña al principio para ayudarle a saltar.
Tome tiempo para dibujar con su niño cuando quiera sacar el papel y los crayones. Dibuje formas grandes y deje que su niño las coloree. Tomen turnos para dibujar.	Cuando su niña esté jugando en el arenero (cajón de arena), vierta un poco de agua sobre la arena. Enseñe a la niña cómo llenar un recipiente con arena mojada y cómo darle vuelta para hacer estructuras o pastelitos de arena.	Ponga uno o dos catálogos viejos en el estante de libros de su niño. Un catálogo es un buen "libro" de fotos para nombrar objetos comunes.	Proporciónele a su niña jabón, una toallita para lavarse y una vasija con agua. Deje que su niña lave un muñeco "sucio", platos de juguete, o ropa de muñeco. Es una buena práctica para aprender a lavarse y secarse las manos.	Haga instrumentos musicales con los huevos de Pascua de plástico o con el envase de plástico en él que vienen las medias de nylon de marca "L'eggs". Llene los huevos con objetos ruidosos como arena, frijoles, o arroz y ciérrelos con cinta adhesiva. Haga 2 huevos para cada sonido. Ayude a su niña a emparejar sonidos y a acomodar los huevos en un cartón de huevos.
Enseñe a su niño cómo hacer serpientes, pelotas, o panqueques de plastilina. Utilice un rodillo para aplanar la plastilina o moldes de galletas para hacer diferentes formas.	A esta edad, a los niños les fascina jugar a imaginarse que son otras personas o cosas y también disfrutan cuando usted lo hace con ellos. Juegue con su niña a ser distintos animales como un perro o un gato. Haga sonidos y movimientos de animales y deje que su niña se imagine que ella es la dueña de la mascota y que la acaricie y alimente.	Su niño empezará a ser capaz de tomar decisiones. Ayúdele a escoger la ropa que quiera ponerse cada día, dándole la opción de elegir entre dos pares de calcetines, dos camisas, etc. Déle opciones a la hora de comer o tomar un bocadillo (ofrézcale dos tipos de bebida, galletas, etc.).	Ayude a su niña a desarrollar sus habilidades auditivas a través de la música. Ponga discos compactos o cassettes de música con ritmo lento y rápido. Las canciones que contienen una variedad de ritmos son excelentes. Enséñele a su niña cómo moverse de manera rápida o lenta al son de la música. (Usted podrá encontrar cassettes o discos compactos para niños en la biblioteca local).	Las cajas tienen infinidad de usos para los niños. Una caja que sea lo suficientemente grande para que su niño se meta puede convertirse en un automóvil. También se pueden cortar aperturas a manera de ventanas y puerta en una caja de electrodomésticos para hacer una casita de juegos. Decorar las cajas con lápices de colores, marcadores, o pinturas puede ser una actividad divertida para hacer juntos.
Juegue a "Seguir al líder" con su niña. Haga que ella copie lo que usted hace: Camine de puntitas, hacia atrás, despacio o rápido, dé pasos grandes y pasos pequeños. Después, cambien de rol y siga usted a su niña.	Al pintar con los dedos, experimente con varios medios. Puede utilizar crema batida sobre una superficie que se pueda lavar (una bandeja para galletas o una mesa con un acabado impermeable como la "formica"). Ayúdele a su niño a extender la crema y a hacer dibujos con sus dedos. Añada colorante para alimentos para darle algo de color.	Las actividades corporales son una parte importante de la vida de los niños. Usted puede crear un juego usando una pelota y dándole instrucciones a su niña para que haga una serie de acciones, tales como "rodar la pelota, patearla, rebotarla, empujarla, lanzarla y agarrarla". Túrnense a la hora de dar instrucciones.	Haga una especie de carrera de obstáculos usando sillas, almohadas, o cajas de cartón grandes. Dígale a su niño que pase por encima, por debajo, en medio, por atrás o enfrente de los obstáculos. Ubique los obstáculos de manera que las piezas estén bien afianzadas y que no se vayan a caer y lastimar a su niño.	Junte objetos grandes y pequeños (pelotas, cubos [bloques], platos) y muéstreselos a su niña, indicándole si son grandes o pequeños. Pídale a su niña que seleccione una pelota grande del grupo y después, todas las pelotas grandes. Haga lo mismo con los objetos pequeños. Otro juego de este tipo consiste en estirar los brazos hacia arriba para hacerse más alto y después ponerse en cuclillas para hacerse más pequeño.

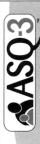

ACTIVIDADES PARA NIÑOS DE ENTRE 30 Y 36 MESES DE EDAD

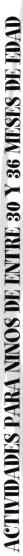

Cuéntele o léale una historia que le resulte familiar a su niño y haga frecuentes pausas para dejar fuera una palabra, pidiéndole a su niño que se la diga. Por ejemplo, Caperucita Roja dijo "Abuelita, qué _____ más grandes tienes".	Enséñele a su niña a dar maromas (volteretas). Primero dé usted una maroma y después ayude a su niña a dar una. Finalmente, deje que lo intente sola. Asegúrese de que no haya muebles cerca con los que se pueda golpear. También podría colocar algunas almohadas en el suelo para asegurarse de que su niña no se lastime.	Coloque una manta vieja sobre una mesa para hacer una tienda de campaña o una casa. Déle una bolsa con comida a su niña para hacer un "picnic". Pídale a su niña que ponga una almohada dentro de la casita para jugar a "acampar" y tomar una siesta. También le puede dar una linterna; éstas son muy divertidas para los niños.	Tome un pedazo de papel que sea lo suficientemente grande como para que su niño no se pueda acostar en él. Haga una línea alrededor del cuerpo de su niño para que quede marcado su contorno (silueta). No se olvide de incluir las manos y los pies. Habla de las partes del cuerpo y escriba las palabras en el papel. Deje que su niño coloree el dibujo. Cuelgue el cartel en el cuarto de su niño.
A esta edad, a muchos niños les interesa crear arte de varias maneras diferentes. Haga un sello usando una papa; primero corte una papa por la mitad y talle con un cuchillo un diseño sencillo en el centro de la papa. Después, ponga pintura en un platito y enseñe a su niña a mojar la papa en la pintura y a imprimir el diseño en un trozo de papel.	Ponga un poco de pintura (con base de agua - témpera) en un bote y añada agua para hacerla más líquida. Ponga unas gotas de esta mezcla en un papel y sople con una pajita (un popote) para mover la pintura a través del papel. También puede llenar un pomo viejo de desodorante con punta de bola ("roll-on") con pintura diluida en agua, para que su niño pueda usarlo como si fuera un crayón y deslizarlo sobre el papel.	Trace objetos sencillos con lápiz y papel. Se pueden usar tazas de diferentes tamaños, cubos, sus propias manos y las manos de su niño. También pueden usar marcadores de punta de fieltro o crayones de colores para hacer los trazos.	Pídale a su niña que le ayude a poner la mesa. Primero, pídale que coloque los platos, luego las tazas, y después las servilletas al lado de cada plato. Esta actividad le permitirá a su niña aprender la correspondencia individual entre las cosas. Enséñele dónde se deben colocar los utensilios.
Junte cajas vacías (de cereal, de comida preparada, o cartones de huevo) y ayude a su niño a crear su propio supermercado.	Ayude a su niña a aprender nuevas palabras para describir objetos en las conversaciones cotidianas. Describa los colores, tamaños, y formas de los objetos (la taza *azul*, la pelota *grande*). Describa también cómo se mueven las cosas (los autos van *rápido*, la tortuga se mueve *lentamente*) y la sensación que producen (el helado es *frío*, la sopa está *caliente*).	Haga sus propios rompecabezas con fotografías cortadas de revistas. Corte fotos que muestren personas de cuerpo completo y pídale a su niño que le ayude a pegar las fotografías en un cartón. Después, corte estas fotografías en tres pedazos, dividiendo la cabeza, el torso y las piernas. Haga los cortes en forma de curva para que sea más interesante volver a unir las partes.	Un buen juego para los viajes en auto es emparejar las cartas de un juego de "Memoria". Muéstrele una carta a su niño y pídale que encuentre una igual.
Corte fotos de revistas y clasifíquelas en dos grupos, por ejemplo: grupos de perros, de comida, de juguetes, o de prendas de vestir. Tenga dos cajas listas y ponga una fotografía de un perro en una y una fotografía de comida en la otra. Haga que su niña ponga fotografías adicionales en la caja correspondiente, ayudándole así a aprender cosas sobre categorías.	Corte un plato de cartón en forma de raqueta y enseñe a su niño cómo usarla para golpear un globo. Vea cuánto tiempo puede mantener su niño el globo en el aire o cuántas veces puede golpearlo para devolvérselo. Esta actividad ayuda a desarrollar la coordinación de todo el cuerpo y la coordinación entre las manos y la vista. Supervise siempre cuidadosamente las actividades de su niño cuando juegue con globos.	Para mejorar la coordinación y el equilibrio, muestre a su niña "cómo caminan los osos" caminando en cuatro patas con las manos y los pies, asegurándose de mantener rectos los brazos y las piernas. Imite el "salto del conejo" agachándose y saltando hacia adelante.	Muéstrele a su niño la "manera de caminar del elefante" y motívelo para que lo/la imite. Incorpore su cuerpo hacia delante poniendo los brazos enfrente con las manos enlazadas a manera de trompa de elefante. Deje que "esta trompa" se balancee libremente de un lado hacia el otro mientras da pasos lentos y pesados. Esta es una actividad excelente para hacerla escuchando música.	Haga un cartel de las cosas favoritas de su niña usando fotografías de revistas viejas. Utilice tijeras y goma para pegar especiales para niños para que su niña pueda hacer esta actividad de forma independiente, pero segura.

ASQ-3™ *User's Guide* by Squires, Twombly, Bricker, & Potter. © 2009 Paul H. Brookes Publishing Co. All rights reserved.

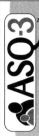

ACTIVIDADES PARA NIÑOS DE ENTRE 36 Y 48 MESES DE EDAD

Haga un álbum de recuerdos "sobre mi niña". Incluya fotos de la familia, hojas de árbol, fotos de revistas de una de las comidas favoritas de su niña y dibujos que ella haga. Ponga estas cosas en un álbum de fotos o péguelas a hojas de papel y engrápelas para crear su propio álbum de recuerdos.	Haga un comedero para pájaros usando mantequilla de cacahuate y alimento para pájaros. Primero, busquen una piñita (de pino) o un pedazo de madera, úntenlo con mantequilla de cacahuate y rocíenlo con el alimento para pájaros. Finalmente, cuélguenlo en un árbol o afuera de una ventana. Cuando su niño observe los pájaros que se acercan al comedero, pídale que le diga cuántos pájaros hay, de qué color son y de qué tamaño.	Cultive una planta con su niña. Llenen tres cuartos de un vasito desechable de papel con tierra y después coloque algunas semillas. Elija semillas que broten rápidamente como frijoles o arvejas. Finalmente, cubran las semillas con tierra para que queden 1/2 pulgada debajo de la tierra. Coloque el vasito en una repisa soleada cerca de la ventana y motive a su niña a regar la planta y a verla crecer.	Antes de ir a la cama, miren juntos una revista o un libro para niños. Pida a su niño que señale las fotografías cuando usted las nombre como, por ejemplo "¿Dónde está el camión?" Juegue con el niño y pídale que señale las fotografías con el codo o con el pie. Pídale que le muestre algo que sea redondo o algo que se mueva rápido.	Jueguen a emparejar dos fotografías que sean iguales. Primero haga dos conjuntos de 10 ó más fotografías. Cada conjunto debe incluir las mismas fotografías, es decir el segundo conjunto debe ser una réplica del primero. Usted puede usar las fotografías de dos ejemplares de la misma revista o las cartas de una baraja. Coloque las fotografías boca arriba y pida a su niña que encuentre dos que sean iguales. Comience con dos conjuntos de fotografías y añada más gradualmente.
Durante la preparación de alimentos o la cena, pueden jugar a ver quién tiene "más o menos" cantidad de un alimento. Pregúntele a su niño quién tiene más "papas" o quién tiene menos. También pueden hacer este juego observando la cantidad de líquido que hay en una taza o vaso. Use dos vasos o tazas iguales y llénelos de jugo o leche, después pregúntele quién tiene más o menos jugo.	Corte unos círculos grandes de papel y muéstreselos a su niña. Hable con ella sobre las cosas que hay en el mundo que tienen una forma "redonda" (una pelota, la luna). Corte los círculos por la mitad y pregúntele si puede hacer que vuelvan a ser redondos. Después, corte los círculos en tres partes, y así sucesivamente.	Durante el baño, juegue a "Simón dice" para enseñarle a su niño los nombres de las partes del cuerpo. Primero, usted puede ser "Simón" y ayudar a su niño a lavarse la parte del cuerpo que "Simón diga". Después deje que su niño sea "Simón". Asegúrese de nombrar cada una de las partes del cuerpo a medida que la lave y déle a su niño la oportunidad de lavarse solito.	Hable del número 3. Lea historias que incluyan el número 3 (Los tres chivitos, Los tres cerditos, Los tres ositos). Incentive a su niña a que cuente hasta 3 usando grupos de 3 objetos similares (piedras, cartas, cubos [bloques]). Hable de que su niña tiene 3 años de edad. Después de que su niña comprenda la idea, pase a los números 4, 5 y así sucesivamente siempre que su niña se muestre interesada.	Saque varios objetos que le resulten familiares a su niño (cepillo, abrigo, plátano, cuchara, libro). Pida a su niño que le muestre qué objetos son para comer y qué objetos se utilizan para salir a la calle. Ayúdele a poner los objetos en grupos que tengan una correspondencia, por ejemplo, "cosas que comemos" y "cosas para vestirse".
Cuando su niña se esté vistiendo, motívela a que practique cómo abrochar y desabrochar los botones y subir y bajar los cierres (cremalleras). Haga un juego, mostrándole a su niña cómo los botones aparecen y desaparecen al abotonarlos o desabotonarlos, o hágale imaginar que el cierre es un tren pequeñito que "que sube y baja" por la vía.	Establezca un lugar para jugar en la casa e invite a dos niños (hermano, hermana o amigo) a jugar con su niña. Es mejor incluir pocos niños al principio y tener varios juguetes del mismo tipo para que no tengan que compartir todo el tiempo. Los títeres o cubos son un buen juguete para esta actividad porque son propicios para que los niños jueguen juntos. Si es necesario, use un reloj con alarma para que cada niño tome turnos iguales con cada juguete.	Practique cómo seguir instrucciones. Pídale a su niño que haga acciones que sean cómicas o un tanto absurdas, por ejemplo, pídale que "toque su codo y después que corra en círculos" o que "busque un libro y lo ponga sobre su cabeza". Déle dos o tres instrucciones seguidas para que él las haga una detrás de la otra.	Escuchen sonidos juntos. Busque un lugar cómodo y acogedor para sentarse con su niño. Permanezcan callados un momento para escuchar los sonidos alrededor. Traten de identificar todos los sonidos que oigan y pídale a su niño que le diga si los sonidos que escucha son fuertes o suaves. Intente hacer esta actividad dentro y fuera de su casa.	Haga un "caminito de aventuras afuera de la casa. Construya este caminito con una manguera, una cuerda, o un pedazo de tiza. Estire la manguera o cuerda o dibuje el caminito siguiendo el contorno de la casa, el contorno de los árboles, o si tienen una banquita, pase la cuerda por debajo de ésta. Camine con su niña a lo largo del camino y ya que pueda hacerlo sola, haga un nuevo camino, o pídale a su niña que ella crea uno nuevo.
Busque pedazos grandes de papel o cartón para que dibuje su niño. Usando crayones, lápices de colores, o marcadores, pídale a su niño que dibuje algo y usted copie lo mismo que él ha dibujado. Después, incentívelo a copiar los dibujos que usted haga, por ejemplo, círculos o líneas rectas.	Haga un collar que se pueda comer, ensartando cereales en forma de anillo como "Cheerios" o "Froot Loops" en un trozo de hilo o estambre. Envuelva un extremo de un trozo de estambre con cinta adhesiva para crear una especie de aguja y facilitar que su niño ensarte el cereal.	Cuando le esté leyendo o contando una historia que le sea familiar a su niña antes de ir a dormir, haga una pausa y deje fuera una palabra. Espere a que su niña le diga la palabra que falta.	Escuche y baile al son de la música con su niña. Usted puede parar la música durante un momento y jugar al juego de "quedarse inmóvil", en el que todos se "quedan inmóviles" o paralizados hasta que la música vuelva a empezar. Intente "quedarse inmóvil" en posiciones cómicas para divertirse.	Haga bufandas largas con retazos de tela, vestidos viejos, o camisas viejas. Use telas ligeras y rompa o córtelas en pedazos largos. Después, juegue con su niño sujetando un extremo de una bufanda y dándole vueltas o corriendo y saltando con él.

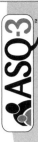
ACTIVIDADES PARA NIÑOS DE ENTRE 48 Y 60 MESES DE EDAD

Jueguen al juego de "quién, qué, y dónde". Pregúntele a su niño *quién* trabaja en una escuela, *qué* hay en una escuela, y *dónde* está la escuela. Hágale preguntas adicionales para que su niño amplíe sus respuestas. Pregúntele sobre otros lugares como, por ejemplo, la biblioteca, la parada del autobús, o la oficina de correos.	Cuando ponga la mesa para comer, jueguen al juego de "qué es lo que no pertenece aquí". Coloque un juguete pequeño u otro objeto al lado del plato y los cubiertos. Vea si su niña puede decirle qué objeto no se usa en la mesa. Usted puede hacer este juego a cualquier hora del día. Por ejemplo, cuando le vaya a cepillar el pelo, ponga un cepillo, un broche para el pelo, un peine, y una pelota en la mesa.	Deje que su niño le ayude a preparar un picnic. Muéstrele los alimentos que puede usar para el picnic (por ejemplo, pan, queso, mantequilla de cacahuate y manzanas). Después, saque las bolsas de plástico para sándwiches y una caja para el almuerzo, una canasta, o una bolsa de papel grande para que su niño empaque la comida. Finalmente, ¡salgan a disfrutar del día con su canasta de picnic!	En un día lluvioso, imagínense que van a abrir una zapatería. Use unos zapatos viejos, papel, lápices, y una silla para sentarse y probarse los zapatos. Usted puede ser el/la cliente. Dígale a su niña que apunte su "pedido" en un papel. Después, ella puede venir a probarse y a "comprar" zapatos. Este es un buen juego para paracticar cómo probarse cosas y comprar.	Jueguen a "adivina lo qué pasará" para fomentar que su niño desarrolle las capacidades de solucionar problemas y de pensar. Por ejemplo, a la hora de bañarlo, pregúntele, "¿qué crees que pase si abro el agua caliente y el agua fría al mismo tiempo?" o "¿qué pasaría si encimara estos cubos (bloques) uno por uno hasta el techo?"
Juegue al "baloncesto de cubeta". Ponga a su niño de pie a una distancia de unos 6 pies (2 metros) de una cubeta grande o de un cesto para la basura, y dígale que tire una pelota de tamaño mediano para intentar hacer una "canasta". Para hacer este juego más divertido en el verano, llene la cubeta de agua afuera.	Escriba el nombre de su niña con frecuencia. Cuando ella termine de hacer un dibujo, asegúrese de escribir su nombre en él, y de nombrar las letras en voz alta a medida que las vaya escribiendo. Si su niña muestra interés, motívela a nombrar y/o a copiar las letras. A lo largo del día, señálele las letras de su nombre en las cajas de cereal, en carteles, y en libros.	Invite a su niño a jugar un juego de contar. En una hoja grande de papel, haga un tablero de juego sencillo, trazando una fila de casillas para hacer el camino. Traiga unos dados y láncelos para decidir cuántas casillas debe avanzar. Cuente con su niño y motívelo a avanzar la ficha de juego casilla por casilla, contando en voz alta cada vez que toque el tablero.	Usando plastilina o arcilla y unos objetos pequeños, (como palitos, botones, palillos de dientes, cuentas de madera y cualquier otro artículo pequeño), haga una persona. Primero forme la cabeza y el cuerpo con la plastilina (o arcilla), y después use los objetos pequeños para ponerle los brazos, las piernas, y los ojos. Hágale preguntas a su niña sobre la persona que está haciendo.	Incentive a su niño a aprender su nombre completo, su dirección, y su número de teléfono. Hágalo como si fuera un juego de cantar o de rimar para que sea divertido. Pídale que repita la información después de que usted se la haya dicho cuando estén de camino en el coche o en el autobús.
Recorte tres círculos pequeños, tres de tamaño mediano, y tres grandes. Coloree cada conjunto de círculos con un color diferente (o use papel de un color diferente para cada conjunto). Su niña puede separar los círculos según el color o la forma. También usted puede preguntarle sobre los diferentes tamaños de los círculos. Por ejemplo, pregúntele a su niña "¿cuál es el más pequeño? Puede intentar este juego también usando los botones que haya quitado de una camisa vieja.	Salga a caminar con su niño, y recoja cosas que encuentre en el camino. Lléveselas a casa y ayude a que su niño las separe por grupo. Por ejemplo, un grupo puede incluir piedras, papel, u hojas de árbol. Estimúlele a hacer una colección de cosas especiales. Busque una caja o un lugar especial donde pueda mostrar la colección.	Juegue a adivinar "qué imagen es". Use una hoja de papel para tapar una de las imágenes en un libro que su niña conozca bien. Poco a poco, vaya moviendo la hoja para destapar la imagen hasta que su niña adivine qué es.	Deje que su niño le ayude a preparar una comida. Puede untar mantequilla de cacahuate y mermelada, cortar usando un cuchillo para mantequilla, servir cereal, y añadir leche (usando un envase pequeño). No le dé nunca ninguna tarea que requiera el uso de la estufa o del horno sin supervisarlo cuidadosamente.	"Escriba" y envíe por correo una carta a un amigo o pariente. Proporciónele a su niña papel, un lápiz o crayones, y un sobre. Déjela dibujar, trazar rayas (garabatos) o escribir; o ella le puede decir a usted lo que quiere escribir. Cuando su niña haya terminado, déjela doblar la carta, meterla al sobre, lamerlo y cerrarlo. Usted puede escribir la dirección. Asegúrese de dejar que su niña decore el sobre si quiere. Después de que su niña haya puesto el sello, ayúdela a echar la carta a un buzón.
Jueguen al "circo". Busque unas viejas prendas de ropa coloridas y ayúdele a su niño a organizar un espectáculo de circo. Coloque una cuerda sobre el suelo para el acto de la cuerda floja. Proporciónele una caja sólida y resistente para que se suba en ella y anuncie los actos. También déle unos objetos divertidos para el acto de magia, y unos animales de peluche para el espectáculo. Fomente que su niño use su imaginación y creatividad a la hora de planificar el espectáculo. ¡No olvide aplaudir!	Tome una baraja y saque las cartas necesarias para hacer cuatro o cinco pares. Coloque las cartas boca arriba y ayúdele a su niña a encontrar los pares. Háblele de por qué las cartas que forman los pares son "iguales" o "diferentes".	Diviértanse haciendo burbujas. La receta es 3/4 de taza de jabón líquido para lavar platos y 8 tazas de agua. Pueden usar una pajita (popote), para soplar las burbujas, o pueden ensartar dos segmentos de pajita en un trozo de estambre y atar los extremos del hilo para hacer un círculo. Sumerja el círculo en la mezcla de jabón. Sáquelo y muévalo lentamente hacia adelante y hacia atrás. Verá unas burbujas grandes y bonitas.	Haga una almohadilla rellena de frijoles para lanzar y atrapar. Llene el dedo gordo de un calcetín o unas medias viejas con 3/4 de taza de frijoles secos. Cosa el otro lado o átelo con una goma elástica. Juegue a "la papa caliente" con su niña, o simplemente pásense la pelota. Enséñele a su niña cómo lanzarla por encima de su hombro y también desde la altura de la cintura.	Imagínense que son diferentes animales. Sugiérale a su niño que use la imaginación para convertirse en gatito. Usted puede preguntarle, "¿qué les gusta comer a los gatitos?" o "¿dónde viven los gatitos?" Siga jugando para ver hasta dónde llega la imaginación.

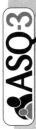

ASQ-3

ACTIVIDADES PARA NIÑOS DE ENTRE 60 Y 66 MESES DE EDAD

Hagan un collage con objetos de la naturaleza. Vayan afuera a recoger hojas, piedritas, y palitos pequeños y péguenlos a una hoja de cartón o papel duro. También puede usar una caja de galletas o de cereal para pegar los objetos del collage.	Para practicar la escritura con su niña, escriba los nombres de amigos, juguetes, o parientes en una hoja. Puede ser que al principio su niña necesite trazar las letras de los nombres por encima. Asegúrese de escribir usando letra de molde grande.	Incentive a su niño a hacer representaciones dramáticas. Ayúdelo a desempeñar los papeles de su rima infantil favorita, de un dibujo animado, o de un cuento. Para el vestuario puede usar prendas de vestir grandes y viejas.	Organice juegos sencillos de pelota como "kickból" (es como el béisbol, pero con una pelota grande que se patea) con su niña. Tome una pelota grande de 8 a 12 pulgadas (20 a 30 centímetros) y hágala rodar lentamente hacia ella. Vea si ella puede darle una patada y correr hasta "primera base".	Cuando le lea cuentos a su niño, deje que él se imagine el final, o pídale que recuente sus historias favoritas con nuevos finales chistosos que él invente.
Deje que su niña le ayude en la cocina haciendo tareas sencillas como machacar papas, hacer tortas (sándwiches) de queso, o servir cereal en un plato hondo. Después, pregúntele si le puede decir el orden de los pasos que usted siguió para cocinar y machacar las papas o para sacar el pan de la despensa y ponerle queso. Siempre vigile cuidadosamente a su niña cuando esté cerca de la estufa caliente.	Jueguen a "20 preguntas". Primero, piense usted en un animal sin decirle a su niño qué animal es. Deje que su niño le haga 20 preguntas, a las que usted tiene que responder "sí" o "no", para tratar de adivinar cuál es el animal. (Puede ser que usted le tenga que ayudar a formular este tipo de pregunta.) Después, deje que su niño piense en un animal y haga usted las 20 preguntas. Use también otras categorías tales como la comida, los juguetes, o las personas.	Hagan un juego de "contar hasta diez" usando los números de las placas que ven cuando están viajando en coche o en autobús. Busquen una placa cuyo número de matrícula contenga el número 1. Después, busquen el 2, el 3, el 4 y así sucesivamente hasta llegar al 10. Cuando su niña pueda encontrar los números en orden del 1 al 10, jueguen contando hacia atrás, comenzando con el número 9, luego el 8, 7, 6 y así sucesivamente hasta llegar al 1.	Juegue al juego de "Caras y gestos". Haga señas y gestos para representar situaciones imaginarias (pantomimas) y tome turnos con su niño adivinando qué acción es. Aquí hay algunas ideas para actuar: 1) comer una pizza caliente que tiene queso derritiéndose en hebras largas; 2) ganar una carrera; 3) encontrar una araña enorme; 4) caminar sobre barro espeso y pegajoso, y 5) dejar huellas al caminar descalzo sobre arena mojada.	Haga un juego sencillo de concentración con dos o tres pares de cartas iguales (dos reyes de corazones, por ejemplo) o haga sus propias cartas con fotografías o anuncios de revista idénticos. Empiece con dos o tres pares de cartas. Póngalas boca abajo y mézclelas. Deje que su niña voltee dos cartas para ver si hacen un par. Si no encuentra un par, vuelva a colocar las cartas boca abajo. Poco a poco puede ir aumentando el número de pares en el juego.
Haga una pequeña carrera de obstáculos dentro o fuera de la casa. Use cajas de cartón para trepar y saltar, ponga palos de escoba entre unas sillas para jugar al "limbo" (pasar por debajo de ellos), y use almohadas para bloquear el camino. Deje que su niño le ayude a diseñar la carrera de obstáculos. Después de que su niño la recorra dos o tres veces para ver cómo se hace, pídale que la haga lo más rápido que pueda. Luego pueden intentar pasar por los obstáculos brincando o saltando.	Después de lavarse las manos, escriban letras y números con budín o en una capa fina de puré de papas extendida sobre una bandeja para hornear galletas o una tabla para cortar alimentos. ¡Se permite chuparse los dedos!	Jueguen al "calcetín misterioso". Ponga un artículo doméstico común adentro de un calcetín. Haga un nudo en la parte superior del calcetín. Pídale a su niña que lo palpe y que adivine lo que hay adentro. Después pídale a ella que ponga otro artículo dentro del calcetín y usted debe adivinar el contenido. Tome turnos con ella para adivinar lo que hay adentro.	Invente rimas con los nombres de los colores. Tomen turnos haciendo rimar un color y una palabra: azul, baúl; rojo, flojo; amarillo, grillo. También pueden hacer rimas con nombres (María, mía; Enrique/meñique). Tomen turnos para hacer las rimas.	Haga un cartel que diga "Yo puedo leer". Recorte algunos nombres que su niño sepa leer—los nombres de restaurantes de comida rápida o los nombres de las cajas de cereal u otros alimentos. Puede escribirlos en trozos de papel (por ejemplo, use el nombre de su niño, sus parientes, o los amigos) y pegarlos al cartel. Añada más nombres al cartel a medida que su niño vaya aprendiendo a leer más nombres.
Jueguen a "¿qué es lo que no pertenece aquí?" Deje que su niña encuentre la palabra que no debe estar en una lista de seis o siete palabras que Ud. diga. Podría ser que la palabra no rime, o que corresponda a una categoría diferente. Algunos ejemplos son: 1) ir, decir, vivir, perro; 2) dar, parar, tomar, caballo; 3) azul, gris, rojo, verde, amarillo, trece; 4) casa, pared, alfombra, sillón, avión. Pídale a su niña que diga tres o cuatro palabras, y que mencione una que no pertenezca a la categoría común.	Juegue al juego de "memoria" con su niño. Ponga cinco o seis objetos comunes que le sean familiares sobre una mesa. Pídale que cierre los ojos. Quite un objeto y revuelva los que quedan. Pregúntele a su niño cuál es el objeto que falta. Tomen turnos descubriendo cuál es el objeto que falta.	Haga unos títeres usando palos de paleta, bolsas de papel, calcetines o cartones de huevo. Puede decorarlos con estambre, lápices, botones y papel de colores. Haga un escenario para los títeres poniendo una mesa pequeña (una mesa de centro o una mesita para jugar a las cartas) sobre su costado. Después, dígale a su niño que se esconda detrás de la mesa y que dé la función de títeres mientras que usted actúa como si fuera el público.	Juegue a "¿dónde está el objeto escondido?" Tome cuatro tazas o vasos opacos (que no sean transparentes). Mientras su niña lo/la está mirando, coloque un objeto pequeño (como una pasa o una pelota) debajo de una de las tazas y mueva todas las tazas de su posición original. Pídale a su niña que intente recordar qué taza tiene el objeto debajo. Tome turnos con su niña para esconder el objeto y para decir dónde está.	Juegue al "sonido misterioso". Seleccione algunos artículos domésticos que produzcan sonidos distintos como, por ejemplo, un reloj, una caja de cereal, una tapadera de metal (colocada sobre una cacerola), y una bolsa de papas fritas. Tápele los ojos a su niño con un pañuelo o una venda y pídale que intente adivinar el objeto que produjo el sonido. Tome turnos con su niño para jugar a este juego.

Index

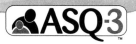

Page numbers followed by *t*, *f*, and *bf* denote tables, figures, and photocopiable blank forms, respectively.

ASQ Ordering Guide

Questionnaires, Online System, Training DVDs, and more

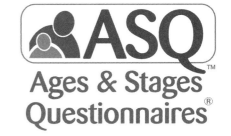

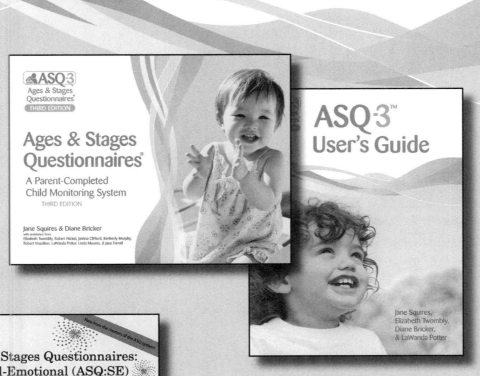

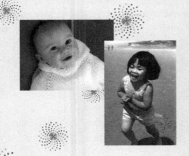

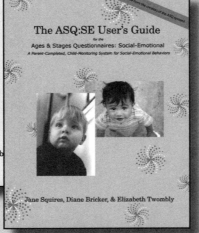

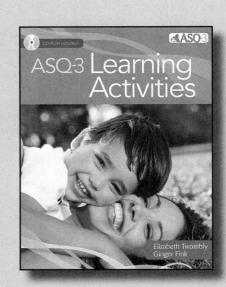

1-800-638-3775   www.agesandstages.com   A product of **BROOKES** PUBLISHING CO

■ Ages & Stages Questionnaires®, *Third Edition* (ASQ-3™)
A Parent-Completed Child Monitoring System

Now enhanced and updated based on extensive user feedback and an unparalleled research sample of more than 15,000 children, ASQ-3™ is the best, most reliable way to identify children from birth to 5 years with developmental delays. The Starter Kit contains everything you need to start screening children with ASQ-3™: 21 paper masters of the questionnaires and scoring sheets, a CD-ROM with printable PDF questionnaires, the ASQ-3™ User's Guide in English, and a FREE ASQ-3™ Quick Start Guide.

Starter Kit with English Questionnaires
US$275.00 • Stock Number: BA-70410
2009 • ISBN 978-1-59857-041-0

Starter Kit with Spanish Questionnaires
US$275.00 • Stock Number: BA-70427
2009 • ISBN 978-1-59857-042-7

Also Sold Separately

ASQ-3™ Questionnaires
Masters of the 21 photocopiable questionnaires and scoring sheets, plus a CD-ROM with printable PDFs, in a handy box.

English—US$225.00 • Stock Number: BA-70021 • 2009 • ISBN 978-1-59857-002-1

Spanish—US$225.00 • Stock Number: BA-70038 • 2009 • ISBN 978-1-59857-003-8 *(Comes with 1 Spanish Quick Start Guide)*

ASQ-3™ User's Guide
Absolutely essential to using ASQ-3™, this revised and redesigned guide provides step-by-step guidance on administering and scoring the questionnaires, setting up a screening system, working with families effectively, and using ASQ-3™ across a wide range of settings.
US$50.00 • Stock Number: BA-70045
2009 • 256 pages • 8.5 x 11 • paperback • ISBN 978-1-59857-004-5

ASQ-3™ Quick Start Guide
Perfect for busy professionals on the go, this lightweight laminated guide to ASQ-3™ keeps administration and scoring basics close at hand. Sold in packages of 5 so everyone in your program can have a copy.
US$24.95 • set of 5, 4 pages each • 8.5 x 11 • gatefold

English—Stock Number: BA-70052 • 2009 • ISBN 978-1-59857-005-2

Spanish—Stock Number: BA-71974 • 2011 • ISBN 978-1-59857-197-4

The Ages & Stages Questionnaires® on a Home Visit (Training DVD)
Get a rare inside look at ASQ as a home visitor guides a family with three children through the items on a questionnaire.
US$49.95 • Stock Number: BA-69711 • 1995 • 20 minutes • ISBN 978-1-55766-971-1

ASQ-3™ Scoring & Referral (Training DVD)
Through footage of ASQ-3™ tasks and close-ups of sample questions and scores, learn how to score the questionnaires accurately and decide if a referral for further assessment is needed.
US$49.95 • Stock Number: BA-70250 • 2004, 2009 • 16 minutes • ISBN 978-1-59857-025-0

■ ASQ Pro
Ideal for single-site programs, this online management option is your key to managing all your ASQ-3™ and ASQ:SE data and ensuring the most accurate results. ASQ Pro gives you automated scoring of questionnaires, easy questionnaire selection, customizable letters to parents, individual child and program reports, and much more. To use ASQ Pro, each site must own print versions of the ASQ-3™ and/or ASQ:SE questionnaires that will be managed in the system.
US$149.95 for annual subscription, plus quarterly billing based on screening volume. For cost per screen, see www.agesandstages.com
Stock Number: BA-70380 • ISBN 978-1-59857-038-0

■ ASQ Enterprise
Developed to meet the needs of multisite programs, ASQ Enterprise gives you all the data management features of ASQ Pro plus advanced rights management and aggregate reporting. To use ASQ Enterprise, each site must own print versions of the ASQ-3™ and/or ASQ:SE questionnaires that will be managed in the system.
US$499.95 for annual subscription, plus quarterly billing based on screening volume. For cost per screen, see www.agesandstages.com
Stock Number: BA-70397 • ISBN 978-1-59857-039-7

■ ASQ Family Access
Online questionnaires for parents! Save time and postage with a secure, customizable web site where parents complete ASQ-3™ and ASQ:SE questionnaires and you access the results electronically. Available for purchase when you buy ASQ Pro or Enterprise.
US$349.95 for annual subscription
Stock Number: BA-70403 • ISBN 978-1-59857-040-3

■ Ages & Stages Questionnaires®: Social-Emotional (ASQ:SE)

A Parent-Completed, Child-Monitoring System for Social-Emotional Behaviors

Field-tested with thousands of families, ASQ:SE accurately identifies children 3–66 months of age who are at risk for social and emotional difficulties and helps professionals determine when children need further assessment. ASQ:SE provides a complete picture of a child's social-emotional development by screening seven key behavioral areas: self-regulation, compliance, communication, adaptive functioning, autonomy, affect, and interaction with people.

The ASQ:SE Starter Kit includes one ASQ:SE box with questionnaires on CD-ROM and paper; plus the ASQ:SE User's Guide in English.

Starter Kit with English Questionnaires
US$225.00 • Stock Number: BA-70120 • 2002 • ISBN 978-1-59857-012-0

Starter Kit with Spanish Questionnaires
US$225.00 • Stock Number: BA-70137 • 2002 • ISBN 978-1-59857-013-7

Also Sold Separately

ASQ:SE Questionnaires
Masters of the 8 photocopiable questionnaires and scoring sheets plus a CD-ROM with printable PDFs, in a handy box.
English—US$175.00 • Stock Number: BA-70229 • 2002 • ISBN 978-1-59857-022-9
Spanish—US$175.00 • Stock Number: BA-70236 • 2002 • ISBN 978-1-59857-023-6

ASQ:SE User's Guide
This essential guide shows you how to work with parents to complete the questionnaires, how to score them, and how to interpret results with sensitivity to children's environmental, cultural, and developmental differences.
US$50.00 • Stock Number: BA-65331
2002 • 192 pages • 8.5 x 11 • spiral-bound • ISBN 978-1-55766-533-1

ASQ:SE in Practice (Training DVD)
Watch a home visitor using ASQ:SE with the family of a 4-year-old boy. You'll see how parents complete the questionnaires (close-ups of sample questions included) and learn about key success factors in working with families, such as establishing trust and ensuring confidentiality.
US$49.95 • Stock Number: BA-69735 • 2004 • 26 minutes • ISBN 978-1-55766-973-5

■ Enhance Your Screening with Other ASQ Products!

ASQ-3™ Learning Activities
Enhance the development of infants and young children with hundreds of fun, fast, and developmentally appropriate learning activities, now in a new edition specially developed to complement ASQ-3™.
English—US$49.95 • Stock Number: BA-72469 • 2012 • 160 pages • 8.5 x 11 • paperback with CD-ROM
ISBN 978-1-59857-246-9

Spanish—US$49.95 • Stock Number: BA-72476 • January 2013 • approx. 160 pages • 8.5 x 11 • paperback with CD-ROM
ISBN 978-1-59857-247-6

ASQ-3™ Materials Kit
This kit contains all of the items you need during any ASQ-3™ screening—no matter which age interval—in one convenient tote bag. Every item is safe, easy to clean, durable, age appropriate, gender neutral, and culturally sensitive.
US$295.00 • Stock Number: BA-70274 • ISBN 978-1-59857-027-4

Learn more at www.agesandstages.com

ORDER FORM

Qty	Stock #	Title	Price
	BA-_ _ _ _ _		
	BA-_ _ _ _ _		
	BA-_ _ _ _ _		
	BA-_ _ _ _ _		

ASQ Discounts

Buy 6 or more copies of the same ASQ family product and SAVE:
6-10 copies: 5%
11-20 copies: 10%
21-50 copies: 15%
51-100 copies: 20%
101-200 copies: 25%
201-500 copies: 30%
501-1000 copies: 35%
1001-2500 copies: 40%
2501+ copies: 45%
(Please note: the ASQ-3™ Materials Kit has a discount limit of 35%. ASQ Pro, ASQ Enterprise, and ASQ Family Access are not discounted.)

Product subtotal (in U.S. dollars) _____

Shipping (see chart at bottom) _____

Order subtotal _____

PA or MD state sales tax or regional sales tax
(for WA state residents) or GST (for CAN residents)* _____

Grand total _____

Convenient ways to order:

CALL toll-free
1-800-638-3775
M-F, 9 a.m. to 6 p.m. ET.

FAX
410-337-8539

MAIL order form to:
Brookes Publishing Co.
P.O. Box 10624
Baltimore, MD 21285-0624

ONLINE
www.brookespublishing.com

Money-back guarantee! Ordering with Brookes is risk-free!
If you are not completely satisfied, you may return products within 30 days for a full credit of the purchase price (unless otherwise indicated). Refunds will be issued for prepaid orders. Items must be returned in unused and resalable condition.

Policies and prices subject to change without notice. Prices may be higher outside the U.S.

❑ Check enclosed (payable to Brookes Publishing Co.)

❑ Purchase Order attached (bill my institution—P.O. MUST be attached)
   We reserve the right to add an additional 2% order processing fee on all orders that require special processing.

❑ Please charge my credit card: ❑ American Express ❑ MasterCard ❑ Visa ❑ Discover

Credit Card #_____ Exp. Date: _____

Security code (3 digit code on back of card, or 4 digit code on front of card for American Express): _ _ _ _

Signature (required with credit card use): _____

Name:_____

Daytime Phone: _____

Organization:_____

Street Address: _____
Complete street address required.   ❑ residential ❑ commercial

City/State/Zip:_____ Country: _____

Shipping & Handling

(For other shipping options and rates, call 1-800-638-3775, in the U.S.A. and Canada, and 410-337-9580, worldwide.)

Continental U.S.A.; U.S.A. territories & protectorates; AK, HI & PR‡

For subtotal of	Add*
US$50.00 and under	$6.50
US$50.01 and over	13%

‡ *AK, HI, and PR please add an additional US$12.00. Orders ship via UPS Air.*
Please call or email for expedited shipping options and rates.

Canada

For subtotal of	Add*
US$70.00 and under	$10.50
US$70.01 and over	15%

Orders for Canada are consolidated for shipping twice each month. For minimum shipping time, please place your orders by the 9th or 24th of each month.

calculate percentage on subtotal

PA and MD residents: Please add state sales tax. WA residents: Please add applicable sales tax by region. Canadian residents: please add your GST. Sales tax should be calculated based on the total order (including shipping) in U.S. dollars. If sales tax is calculated incorrectly, Customer Service will correct it prior to processing your order and the adjusted total will appear on your invoice.

❑ Yes! I want to receive the ASQ News & Updates e-newsletter! My e-mail will not be shared with any other party.

ABOUT YOU
Write in your title and check area of specialty: _____

❑ Birth to Five ❑ K–12 ❑ 4-year College/Graduate ❑ Community College/Vocational ❑ Clinical/Medical ❑ Community Services ❑ Association/Foundation

YOUR LIST CODE IS BA

7/12